Primer
of Biostatistics

Primer
of Biostatistics

SECOND EDITION

Stanton A. Glantz, Ph.D.
Professor of Medicine
Member, Cardiovascular Research Institute
University of California, San Francisco

MCGRAW-HILL INFORMATION SERVICES COMPANY
HEALTH PROFESSIONS DIVISION

New York St. Louis San Francisco Colorado Springs Auckland Bogotá
Hamburg Lisbon London Madrid Mexico Milan Montreal New Delhi
Panama Paris San Juan São Paulo Singapore Sydney Tokyo Toronto

This book was set in Press Roman.
The editors were Beth Kaufman Barry and Julia White; the production
supervisor was Thomas J. LoPinto.
The cover was designed by Edward R. Schultheis.
The Book Press, Inc. was printer and binder.

PRIMER OF BIOSTATISTICS

5 6 7 8 9 10 11   BKP BKP   9 0 9 8 7 6 5 4 3 2 1 0

ISBN 0-07-023372-1

Library of Congress Cataloging-in-Publication Data
Glantz, Stanton A.
    Primer of biostatistics.

    Bibliography: p.
    Includes index.
    1. Medical statistics.   2. Biometry.   I. Title.
RA409.G55   1987   610'.72   86-21329
ISBN 0-07-023372-1

To Marsha Kramar Glantz

Hunches and intuitive impressions are essential for getting the work started, but it is only through the quality of the numbers at the end that the truth can be told.

Lewis Thomas*
Memorial Sloan-Kettering Cancer Center

*L. Thomas, "Biostatistics in Medicine," *Science* **198**:675, 1977. Copyright 1977 by the American Association for the Advancement of Science.

Contents

Preface

Over the last few years, many friends and colleagues have come to me for advice and explanations about biostatistics. Since most of them had less knowledge of statistics than I did, I tried to learn what I needed to help them. The need to develop quick and intuitive, yet correct, explanations of the various tests and procedures slowly evolved into a set of stock explanations and a two-hour slide show on common statistical errors in the biomedical literature and how to cope with them. The success of this slide show led many people to suggest that I expand it into an introductory book on biostatistics.

As a result, this book is oriented as much to the individual reader–be he student, postdoctoral research fellow, professor, or practitioner–as to the student attending formal lectures.

This book can be used as a text at many levels. It has been the required text for the biostatistics portion of the epidemiology and biostatistics course required of all medical students at the University of California, San Francisco. This course covers the material in the first eight chapters in eight one-hour lectures. The material is discussed along with other epidemiology in an additional problem session each week. The book is also used for a more abbreviated set of lectures on biostatistics (covering the first three chapters) given to our dental students. In addition, it has served me (and others) well in a one quarter four unit course in which we cover the entire book in depth. This course meets for three lecture hours and has a one hour problem session. It is attended by a wide variety of students, from undergraduates through graduate students and postdoctoral fellows, as well as an occasional faculty member.

Since this book includes the technical material covered in any introductory statistics course, it is suitable as either the primary or supplementary text for a general undergraduate introductory statistics course (which is essentially the level at which this material is taught in medical schools), especially for a teacher seeking a way to make statistics relevant to students majoring in the life sciences.

This book differs from other introductory texts on biostatistics in several ways, and it is these differences which seem to account for the book's popularity.

First, it is based on the premise that much of what is published in the biomedical literature uses dubious statistical practices, so that a reader who takes what he reads at face value may often be absorbing erroneous information. Most of the errors (at least as they relate to statistical inference) center on misuse of the t test, probably because the people doing the research were unfamiliar with anything else. The t test is usually the first procedure presented in a statistics book that will yield the highly prized P value. Analysis of variance, if presented at all, is deferred to the end of the book to be ignored or rushed through at the end of the term. Since so much is published that should probably be analyzed with analysis of variance, and since analysis of variance is really the paradigm of all parametric statistical tests, I present it first, then discuss the t test as a special case.

Second, in keeping with the problems I see in the literature, there is a discussion of multiple comparison testing.

Third, the book is organized around hypothesis testing and estimation of the size of treatment effects, as opposed to the more traditional (and logical from a theory of statistics perspective) organization that goes from one-sample to two-sample to general k-sample estimation and hypotheses testing procedures. I believe my approach goes directly to the kinds of problems one most commonly encounters when reading about or doing biomedical research.

The examples are mostly based on interesting studies from the literature and are reasonably true to the original data. I have, however, taken some liberty in recreating the raw data to simplify the statistical problems (for example, making the sample sizes equal) so that I could focus on the important intuitive ideas behind the statistical procedures rather than getting involved in the algebra and arithmetic. When the text only discusses the case of equal sample sizes, the formulas for the more general unequal sample size case are included in an appendix.

When I wrote the first edition of this book, I anticipated that it would serve as a *primer*, a first book, that would introduce people to biostatistics before they went on to read more traditional texts. While the book has enjoyed great success as a text, I discovered that many researchers found its organization and perspective so appealing that they were using it as a reference. This created something of a problem for me because I had purposely selected (on didactic grounds) to present only the simplest of the multiple-comparisons testing procedures–the Bonferroni *t* test–despite the fact that there are better techniques available. In doing so, I have inadvertently popularized a method for treating multiple comparisons that is often too conservative. This edition corrects this oversight by adding a section on the more powerful Student-Newman-Kuels test.

For this new edition, I have revised many of the examples, problems, and figures to simplify and tighten them, and have rewritten sections of the text to clear up ambiguities that many students and other readers brought to my attention, especially in the chapter on statistical power. I have also added new problems, based on real examples taken from scientific papers published in recent years to expand the range of disciplines represented in the examples.

It is worth mentioning a few items I did not add. Some people suggested that I add an explicit discussion of probability calculus and expected values, rather than the implicit discussion of them in the existing text. Others suggested that I make the distinction between P and α more precise. (I purposefully blurred this distinction in the first edition.) I also was tempted to use the platform this book has created within the research community to popularize multivariate statistical methods–in particular multiple regression–within the biomedical community. These methods have been applied widely with good results in the social sciences and I have found them very useful in my work on cardiac function. I decided against making these changes, however, because they would have fundamentally changed the scope and tone of the book, which are the keys to its success.

As with all books, there are many people who deserve thanks. Julien Hoffman gave me the first really clear and practically oriented course in biostatistics that allowed me to stay one step ahead of the people who came to me for expert help. His continuing interest and discussion of statistical issues has helped me learn enough to even think of writing this book. Philip Wilkinson and Marion Nestle suggested some of the best examples and also offered very useful criticism of the manuscript. Mary Giammona offered many useful criticisms from a student's point of view and helped develop the original problem sets. Bryan Slinker helped develop the new problems in the second edition. Virginia Ernster and

Susan Sacks not only offered many helpful suggestions, but also unleashed their 300 first- and second-year medical students on the manuscript for the first edition when they graciously offered to use it as the required text for their course. Bryan Slinker and Ken Resser, who served as teaching assistants to me in the course I taught from this book, offered many insightful criticisms of the first edition and concrete suggestions on how to sharpen the explanations, examples, and problems in the book. Finally, I thank the many others who have used the book, both as students and as teachers of biostatistics, who took the time to write me questions, comments and suggestions on how to improve it. I have done my best to heed their advice in preparing this second edition.

I thank the National Institutes of Health for honoring me with a Research Career Development Award that not only gave me the freedom to develop my scientific ideas but also to engage in the efforts to improve the use of statistical techniques in biomedical research that led to this book.

Finally, I thank the people who helped me convert my first draft into a finished manuscript. Mary Hurtado typed the manuscript with amazing speed and accuracy. Thomas Sumner, Sonja Bock, and Mike Matrigali helped with the final text-editing with UNIX. Dale Johnson prepared the illustrations.

Many of the pictures in this book are direct descendants of my slides. In fact, as you read this book, you would do best to think of it as a slide show that has been set to print. Most people who attend my slide show leave more critical of what they read in the biomedical literature. After I gave it to the MD-PhD candidates at the University of California, San Francisco, I heard that the candidates gave every subsequent speaker a hard time about misuse of the standard error of the mean as a summary statistic and abuse of t tests. Nothing could be more flattering or satisfying to me. Hopefully, this book will make more people more critical and help improve the quality of the biomedical literature and, ultimately, the care of people.

Stanton A. Glantz

Primer
of Biostatistics

Chapter 1

Biostatistics and Clinical Practice

In an ideal world, editors of medical journals would do such an excellent job of ensuring the quality and accuracy of the statistical methods of the papers they publish that readers with no personal interest in this aspect of the research work could simply take it for granted that anything published was correct. If past history is any guide, however, we will probably never even approach that ideal. In the meantime, consumers of the medical literature—practicing physicians and nurses, biomedical researchers, and health planners—must be able to assess statistical methods on their own in order to judge the strength of the arguments for or against the specific diagnostic test or therapy under study. As discussed below, these skills will become more important as financial constraints on medical practice grow.

THE CHANGING MEDICAL ENVIRONMENT

The practice of medicine, like the delivery of all medical services, is entering a new era. Until the second quarter of this century, medical treatment had little positive effect on when, or even whether, sick people recovered. With the discovery of ways to reverse the biochemical deficiencies that caused some diseases and the development of anti-bacterial drugs, it became possible to cure sick people. These early successes and the therapeutic optimism they engendered stimulated the medical research community to develop a host of more powerful agents to treat heart disease, cancer, neurologic disorders, and other ailments. These successes led society to continue increasing the amount of resources devoted to the delivery of medical services. In 1984 the United States spent $387 billion (10.6 percent of the gross national product) on medical services. In addition, both the absolute amount of money and the fraction of the gross national product devoted to the medical sector have been growing rapidly (Fig. 1-1). If present trends were to continue, the medical industry would consume 20 percent of the gross national product by the year 2000. Today, many govern-

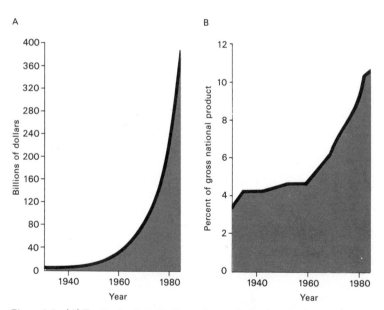

Figure 1-1 (A) Total annual expenditures for medical services in the United States between 1930 and 1984. (B) Expenditures for medical services as a percentage of the gross national product. (*From K. Levitt, H. Lazenby, D. R. Waldo, L. M. Davidoff, "National Health Expenditures, 1984," Health Care Fin. Rev., 7:1–35, 1985.*)

ment and business leaders view this continuing explosion with concern. Containing medical care costs has become a major focus of activity for both state and federal governments as well as the private sector.

During the period of rapid growth that is probably ending, there were ample resources to enable physicians and other health care providers to try tests, procedures, and therapies with little or no restriction on their use. As a result, much of what is considered good medical practice developed without firm evidence demonstrating that these practices actually help the patient. Even for effective therapies, there has been relatively little systematic evaluation of precisely which patients these therapies help.* In addition to wasting money, these practices regularly expose people to powerful drugs, surgery, or other interventions with potentially dangerous side effects in cases where such treatment does not do the patient any good.

What does this have to do with biostatistics?

As the resources available to provide medical care grow more slowly, health professionals will have to identify more clearly which tests, procedures, and therapies are of demonstrated value. In addition to assessing whether or not one intervention or another made a difference, it will become important to assess how great the difference was. Such knowledge will play a growing role in decisions on how to allocate medical resources among potential health care providers and their patients. These issues are, at their heart, statistical issues. Because of factors such as the natural biological variability between individual patients and the placebo effect,† one usually cannot conclude that some therapy was beneficial on the basis of simple experience. For example, about one-third of people given placebos in place of pain killers experience relief. Biostatistics provides the tools for turning clinical and laboratory experience into quantitative statements about whether and by how much a treatment or procedure affected a group of patients.

In addition to studies of procedures and therapies, researchers are

---

*A. L. Cochrane, *Effectiveness and Efficiency: Random Reflections on Health Services,* Nuffield Provincial Hospitals Trust, London, 1972.

†The placebo effect is a response attributable to therapy per se as opposed to the therapy's specific properties. Examples of placebos are an injection of saline, a sugar pill, and surgically opening and closing without performing any specific surgical procedure.

beginning to study how physicians, nurses, and other health care professionals go about their work. For example, one study* demonstrated that patients with uncomplicated pyelonephritis, a common kidney infection, who were treated in accordance with the guidelines in the *Physicians' Desk Reference* remained in the hospital an average of 2 days less than those who were not treated appropriately. Since hospitalization costs constitute a sizable element of total medical care expenditures, it would seem desirable to minimize the length of stay when it does not affect the patient's recovery adversely. Traditionally, there have been few restrictions on how individual physicians prescribed drugs. This study suggests that steps making physicians follow recommended prescribing patterns more closely could significantly reduce hospitalization and save money without harming the patient. Such evidence could be used to support efforts to restrict the individual physician's freedom in using prescription drugs.

Hence, evidence collected and analyzed using biostatistical methods can potentially affect not only how physicians choose to practice medicine but what choices are open to them. Intelligent participation in these decisions requires an understanding of biostatistical methods and models that will permit one to assess the quality of the evidence and the analysis of that evidence used to support one position or another.

Clinicians have not, by and large, participated in debates on these quantitative questions, probably because the issues appear too technical and seem to have little impact on their day-to-day activities. As pressure for more effective use of medical resources grows, clinicians will have to be able to make more informed judgments about claims of medical efficacy so that they can participate more intelligently in the debate on how to allocate medical resources. These judgments will be based in large part on statistical reasoning.

WHAT DO STATISTICAL PROCEDURES TELL YOU?

Suppose researchers believe that administering some drug increases urine production in proportion to the dose and to study it they give

*D. E. Knapp, D. A. Knapp, M. K. Speedie, D. M. Yaeger, and C. L. Baker, "Relationship of Inappropriate Drug Prescribing to Increased Length of Hospital Stay," *Am. J. Hosp. Pharm.*, 36:1334–1337, 1979. This study will be discussed in detail in Chaps. 3 to 5.

different doses of the drug to five different people, plotting their urine production against the dose of drug. The resulting data, shown in Fig. 1-2*A*, reveal a strong relationship between the drug dose and daily urine production in the five people who were studied. This result would probably lead the investigators to publish a paper stating that the drug was an effective diuretic.

The only statement that can be made with absolute certainty is that as the drug dose increased, so did urine production *in the five people in the study.* The real question of interest, however, is: How is the drug likely to affect all people who receive it? The assertion that the drug is effective requires a leap of faith from the limited experience shown in Fig. 1-2*A* to all people. Of course, one cannot know in advance how all people will respond to the drug.

Now, pretend that we knew how every person who would ever

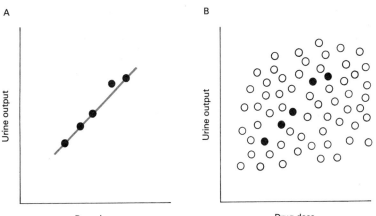

Figure 1-2 (*A*) Results of an experiment in which researchers administered five different doses of a drug to five different people and measured their daily urine production. Output increased as the dose of drug increased in these five people, suggesting that the drug is an effective diuretic in all people similar to those tested. (*B*) If the researchers had been able to administer the drug to all people and measure their daily urine output, it would have been clear that there is no relationship between the dose of drug and urine output. The five specific individuals who happened to be selected for the study in panel *A* are shown as shaded points. It is possible, but not likely, to obtain such an unrepresentative sample that leads one to believe that there is a relationship between the two variables when there is none. A set of statistical procedures called tests of hypotheses permits one to estimate the chance of getting such an unrepresentative sample.

receive the drug would respond. Figure 1-2*B* shows this information. There is no systematic relationship between the drug dose and urine production! The drug is not an effective diuretic.

How could we have been led so far astray? The shaded points in Fig. 1-2*B* represent the specific individuals who happened to be studied to obtain the results shown in Fig. 1-2*A*. While they are all members of the population of people we are interested in studying, the five specific individuals we happened to study, taken as a group, were not really representative of how the entire population of people responds to the drug.

Looking at Fig. 1-2*B* should convince you that obtaining such an unrepresentative sample of people, though possible, is not very likely. One set of statistical procedures, called *tests of hypotheses,* permits you to estimate the likelihood of concluding that two things are related as Fig. 1-2*A* suggests when the relationship is really due to bad luck in selecting people for study and not a true effect of the drug investigated. In this example, we will be able to estimate that such a sample of people should turn up in a study of the drug only about 5 times in 1000 when the drug actually has no effect.

Of course it is important to realize that although biostatistics is a branch of mathematics, there can be honest differences of opinion about the best way to analyze a problem. This fact arises because all statistical methods are based on relatively simple mathematical models of reality, so the results of the statistical tests are accurate only to the extent that the reality and the mathematical model underlying the statistical test are in reasonable agreement.

WHY NOT DEPEND ON THE JOURNALS?

Aside from direct personal experience, most health care professionals rely on medical journals to keep them informed about the current concepts on how to diagnose and treat their patients. Since few members of the clinical or biomedical research community are conversant in the use and interpretation of biostatistics, most readers assume that when an article appears in a journal, the reviewers and editors have scrutinized every aspect of the manuscript, including the use of statistics. Unfortunately, this is not so.

Figure 1-3 shows the results of four critical reviews of the use of

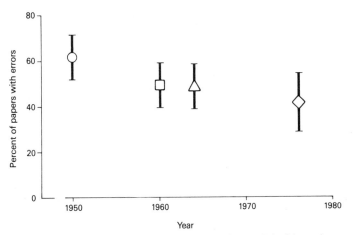

Figure 1-3 Percentage of original research articles published in various general medical journals between 1950 and 1976 that contained errors in their use of statistical methods when interpreting their results. The points represent the percentages reported in articles reviewing a random sample of papers published each year; the vertical lines give an indication of the range, called a confidence interval, that probably contained the percentage of all articles published that year with errors.

statistical methods in the general medical literature conducted between 1950 and 1976.* The points in the figure show the percentages of articles containing errors. Since each reviewer examined only a sample of all articles being published at the time, the percentages of reviewed

*O. B. Ross, Jr. ("Use of Controls in Medical Research," *JAMA*, 145:72–75, 1951) evaluated 100 papers published in *Journal of the American Medical Association, American Journal of Medicine, Annals of Internal Medicine, Archives of Neurology and Psychiatry,* and *American Journal of Medical Sciences* during 1950. R. F. Badgley ("An Assessment of Research Methods Reported in 103 Scientific Articles from Two Canadian Medical Journals," *Can. M.A.J.*, 85:246–250, 1961) evaluated 103 papers published in the *Canadian Medical Association Journal* and *Canadian Journal of Public Health* during 1960. S. Schor and I. Karten ("Statistical Evaluation of Medical Journal Manuscripts," *JAMA*, 195: 1123–1128, 1966) evaluated 295 papers published in *Annals of Internal Medicine, New England Journal of Medicine, Archives of Surgery, American Journal of Medicine, Journal of Clinical Investigation, American Archives of Neurology, Archives of Pathology,* and *Archives of Internal Medicine* during 1964. S. Gore, I. G. Jones, and E. C. Rytter ["Misuses of Statistical Methods: Critical Assessment of Articles in B.M.J. from January to March, 1976," *Br. Med. J.*, 1(6053):85–87, 1977] evaluated 77 papers published in the *British Medical Journal* in 1976.

articles containing errors are only estimates of the true percentage of articles containing errors in the literature at the time. The vertical bars give a range, called a *confidence interval,* which is very likely to contain the true percentage. Computing confidence intervals is another statistical procedure we will study. The confidence intervals in Fig. 1-3 show that critical reviewers of the biomedical literature have consistently found that about half the articles used incorrect statistical methods.

When confronted with this observation—or the confusion that arises when two seemingly comparable articles arrive at different conclusions—people often conclude that statistical analyses are maneuverable to one's needs, or are meaningless, or are too difficult to understand.

Unfortunately, except when a statistical procedure merely confirms an obvious effect (or the paper includes the raw data), a reader cannot tell whether the data in fact support the author's conclusions or not. Ironically, the errors rarely involve sophisticated issues that provoke debate between professional statisticians but are simple mistakes, such as neglecting to include a control group, not allocating treatments to subjects at random, or misusing elementary tests of hypotheses. These errors generally bias the study on behalf of the treatments.

The existence of errors in experimental design and misuse of elementary statistical techniques in a substantial fraction of published papers is especially important in clinical studies. These errors may lead investigators to report a treatment or diagnostic test to be of statistically demonstrated value when, in fact, the available data fail to support this conclusion. Physicians who believe that a treatment has been proved effective on the basis of publication in a reputable journal may use it for their patients. Because all medical procedures involve some risk, discomfort, or cost, people treated on the basis of erroneous research reports gain no benefit and may be harmed. On the other hand, errors could produce unnecessary delay in the use of helpful treatments. Scientific studies which document the effectiveness of medical procedures will become even more important as efforts grow to control medical costs without sacrificing quality. Such studies must be designed and interpreted correctly.

In addition to indirect costs, there are significant direct costs associated with these errors: money is spent, animals may be sacrificed, and human subjects may be put at risk to collect data which are not interpreted correctly.

WHY HAS THE PROBLEM PERSISTED?

Because so many people are making these errors, there is little peer pressure on academic investigators to use statistical techniques carefully. In fact, one rarely hears a word of criticism. Quite the contrary, some investigators fear that their colleagues—and especially reviewers—will view a correct analysis as unnecessarily theoretical and complicated.

The journals are the major force for quality control in scientific work. Some journals have recognized that the regular reviewers often are not competent to review the use of elementary statistics in papers submitted for publication, and these journals have modified their refereeing process accordingly. Generally, they have someone familiar with statistical methods review manuscripts before they are accepted for publication. Most editors, however, apparently assume that the reviewers will examine the statistical methodology in a paper with the same level of care that they examine the clinical protocol or experimental preparation. If this assumption were correct, one would expect all papers to describe, in detail as explicit as the description of the protocol or preparation, how the authors have analyzed their data. Yet, one-third (128 of 389) of the statistical procedures used to test hypotheses in six leading medical journals during 1973 were not even identified.* It is hard to believe that the reviewers examined the methods of data analysis with the same diligence with which they evaluated the experiment used to collect the data.

In short, to read the medical literature intelligently, you will have to be able to understand and evaluate the use of the statistical methods used to analyze the experimental results as well as the laboratory methods used to collect the data. Fortunately, the basic ideas needed to be an intelligent reader—and, indeed, to be an intelligent investigator—are quite simple. The next chapter begins our discussion of these ideas and methods.

*A. R. Feinstein, "Clinical Biostatistics, IIV: Survey of the Statistical Procedures in General Medical Journals," *Clin. Pharm. Therap.,* 15:97–107, 1974.

How to Summarize Data

An investigator collecting data generally has two goals: to obtain descriptive information about the population from which the sample was drawn and to test hypotheses about that population. We focus here on the first goal: to summarize data collected on a single variable in a way that best describes the larger, unobserved population.

When the value of the variable associated with any given individual is more likely to fall near the mean (average) value for all individuals in the population under study than far from it and equally likely to be above the mean and below it, the *mean* and *standard deviation* for the sample observations describe the location of, and amount of variability among, members of the population. When the value of the variable is more likely than not to fall below (or above) the mean, one should report the *median* and values of at least two other percentiles.

To understand these rules, assume that we observe *all* members of the population, not only a limited (ideally representative) sample as in an experiment.

For example, suppose we wish to study the height of Martians and to avoid any guesswork, we visit Mars and measure the entire population—all 200 of them. Figure 2-1 shows the resulting data with each Martian's height rounded to the nearest centimeter and represented by a circle. There is a *distribution* of heights of the Martian population. Most Martians are between about 35 and 45 cm tall, and only a few (10 out of 200) are 30 cm or shorter or 50 cm or taller.

Having successfully completed this project and demonstrated the methodology, we submit a proposal to measure the height of Venusians. Our record of good work assures funding, and we proceed to make the measurements. Following the same conservative approach, we measure the heights of *all* 150 Venusians. Figure 2-2 shows the measured heights for the entire population of Venus, using the same presentation as Fig. 2-1. As on Mars, there is a distribution of heights among members of the population, and all Venusians are around 15 cm tall, almost all of them being taller than 10 cm and shorter than 20 cm.

Comparing Figs. 2-1 and 2-2 demonstrates that Venusians are shorter than Martians and that the variability of heights within the Venusian population is smaller. Whereas almost all (194 of 200) the Martians' heights fell in a range 20 cm wide (30 to 50 cm), the analogous range for Venusians (144 of 150) is only 10 cm (10 to 20 cm). Despite these

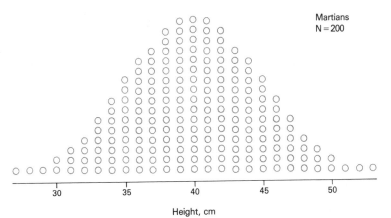

Figure 2-1 Distribution of heights of 200 Martians, with each Martian's height represented by a single circle. Notice that any individual Martian is more likely to have a height near the mean height of the population (40 cm) than far from it and is equally likely to be shorter or taller than average.

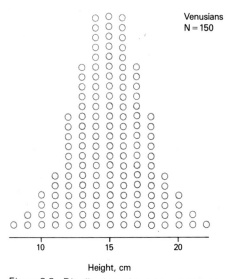

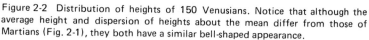

Height, cm

Figure 2-2 Distribution of heights of 150 Venusians. Notice that although the average height and dispersion of heights about the mean differ from those of Martians (Fig. 2-1), they both have a similar bell-shaped appearance.

differences, there are important similarities between these two populations. In both, any given member is more likely to be near the middle of the population than far from it and equally likely to be shorter or taller than average. In fact, despite the differences in population size, average height, and variability, the *shapes* of the distributions of heights of the inhabitants of both planets are almost identical. A most striking result!

We can now reduce all this information to a few numbers, called *parameters* of the distribution. Since the shapes of the two distributions are similar, we need only describe how they differ; we do this by computing the *mean* height and the *variability* of heights about the mean.

THE MEAN

To indicate the location along the height scale, define the *population mean* to be the average height of all members of the population. Population means are often denoted by μ, the Greek letter mu. When the population is made up of discrete members,

$$\text{Population mean} = \frac{\text{sum of values, e.g., heights, for each member of population}}{\text{number of population members}}$$

The equivalent mathematical statement is

$$\mu = \frac{\Sigma X}{N}$$

in which Σ, Greek capital sigma, indicates the sum of the value of the variable X for all N members of the population. Applying this definition to the data in Figs. 2-1 and 2-2 yields the result that the mean height of Martians is 40 cm and the mean height of Venusians is 15 cm. These numbers summarize the qualitative conclusion that the distribution of heights of Martians is higher than the distribution of heights of Venusians.

MEASURES OF VARIABILITY

Next, we need a measure of dispersion about the mean. A value an equal distance above or below the mean should contribute the same amount to our index of variability, even though in one case the deviation from the mean is positive and in the other it is negative. Squaring a number makes it positive, so let us describe the variability of a population about the mean by computing the *average squared deviation from the mean.* The average squared deviation from the mean is larger when there is more variability among members of the population (compare the Martians and Venusians). It is called the *population variance* and is denoted by σ^2, the square of the lower case Greek sigma. Its precise definition for populations made up of discrete individuals is

$$\text{Population variance} = \frac{\text{sum of (value associated with member of population - population mean)}^2}{\text{number of population members}}$$

The equivalent mathematical statement is

$$\sigma^2 = \frac{\Sigma(X - \mu)^2}{N}$$

Note that the units of variance are the square of the units of the variable of interest. In particular, the variance of Martian heights is 25 cm² and the variance of Venusian heights is 6.3 cm². These numbers summarize the qualitative conclusion that there is more variability in heights of Martians than in heights of Venusians.

Since variances are often hard to visualize, it is more common to present the square root of the variance, which we might call the *square root of the average squared deviation from the mean*. Since that is quite a mouthful, this quantity has been named the *standard deviation σ*. Therefore, by definition,

Population standard deviation

$$= \sqrt{\text{population variance}}$$

$$= \sqrt{\frac{\begin{array}{c}\text{sum of (value associated with member} \\ \text{of population - population mean)}^2\end{array}}{\text{number of population members}}}$$

or, mathematically,

$$\sigma = \sqrt{\sigma^2} = \sqrt{\frac{\Sigma(X - \mu)^2}{N}}$$

where the symbols are defined as before. Note that the standard deviation has the same units as the original observations. For example, the standard deviation of Martian heights is 5 cm, and the standard deviation of Venusian heights is 2.5 cm.

THE NORMAL DISTRIBUTION

Table 2-1 summarizes what we found out about Martians and Venusians. The three numbers in the table tell a great deal: the population size, the mean height, and how much the heights vary about the mean. The distributions of heights on both planets have a similar shape, so that *roughly 68 percent of the heights fall within 1 standard deviation from the mean and roughly 95 percent within 2 standard deviations from the mean.* This pattern occurs so often that mathematicians have studied it and found that if the observed measurement is the sum of many independent small random factors, the resulting measurements will take on

Table 2-1   Population Parameters for Heights of Martians and Venusians

	Size of population	Population mean, cm	Population standard deviation, cm
Martians	200	40	5.0
Venusians	150	15	2.5

values that are distributed like the heights we observed on both Mars and Venus. This distribution is called the *normal (or gaussian) distribution.*

Its height at any given value of X is

$$\frac{1}{\sigma\sqrt{2\pi}}\exp\left[-\frac{1}{2}\left(\frac{X-\mu}{\sigma}\right)^2\right]$$

Note that the distribution is completely defined by the population mean μ and population standard deviation σ. Therefore, the information given in Table 2-1 is not just a good abstract of the data, it is *all* the information one needs to describe the population fully *if the distribution of values follows a normal distribution.*

PERCENTILES

Armed with this theoretical breakthrough, we renew our grant by proposing not only to measure the heights of all Jupiter's inhabitants but also to compute the mean and standard deviation of the heights of all Jovians. The resulting data show the mean height to be 37.6 cm and the standard deviation of heights to be 4.5 cm. By comparison with Table 2-1, Jovians appear quite similar in height to Martians, since these two parameters completely specify a normal distribution.

The raw data, however, tell a different story. Figure 2-3A shows that, unlike those living on the other two planets, a given Jovian is not equally likely to have a height above average as below average; the distribution of heights of all population members is no longer symmetric but *skewed.* The few individuals who are much taller than the rest increase the mean and standard deviation in a way that led us to think that most of the heights were higher than they actually are and that the

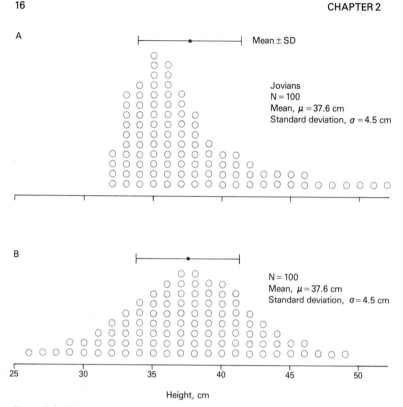

Figure 2-3 When the population values are not distributed symmetrically about the mean, reporting the mean and standard deviation can give the reader an inaccurate impression of the distribution of values in the population. Panel *A* shows the true distribution of the heights of the 100 Jovians (note that it is skewed toward taller heights). Panel *B* shows a normally distributed population with 100 members and the same mean and standard deviation as in panel *A*. Despite this, the distribution of heights in the two populations is quite different.

variability of heights was greater than it actually is. Specifically, Fig. 2-3*B* shows a population of 100 individuals whose heights are distributed according to a normal or gaussian distribution with the same mean and standard deviation as the 100 Jovians in Fig. 2-3*A*. It is quite different. So, although we can compute the mean and standard deviation of heights of Jupiter's—or, for that matter, any—population, these two numbers do not summarize the distribution of heights nearly so well as they did when the heights in the population followed a normal distribution.

An alternative approach which better describes such data is to report the *median*. The median is the value that half the members of the population fall below and half above. Figure 2-4*A* shows that half the Jovians are taller than 36 cm; 36 cm is the median. Since 50 percent of the population values fall below the median, it is also called the *50th percentile*.

To give some indication of the dispersion of heights in the population, report the value which separates the lowest (shortest) 25 percent of the population from the rest and the value which separates the highest (tallest) 25 percent of the population from the lower 75 percent of the population. These two points are called the *25th* and *75th percentile* points, respectively. For the Jovians, Fig. 2-4*B* shows that these percentiles are 34 and 40 cm. While these three numbers (the 25, 50, and 75 percentile points, 34, 36, and 40 cm) do not precisely describe the distribution of heights, they do indicate what the range of heights is and that there are a few very tall Jovians but not many very short ones.

Although these percentiles are often used, one could equally well report the 5th and 95th percentile points, or, for that matter, report the 5, 25, 50, 75, and 95 percentile points.

Computing the percentile points of a population is a good way to see how close to a normal distribution it is. Recall that we said that in a population which exhibits a normal distribution of values, about 95 percent of the population members fall within 2 standard deviations of the mean and about 68 percent fall within 1 standard deviation of the mean. Figure 2-5 shows that, for a normal distribution, the values of the associated percentile points are:

2.5th percentile	mean − 2 standard deviations
16th percentile	mean − 1 standard deviation
50th percentile (median)	mean
84th percentile	mean + 1 standard deviation
97.5th percentile	mean + 2 standard deviations

If the values associated with the percentiles are not too different from what one would expect on the basis of the mean and standard deviation, the normal distribution is a good approximation to the true population and then the mean and standard deviation describe the population adequately.

Why care whether or not the normal distribution is a good approxi-

A

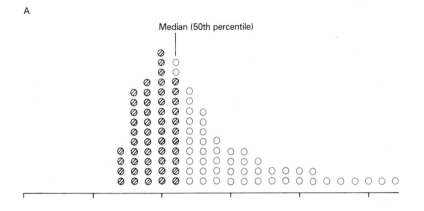

B

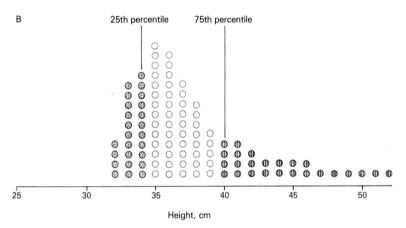

Height, cm

Figure 2-4 One way to describe a skewed distribution is with percentiles. The median is the point which divides the population in half. Panel *A* shows that 36 cm is the median height on Jupiter. Panel *B* shows the 25th and 75th percentiles, the points locating the lowest and highest quarter of the heights, respectively. The fact that the 25th percentile is closer to the mean than the 75th percentile indicates that the distribution is skewed toward higher values.

mation? Because many of the statistical procedures used to test hypotheses—including the ones we will develop in Chaps. 3, 4, and 9— require that the population follow a normal distribution at least approximately for the tests to be reliable. (Chapter 10 presents alternative tests that do not require this assumption.)

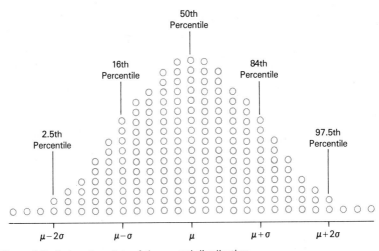

Figure 2-5 Percentile points of the normal distribution.

HOW TO MAKE ESTIMATES FROM A LIMITED SAMPLE

So far, everything we have done has been exact because we followed the conservative course of examining every single member of the population. Usually it is physically or fiscally impossible to do this, and we are limited to examining a *sample* of *n* individuals drawn from the population in the hope that it is representative of the complete population. Without knowledge of the entire population, we can no longer know the population mean μ and population standard deviation σ. Nevertheless, we can estimate them from the sample. The estimate of the population mean is called the *sample mean* and is defined analogously to the population mean:

$$\text{Sample mean} = \frac{\text{sum of values, e.g., heights, of each observation in sample}}{\text{number of observations in sample}}$$

The equivalent mathematical statement is

$$\bar{X} = \frac{\Sigma X}{n}$$

in which the bar over the X denotes that it is the mean of the n observations of X.

The estimate of the population standard deviation is called the *sample standard deviation s* and is defined by

$$\text{Sample standard deviation} = \sqrt{\frac{\text{sum of (value of observation in the sample - sample mean)}^2}{\text{number of observations in sample - 1}}}$$

or, mathematically,*

$$s = \sqrt{\frac{\Sigma(X - \bar{X})^2}{n - 1}}$$

(The standard deviation is also often denoted SD.) This definition differs from the definition of the population standard deviation σ in two ways: (1) the population mean μ has been replaced by our estimate of it, the sample mean $\bar{X}$, and (2) we compute the "average" squared deviation of a sample by dividing by $n - 1$ rather than n. The precise reason for this requires substantial mathematical arguments, but we can present the following intuitive justification. The sample will never show as much variability as the entire population and dividing by $n - 1$ instead of n compensates for the resultant tendency to underestimate the population standard deviation.

In conclusion, when there is no evidence that the sample was not drawn from a normal distribution, summarize data with the sample mean and sample standard deviation, the best estimates of the population mean and population standard deviation, because these two parameters completely define the normal distribution. When there is evidence that the population under study does not follow a normal distribution, summarize data with the median and upper and lower percentiles.

---

*All equations in the text will be presented in the form most conducive to understanding statistical concepts. Often there is another, mathematically equivalent, form of the equation which is more suitable for computation. These forms are tabulated in Appendix A.

HOW GOOD ARE THESE ESTIMATES?

The mean and standard deviation computed from a random sample are estimates of the mean and standard deviation of the entire population from which the sample was drawn. There is nothing special about the specific random sample used to compute these statistics, and different random samples will yield slightly different estimates of the true population mean and standard deviation. To quantitate how accurate these estimates are likely to be, we can compute their *standard errors*. It is possible to compute a standard error for any statistic, but here we shall focus on the *standard error of the mean*. This statistic quantifies the certainty with which the mean computed from a random sample estimates the true mean of the population from which the sample was drawn.

What is the standard error of the mean?

Figure 2-6*A* shows the same population of Martian heights we considered before. Since we have complete knowledge of every Martian's height, we will use this example to explore how accurately statistics computed from a random sample describe the entire population. Suppose that we draw a random sample of 10 Martians from the entire population of 200, then compute the sample mean and sample standard deviation. The 10 Martians in the sample are indicated by solid circles in Fig. 2-6*A*. Figure 2-6*B* shows the results of this random sample as it might be reported in a journal article, together with the sample mean ($\overline{X}$ = 41.5 cm) and sample standard deviation (s = 3.8 cm). The values are close, but not equal, to the population mean (μ = 40 cm) and standard deviation (σ = 5 cm).

There is nothing special about this sample—after all, it was drawn at random—so let us consider a second random sample of 10 Martians from the same population of 200. Figure 2-6*C* shows the results of this sample, with the specific Martians identified in Fig. 2-6*A* as hatched circles. While the mean and standard deviation, 36 and 5 cm, of this second random sample are also similar to the mean and standard deviation of the whole population, they are not the same. Likewise, they are also similar, but not identical, to those from the first sample.

Figure 2-6*D* shows a third random sample of 10 Martians, identified in Fig. 2-6*A* with circles containing dots. This sample leads to estimates of 40 and 5 cm for the mean and standard deviation.

Now, we make an important change in emphasis. Instead of con-

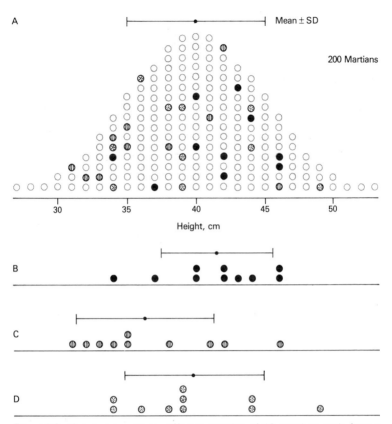

Figure 2-6 If one draws three different samples of 10 members each from a single population, one will obtain three different estimates of the population mean and standard deviation.

centrating on the population of all 200 Martians, let us examine the *means of all possible random samples of 10 Martians.* We have already found three possible values for this mean, 41.5, 36, and 40 cm, and there are many more possibilities. Figure 2-7 shows these three means, plotted as circles, just as we plotted the individual heights, using the same symbols as Fig. 2-6. To better understand the amount of variability in the means of samples of 10 Martians, let us draw another 22 random samples of 10 Martians each and compute the mean of each sample. These additional means are plotted on Fig. 2-7 as open circles.

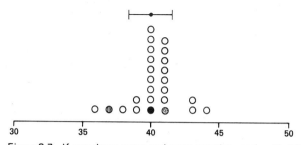

Figure 2-7 If one draws more and more samples—each with 10 members—from a single population, one obtains the population of all possible sample means. This figure illustrates the means of 25 samples of 10 Martians each drawn from the population of 200 Martians shown in Figs. 2-1 and 2-6A. The means of the three specific samples shown in Fig. 2-6 are shown using circles filled with corresponding patterns. This new population of all possible sample means will be normally distributed regardless of the nature of the original population; its mean will equal the mean of the original population; its standard deviation is called the standard error of the mean.

Now that we have drawn 25 random samples of 10 Martians each, have we exhausted the entire population of 200 Martians? No. There are more than 10^{16} different ways to select 10 Martians at random from the population of 200 Martians.

Look at Fig. 2-7. The collection of the means of 25 random samples, each of 10 Martians, has a roughly bell-shaped distribution which is similar to the normal distribution. When the variable of interest is the sum of many other variables, its distribution will tend to be normal, regardless of the distributions of the variables used to form the sum. Since the sample mean is just such a sum, its distribution will tend to be normal, with the approximation improving as the sample size increases. (If the sample were drawn from a normally distributed population, the distribution of the sample means would have a normal distribution regardless of the sample size.) Therefore, it makes sense to describe the data in Fig. 2-7 by computing their mean and standard deviation. Since the mean value of the 25 points in Fig. 2-7 is the mean of the means of 25 samples, we will denote it $\bar{X}_{\bar{X}}$. The standard deviation is the *standard deviation of the means* of 25 independent random samples of 10 Martians each, and so we will denote it $s_{\bar{X}}$. Using the formulas for mean and standard deviation presented earlier, we compute $\bar{X}_{\bar{X}} = 40$ cm and $s_{\bar{X}} = 1.6$ cm.

The mean of the sample means $\bar{X}_{\bar{X}}$ is (within measurement and rounding error) equal to the mean height μ of the entire population of 200 Martians from which we drew the random samples. This is quite a remarkable result, since $\bar{X}_{\bar{X}}$ is *not* the mean of a sample drawn directly from the original population of 200 Martians; $\bar{X}_{\bar{X}}$ is the mean of 25 random samples of size 10 drawn from the *population consisting of all 10^{16} possible values of the mean of random samples of size 10 drawn from the original population of 200 Martians.*

Is $s_{\bar{X}}$ equal to the standard deviation σ of the population of 200 Martians? No. In fact, it is quite a bit smaller; the standard deviation of the collection of sample means $s_{\bar{X}}$ is 1.6 cm while the standard deviation for the whole population is 5 cm. Just as the standard deviation of the original sample of 10 Martians s is an estimate of the variability of Martians' heights, $s_{\bar{X}}$ is an estimate of the *variability of possible values of means of samples of 10 Martians.* Since when one computes the mean, extreme values tend to balance each other, there will be less variability in the values of the sample means than in the original population. $s_{\bar{X}}$ is a measure of the precision with which a sample mean $\bar{X}$ estimates the population mean μ. We might name $s_{\bar{X}}$ "the standard deviation of means of random samples of size 10 drawn from the original population." To be brief, statisticians have coined a shorter name, the *standard error of the mean* (SEM).

Since the certainty with which we can estimate the mean increases as the sample size increases, the standard error of the mean decreases as the sample size increases. Conversely, the more variability in the original population, the more variability will appear in possible mean values of samples; therefore, the standard error of the mean increases as the population standard deviation increases. The true standard error of the mean of samples of size n drawn from a population with standard deviation σ is*

$$\sigma_{\bar{X}} = \frac{\sigma}{\sqrt{n}}$$

The best estimate of $\sigma_{\bar{X}}$ from a single sample is

$$s_{\bar{X}} = \frac{s}{\sqrt{n}}$$

where s is the sample standard deviation.

*This equation is derived in Chap. 4.

Since the possible values of the sample mean tend to follow a normal distribution, the true (and unobserved) mean of the original population will lie within 2 standard errors of the sample mean about 95 percent of the time.

As already noted, mathematicians have shown that the distribution of mean values will always approximately follow a normal distribution *regardless* of how the population from which the original samples were drawn is distributed. We have developed what statisticians call the *central-limit theorem.* It says:

- *The distribution of sample means will be approximately normal regardless of the distribution of values in the original population from which the samples were drawn.*
- *The mean value of the collection of all possible sample means will equal the mean of the original population.*
- *The standard deviation of the collection of all possible means of samples of a given size, called the standard error of the mean, depends on both the standard deviation of the original population and the size of the sample.*

Figure 2-8 illustrates the relationship between the sample mean, the sample standard deviation, and the standard error of the mean and how they vary with sample size as we measure more and more Martians.* As we add more Martians to our sample, the sample mean $\bar{X}$ and standard deviation s estimate the population mean μ and standard deviation σ with increasing precision. This increase in the precision with which the sample mean estimates the population mean is reflected by the smaller standard error of the mean with larger sample sizes. Therefore, the standard error of the mean tells not about variability in the original population, as the standard deviation does, but about the certainty with which a sample mean estimates the true population mean.

The *standard deviation* and *standard error of the mean* measure two very different things and are often confused. Most medical investigators summarize their data with the standard error of the mean because

*Figure 2-8 was obtained by selecting two Martians from Fig. 2-1 at random, then computing $\bar{X}$, s, and $s_{\bar{X}}$. Then one more Martian was selected and the computations done again. Then, a fourth, a fifth, and so on, always adding to the sample already drawn. Had we selected different random samples or the same samples in a different order, Fig. 2-8 would have been different.

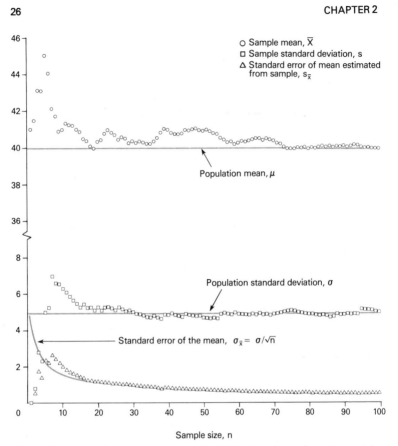

Figure 2-8 As the size of a random sample of Martians drawn from the population depicted in Fig. 2-1 grows, the precision with which the sample mean and sample standard deviation, $\bar{X}$ and s, estimate the true population mean and standard deviation, μ and σ, increases. This increasing precision appears in two ways: (1) the difference between the statistics computed from the sample (the points) moves closer to the true population values (the lines), and (2) the size of the standard error of the mean decreases.

it is always smaller than the standard deviation. It makes their data look better. However, unlike the standard deviation, which quantifies the *variability in the population*, the standard error of the mean quantifies *uncertainty in the estimate of the mean*. Since readers are generally interested in knowing about the population, data should never be summarized with the standard error of the mean.

To understand the difference between the standard deviation and standard error of the mean and why one ought to summarize data using the standard deviation, suppose that in a sample of 20 patients an investigator reports that the mean cardiac output was 5.0 L/min with a standard deviation of 1 L/min. Since about 95 percent of all population members fall within about 2 standard deviations of the mean, this report would tell you that, assuming that the population of interest followed a normal distribution, it would be unusual to observe a cardiac output below about 3 or above about 7 L/min. Thus, you have a quick summary of the population described in the paper and a range against which to compare specific patients you examine. Unfortunately, it is unlikely that these numbers would be reported, the investigator being more likely to say that the cardiac output was 5.0 ± .22 (SEM) L/min. If you confuse the standard error of the mean with the standard deviation, you would believe the range of most of the population was narrow indeed—4.36 to 5.44 L/min. These values describe the range which, with about 95 percent confidence, contains the mean cardiac output of the entire population from which the sample of 20 patients was drawn. (Chapter 7 discusses these ideas in detail.) In practice, one generally wants to compare a specific patient's cardiac output not only with the population mean but with the spread in the population taken as a whole.

SUMMARY

When a population follows a normal distribution, we can describe its location and variability completely with two parameters, the mean and standard deviation. When the population does not follow a normal distribution at least roughly, it is more informative to describe it with the median and other percentiles. Since one can rarely observe all members of a population, we will estimate these parameters from a sample drawn at random from the population. The standard error quantifies the precision of these estimates. For example, the standard error of the mean quantifies the precision with which the sample mean estimates the population mean.

In addition to being useful for describing a population or sample, these numbers can be used to estimate how compatible measurements are with clinical or scientific assertions that an intervention affected some variable. We now turn our attention to this problem.

2-1 Find the mean, median, standard deviation, and 25th and 75th percentiles of the following observations: 0, 0, 0, 1, 1, 1, 1, 1, 1, 1, 1, 1, 1, 1, 1, 2, 2, 2, 2, 3, 3, 3, 3, 4, 4, 5, 5, 5, 5, 6, 7, 9, 10, 11. Do these data seem to be drawn from a normally distributed population? Why or why not? (These numbers are clinical severity scores for people afflicted with sickle-cell anemia. This study will be analyzed in detail in Prob. 8-4. The data are from R. Hebbel et al., "Erythrocyte Adherence to Endothelium in Sickle-Cell Anemia: A Possible Determinant of Disease Severity," *N. Engl. J. Med.,* **302**: 992–995, 1980. Used by permission.)

2-2 Find the mean, median, standard deviation, and 25th and 75th percentiles of the following observations: 289, 203, 359, 243, 232, 210, 251, 246, 224, 239, 220, 211. Do these data seem to be drawn from a normally distributed population? Why or why not? (These numbers are how many seconds 12 people with heart disease could exercise before smoking a cigarette. This study will be analyzed fully in Prob. 9-5. The data are from W. Aronow, "Effect of Nonnicotine Cigarettes and Carbon Monoxide on Angina," *Circulation,* **61**:262–265, 1979. By permission of the American Heart Association, Inc.)

2-3 Find the mean, median, standard deviation, and 25th and 75th percentiles of the following observations: 1.2, 1.4, 1.6, 1.7, 1.7, 1.8, 2.2, 2.3, 2.4, 6.4, 19.0, 23.6. Do these data seem to be drawn from a normally distributed population? Why or why not? (These numbers quantitate the amount of leakage of a fluorescent dye from the blood stream into the eye in patients with abnormal retinas. The data are from G. A. Fishman et al., "Blood-Retinal Barrier Function in Patients with Cone or Cone-Rod Dystrophy," *Arch. Ophthalmol.* **104**:545–548, 1986.)

2-4 Sketch the distribution of all possible values of the number on the upright face of a die. What is the mean of this population of possible values?

2-5 Roll a *pair* of dice and note the numbers on each of the upright faces. These two numbers can be considered a sample of size 2 drawn from the population described in Prob. 2-3. This sample can be averaged. What does this average estimate? Repeat this procedure 20 times and plot the averages observed after each roll. What is this distribution? Compute its mean and standard deviation. What do they represent?

2-6 Robert Fletcher and Suzanne Fletcher ("Clinical Research in General Medical Journals: A 30-Year Perspective," *N. Engl. J. Med.,* **301**:180–183, 1979, used by permission) studied the characteristics of 612 randomly selected articles published in the *Journal of the American Medical Association, New England Journal of Medicine,* and *Lancet* since 1946. One of the attributes they examined was the number of authors; they found:

Year	No. of articles examined	Mean no. of authors	SD
1946	151	2.0	1.4
1956	149	2.3	1.6
1966	157	2.8	1.2
1976	155	4.9	7.3

Sketch the populations of numbers of authors for each of these years. How closely do you expect the normal distribution to approximate the actual population of all authors in each of these years? Why? Estimate the certainty with which these samples permit you to estimate the true mean number of authors for all articles published in comparable journals each year.

How to Test for Differences between Groups

Statistical methods are used to summarize data and test hypotheses with those data. Chapter 2 discussed how to use the mean, standard deviation, median, and percentiles to summarize data and how to use the standard error of the mean to estimate the precision with which a sample mean estimates the population mean. Now we turn our attention to how to use data to test scientific hypotheses. The statistical techniques used to perform such tests are called *tests of significance;* they yield the highly prized *P value.* We now develop procedures to test the hypothesis that, on the average, different treatments all affect some variable identically. Specifically, we will develop a procedure to test the hypothesis that diet has no effect on the mean cardiac output of people living in a small town. Statisticians call this hypothesis of no effect the *null hypothesis.*

The resulting test can be generalized to analyze data obtained in experiments involving any number of treatments. In addition, it is the archetype for a whole class of related procedures known as *analysis of variance.*

THE GENERAL APPROACH

To begin our experiment, we randomly select four groups of seven people each from a small town with 200 healthy adult inhabitants. All participants give informed consent. People in the control group continue eating normally; people in the second group eat only spaghetti; people in the third group eat only steak; and people in the fourth group eat only fruit and nuts. After 1 month, each person is catheterized and his cardiac output is measured.

As with most tests of significance, we begin with the hypothesis that all treatments (diets) have the same effect (on cardiac output). Since the study includes a control group (as experiments generally should), this hypothesis is equivalent to the hypothesis that diet has no effect on cardiac output. Figure 3-1 shows the distribution of cardiac outputs for the entire population, with each individual's cardiac output represented by a circle. The specific individuals who were randomly selected for each diet are indicated by shaded circles, with different shading for different diets. Figure 3-1 shows that the hypothesis is, in fact, true. Unfortunately, as investigators we cannot observe the entire population and are left with the problem of deciding whether or not

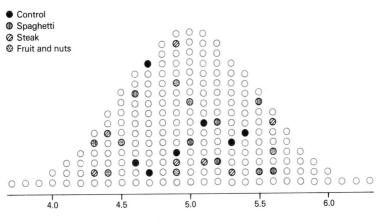

Cardiac output, liters/min

Figure 3-1 The values of cardiac output associated with all 200 members of the population of a small town. Since diet does not affect cardiac output, the four groups of seven people each selected at random to participate in our experiment (control, spaghetti, steak, fruit and nuts) simply represent four random samples drawn from a single population.

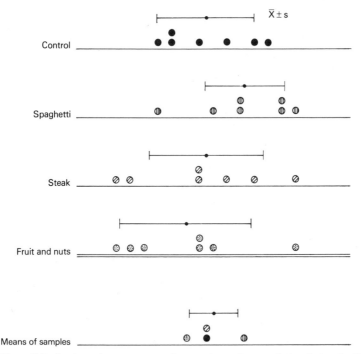

Figure 3-2 An investigator cannot observe the entire population but only the four samples selected at random for treatment. This figure shows the same four groups of individuals as in Fig. 3-1 with their means and standard deviations as they would appear to the investigator. The question facing the investigator is: Are the observed differences due to the different diets or simply random variation? The figure also shows the collection of sample means together with their standard deviation, which is an estimate of the standard error of the mean.

it is true from the limited data shown in Fig. 3-2. There are obviously differences between the samples; the question is: *Are these differences due to the fact that the different groups of people ate differently or are these differences simply a reflection of the random variation in cardiac output between individuals?*

To use the data in Fig. 3-2 to address this question, we proceed under the assumption that the hypothesis that diet has no effect on cardiac output is correct. Since we assume that it does not matter which diet any particular individual ate, we *assume* that the four experimental groups of seven people each are four random samples of size

7 *drawn from a single population* of 200 individuals. Since the samples are drawn at random from a population with some variance, we expect the samples to have different means and standard deviations, but *if our hypothesis that the diet has no effect on cardiac output is true,* the observed differences are simply due to random sampling.

Forget about statistics for a moment. What is it about different samples that leads you to believe that they are representative samples drawn from different populations? Figures 3-2 to 3-4 show three different possible sets of samples of some variable of interest. Simply looking at these pictures makes most people think that the four samples in Fig. 3-2 were all drawn from a single population, while the samples in Figs. 3-3 and 3-4 were not. Why? The variability within each sample, quantified with the standard deviation, is approximately the same. In Fig. 3-2 the variability in the mean values of the samples is consistent with the variability one observes within the individual samples. In contrast, in Figs. 3-3 and 3-4 the variability among sample means is much larger than one would expect from the variability within each sample. Notice that we reach this conclusion whether all (Fig. 3-3) or only one (Fig. 3-4) of the sample means appear to differ from the others.

Now let us formalize this analysis of variability to analyze our diet experiment. The standard deviation or its square, the variance, is a good measure of variability. We will use the variance to construct a procedure to test the hypothesis that diet does not affect cardiac output.

Chapter 2 showed that two population parameters—the mean and standard deviation (or, equivalently, the variance)—completely describe a normally distributed population. Therefore, we will use our raw data to compute these parameters and then base our analysis on their values rather than on the raw data directly. Since the procedures we will now develop are based on these parameters, they are called *parametric statistical methods.* Because these methods assume that the population from which the samples were drawn can be completely described by these parameters, they are valid only when the real population approximately follows the normal distribution. Other procedures, called *nonparametric statistical methods,* are based on frequencies, ranks, or percentiles and do not require this assumption.* Parametric methods generally provide more information about the treatment being

*We will study these procedures in Chaps. 5, 8, and 10.

studied and are more likely to detect a real treatment effect when the underlying population is normally distributed.

We will estimate the parameter population variance in two different ways: (1) The standard deviation or variance computed from each sample is an estimate of the standard deviation or variance of the entire population. Since each of these estimates of the population variance is computed from within each sample group, the estimates will not be affected by any differences in the mean values of different groups. (2) We will use the values of the means of each sample to determine a second estimate of the population variance. In this case, the differences between the means will obviously affect the resulting estimate of the population variance. If all the samples were, in fact, drawn from the same population (i.e., the diet had no effect), these two different ways to estimate the population variance should yield approximately the same number. When they do, we will conclude that the samples were likely to have been drawn from a single population; otherwise, we will reject this hypothesis and conclude that at least one of the samples was drawn from a different population. In our experiment, rejecting the original hypothesis would lead to the conclusion that diet *does* alter cardiac output.

TWO DIFFERENT ESTIMATES OF THE POPULATION VARIANCE

How shall we estimate the population variance from the four sample variances? When the hypothesis that the diet does not affect cardiac output is true, the variance of each sample of seven people, regardless of what they ate, is an equally good estimate of the population variance, so we simply average our four estimates of *variance within the treatment groups*

Average variance in cardiac output within treatment groups = $\frac{1}{4}$(variance in cardiac output of controls + variance in cardiac output of spaghetti eaters + variance in cardiac output of steak eaters + variance in cardiac output of fruit and nut eaters)

The mathematical equivalent is

$$s_{\text{wit}}^2 = \tfrac{1}{4}(s_{\text{con}}^2 + s_{\text{spa}}^2 + s_{\text{st}}^2 + s_{\text{f}}^2)$$

where s^2 represents variance. The variance of each sample is computed with respect to the mean of that sample. Therefore, the population variance estimated from within the groups, *the within-groups variance* s_{wit}^2, will be the same whether or not diet altered cardiac output.

Next we estimate the population variance from the means of the samples. Since we have hypothesized that all four samples were drawn from a single population, the standard deviation of the four sample means will approximate the standard error of the mean. Recall that the standard error of the mean $\sigma_{\bar{X}}$ is related to the sample size n (in this case 7) and the population standard deviation σ according to

$$\sigma_{\bar{X}} = \frac{\sigma}{\sqrt{n}}$$

Therefore, the true population variance σ^2 is related to the sample size and standard error of the mean according to

$$\sigma^2 = n\sigma_{\bar{X}}^2$$

We use this relationship to estimate the population variance from the variability between the sample means using

$$s_{\text{bet}}^2 = ns_{\bar{X}}^2$$

where s_{bet}^2 is the estimate of the population variance computed from between the sample means and $s_{\bar{X}}$ is the standard deviation of the means of the four sample groups, the standard error of the mean. This estimate of the population variance computed from between the group means is often called the *between-groups variance.*

If the hypothesis that all four samples were drawn from the same population is true (i.e., that diet does not affect cardiac output), the within-groups variance and between-groups variance are both estimates of the same population variance and so should be about equal. Therefore, we will compute the following ratio, called the F-test statistic,

$$F = \frac{\text{population variance estimated from sample means}}{\begin{array}{c}\text{population variance estimated as average}\\\text{of sample variances}\end{array}}$$

$$F = \frac{s^2_{\text{bet}}}{s^2_{\text{wit}}}$$

Since both the numerator and the denominator are estimates of the same population variance σ^2, F should be about $\sigma^2/\sigma^2 = 1$. For the four random samples in Fig. 3-2, $F = 1.4$. Since F is about equal to 1, we conclude that the data in Fig. 3-2 are not inconsistent with the

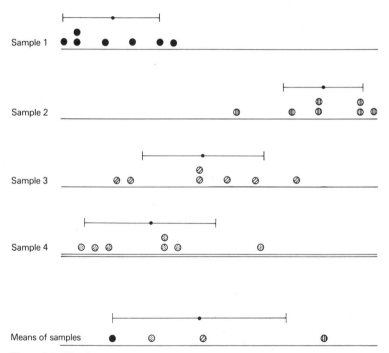

Figure 3-3 The four samples shown are identical to those in Fig. 3-2 except that the variability in the mean values has been increased substantially. The samples now appear to differ from each other because the variability between the sample means is larger than one would expect from the variability within each sample. Compare the relative variability in mean values with the variability within the sample groups with that seen in Fig. 3-2.

hypothesis that diet does not affect cardiac output and we continue to accept that hypothesis.

Now we have a rule for deciding when to reject the hypothesis that all the samples were drawn from the same population:

If F is a big number, the variability between the sample means is larger than expected from the variability within the samples, so reject the hypothesis that all the samples were drawn from the same population.

This quantitative statement formalizes the qualitative logic we used when discussing Figs. 3-2 to 3-4. The F associated with Fig. 3-3 is 68.0, and that associated with Fig. 3-4 is 24.5.

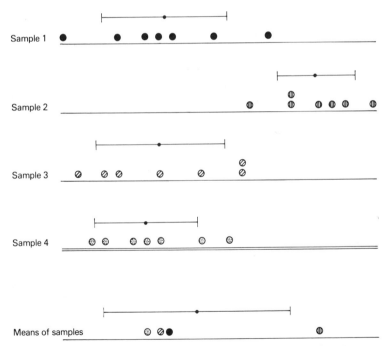

Figure 3-4   When the mean of even one of the samples (sample 2) differs substantially from the other samples, the variability computed from within the means is substantially larger than one would expect from examining the variability within the groups.

WHAT IS A "BIG" F?

The exact value of F one computes depends on which individuals were drawn for the random samples. For example, Fig. 3-5 shows yet another set of four samples of seven people drawn from the population of 200 people in Fig. 3-1. In this example $F = .5$. Suppose we repeated our experiment 200 times on the same population. Each time we would draw four different samples of people and—even if the diet had no effect on cardiac output—get slightly different values for F due to random variation. Figure 3-6A shows the result of this procedure, with the resulting F's rounded to one decimal place and represented with a circle; the two dark circles represent the values of F computed from the data in Figs. 3-2 and 3-5. The exact shapes of the distribution of

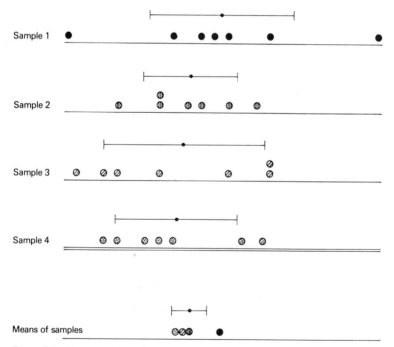

Figure 3-5 Four samples of seven members each drawn from the population shown in Fig. 3-1. Note that the variability in sample means is consistent with the variability within each of the samples. $F = .5$.

values of F depends on how many samples were drawn, the size of each sample, and the distribution of the population from which the samples were drawn.

As expected, most of the computed F's are around 1 (that is, between 0 and 2), but a few are much larger. Thus, even though most experiments will produce relatively small values of F, it is possible that, by sheer bad luck, one could select random samples which are not good representatives of the whole population. The result is an occasional relatively large value for F even though the treatment had no effect. Figure 3-6B shows, however, that such values are unlikely. Only 5 percent of the 200 experiments (10 experiments) produced F values equal to or greater than 3.0. We now have a tentative estimate of what to call a "big" value for F. Since F exceeded 3.0 only 10 out of 200 times *when all the samples were drawn from the same population,* we might decide that F is big when it exceeds 3.0 and reject the hypothesis that all the samples were drawn from the same population (i.e., that the treatment had no effect). In deciding to reject the hypothesis of no effect when F is big, we accept the risk of erroneously rejecting this hypothesis 5 percent of the time because F will be 3.0 or greater about 5 percent of the time, even when the treatment does not alter mean response.

When we obtain such a "big" F, we reject the original hypothesis that all the means are the same and report $P < .05$. $P < .05$ means that there is less than a 5 percent chance of getting a value of F as big or bigger than the computed value if the original hypothesis were true (i.e., diet did not affect cardiac output).

The critical value of F should be selected not on the basis of just 200 experiments but all 10^{42} possible experiments. Suppose we did all 10^{42} experiments and computed the corresponding F values, then plotted the results, just as we did for Fig. 3-6B. Figure 3-6C shows the result with grains of sand to represent each observed F value. The darker sand indicates the biggest 5 percent of the F values. Notice how similar it is to Fig. 3-6B. This similarity should not surprise you, since the results in panel B are just a random sample of the population in panel C. Finally, recall that everything so far has been based on an original population containing only 200 members. In reality, populations are usually much larger, so that there can be many more than 10^{42} possible values of F. Often, there are essentially an infinite num-

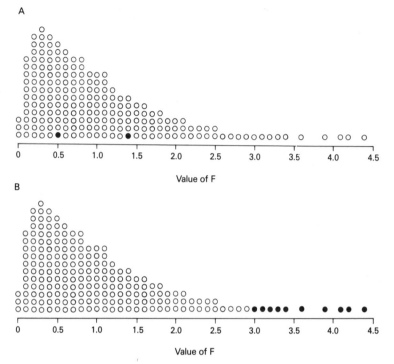

Figure 3-6 (*A*) Values of *F* computed from 200 experiments involving four samples, each of size 7, drawn from the population in Fig. 3-1. (*B*) We expect *F* to exceed 3.0 only 5 percent of the time when all samples were, in fact, drawn from a single population. (*C*) Results of computing the *F* ratio for all possible samples drawn from the original population. The 5 percent of most extreme *F* values are shown darker than the rest. (*D*) The *F* distribution one would obtain when sampling an infinite population. In this case, the cutoff value for considering *F* to be "big" is that value of *F* which subtends the upper 5 percent of the total area under the curve.

ber of possible experiments. In terms of Fig. 3-6*C*, it is as if all the grains of sand melted together to yield the continuous line in Fig. 3-6*D*.

Therefore, *areas under the curve* are analogous to the fractions of total number of circles or grains of sand in panels *B* and *C*. Since the shaded region in Fig. 3-6*D* represents 5 percent of the total area under the curve, it can be used to compute that the cutoff point for a "big" *F* with the number of samples and sample size in this study is 3.01. This and other cutoff values that correspond to $P < .05$ and $P < .01$ are listed in Table 3-1.

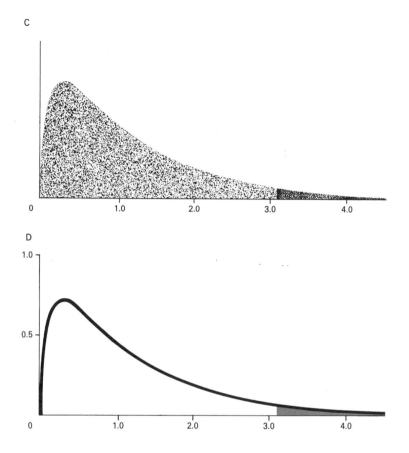

To construct these tables, mathematicians have assumed four things about the underlying population that must be at least approximately satisfied for the tables to be applicable to real data:

- Each sample must be independent of the other samples.
- Each sample must be randomly selected from the population being studied.
- The populations from which the samples were drawn must be normally distributed.*

*This is another reason parametric statistical methods require data from normally distributed populations.

Table 3-1 Critical Values of F Corresponding to $P < .05$ (Lightface) and $P < .01$ (Boldface)

ν_d	1	2	3	4	5	6	7	8	9	10	11	12	14	16	20	24	30	40	50	75	100	200	500	∞
1	161	200	216	225	230	234	237	239	241	242	243	244	245	246	248	249	250	251	252	253	253	254	254	254
	4052	**4999**	**5403**	**5625**	**5764**	**5859**	**5928**	**5981**	**6022**	**6056**	**6082**	**6106**	**6142**	**6169**	**6208**	**6234**	**6261**	**6286**	**6302**	**6323**	**6334**	**6352**	**6361**	**6366**
2	18.51	19.00	19.16	19.25	19.30	19.33	19.36	19.37	19.38	19.39	19.40	19.41	19.42	19.43	19.44	19.45	19.46	19.47	19.47	19.48	19.49	19.49	19.50	19.50
	98.49	**99.00**	**99.17**	**99.25**	**99.30**	**99.33**	**99.36**	**99.37**	**99.39**	**99.40**	**99.41**	**99.42**	**99.43**	**99.44**	**99.45**	**99.46**	**99.47**	**99.48**	**99.48**	**99.49**	**99.49**	**99.49**	**99.50**	**99.50**
3	10.13	9.55	9.28	9.12	9.01	8.94	8.88	8.84	8.81	8.78	8.76	8.74	8.71	8.69	8.66	8.64	8.62	8.60	8.58	8.57	8.56	8.54	8.54	8.53
	34.12	**30.82**	**29.46**	**28.71**	**28.24**	**27.91**	**27.67**	**27.49**	**27.34**	**27.23**	**27.13**	**27.05**	**26.92**	**26.83**	**26.69**	**26.60**	**26.50**	**26.41**	**26.35**	**26.27**	**26.23**	**26.18**	**26.14**	**26.12**
4	7.71	6.94	6.59	6.39	6.26	6.16	6.09	6.04	6.00	5.96	5.93	5.91	5.87	5.84	5.80	5.77	5.74	5.71	5.70	5.68	5.66	5.65	5.64	5.63
	21.20	**18.00**	**16.69**	**15.98**	**15.52**	**15.21**	**14.98**	**14.80**	**14.66**	**14.54**	**14.45**	**14.37**	**14.24**	**14.15**	**14.02**	**13.93**	**13.83**	**13.74**	**13.69**	**13.61**	**13.57**	**13.52**	**13.48**	**13.46**
5	6.61	5.79	5.41	5.19	5.05	4.95	4.88	4.82	4.78	4.74	4.70	4.68	4.64	4.60	4.56	4.53	4.50	4.46	4.44	4.42	4.40	4.38	4.37	4.36
	16.26	**13.27**	**12.06**	**11.39**	**10.97**	**10.67**	**10.45**	**10.29**	**10.15**	**10.05**	**9.96**	**9.89**	**9.77**	**9.68**	**9.55**	**9.47**	**9.38**	**9.29**	**9.24**	**9.17**	**9.13**	**9.07**	**9.04**	**9.02**
6	5.99	5.14	4.76	4.53	4.39	4.28	4.21	4.15	4.10	4.06	4.03	4.00	3.96	3.92	3.87	3.84	3.81	3.77	3.75	3.72	3.71	3.69	3.68	3.67
	13.74	**10.92**	**9.78**	**9.15**	**8.75**	**8.47**	**8.26**	**8.10**	**7.98**	**7.87**	**7.79**	**7.72**	**7.60**	**7.52**	**7.39**	**7.31**	**7.23**	**7.14**	**7.09**	**7.02**	**6.99**	**6.94**	**6.90**	**6.88**
7	5.59	4.74	4.35	4.12	3.97	3.87	3.79	3.73	3.68	3.63	3.60	3.57	3.52	3.49	3.44	3.41	3.38	3.34	3.32	3.29	3.28	3.25	3.24	3.23
	12.25	**9.55**	**8.45**	**7.85**	**7.46**	**7.19**	**7.00**	**6.84**	**6.71**	**6.62**	**6.54**	**6.47**	**6.35**	**6.27**	**6.15**	**6.07**	**5.98**	**5.90**	**5.85**	**5.78**	**5.75**	**5.70**	**5.67**	**5.65**
8	5.32	4.46	4.07	3.84	3.69	3.58	3.50	3.44	3.39	3.34	3.31	3.28	3.23	3.20	3.15	3.12	3.08	3.05	3.03	3.00	2.98	2.96	2.94	2.93
	11.26	**8.65**	**7.59**	**7.01**	**6.63**	**6.37**	**6.19**	**6.03**	**5.91**	**5.82**	**5.74**	**5.67**	**5.56**	**5.48**	**5.36**	**5.28**	**5.20**	**5.11**	**5.06**	**5.00**	**4.96**	**4.91**	**4.88**	**4.86**
9	5.12	4.26	3.86	3.63	3.48	3.37	3.29	3.23	3.18	3.13	3.10	3.07	3.02	2.98	2.93	2.90	2.86	2.82	2.80	2.77	2.76	2.73	2.72	2.71
	10.56	**8.02**	**6.99**	**6.42**	**6.06**	**5.80**	**5.62**	**5.47**	**5.35**	**5.26**	**5.18**	**5.11**	**5.00**	**4.92**	**4.80**	**4.73**	**4.64**	**4.56**	**4.51**	**4.45**	**4.41**	**4.36**	**4.33**	**4.31**
10	4.96	4.10	3.71	3.48	3.33	3.22	3.14	3.07	3.02	2.97	2.94	2.91	2.86	2.82	2.77	2.74	2.70	2.67	2.64	2.61	2.59	2.56	2.55	2.54
	10.04	**7.56**	**6.55**	**5.99**	**5.64**	**5.39**	**5.21**	**5.06**	**4.95**	**4.85**	**4.78**	**4.71**	**4.60**	**4.52**	**4.41**	**4.33**	**4.25**	**4.17**	**4.12**	**4.05**	**4.01**	**3.96**	**3.93**	**3.91**
11	4.84	3.98	3.59	3.36	3.20	3.09	3.01	2.95	2.90	2.86	2.82	2.79	2.74	2.70	2.65	2.61	2.57	2.53	2.50	2.47	2.45	2.42	2.41	2.40
	9.65	**7.20**	**6.22**	**5.67**	**5.32**	**5.07**	**4.88**	**4.74**	**4.63**	**4.54**	**4.46**	**4.40**	**4.29**	**4.21**	**4.10**	**4.02**	**3.94**	**3.86**	**3.80**	**3.74**	**3.70**	**3.66**	**3.62**	**3.60**
12	4.75	3.88	3.49	3.26	3.11	3.00	2.92	2.85	2.80	2.76	2.72	2.69	2.64	2.60	2.54	2.50	2.46	2.42	2.40	2.36	2.35	2.32	2.31	2.30
	9.33	**6.93**	**5.95**	**5.41**	**5.06**	**4.82**	**4.65**	**4.50**	**4.39**	**4.30**	**4.22**	**4.16**	**4.05**	**3.98**	**3.86**	**3.78**	**3.70**	**3.61**	**3.56**	**3.49**	**3.46**	**3.41**	**3.38**	**3.36**
13	4.67	3.80	3.41	3.18	3.02	2.92	2.84	2.77	2.72	2.67	2.63	2.60	2.55	2.51	2.46	2.42	2.38	2.34	2.32	2.28	2.26	2.24	2.22	2.21
	9.07	**6.70**	**5.74**	**5.20**	**4.86**	**4.62**	**4.44**	**4.30**	**4.19**	**4.10**	**4.02**	**3.96**	**3.85**	**3.78**	**3.67**	**3.59**	**3.51**	**3.42**	**3.37**	**3.30**	**3.27**	**3.21**	**3.18**	**3.16**
14	4.60	3.74	3.34	3.11	2.96	2.85	2.77	2.70	2.65	2.60	2.56	2.53	2.48	2.44	2.39	2.35	2.31	2.27	2.24	2.21	2.19	2.16	2.14	2.13
	8.86	**6.51**	**5.56**	**5.03**	**4.69**	**4.46**	**4.28**	**4.14**	**4.03**	**3.94**	**3.86**	**3.80**	**3.70**	**3.62**	**3.51**	**3.43**	**3.34**	**3.26**	**3.21**	**3.14**	**3.11**	**3.06**	**3.02**	**3.00**
15	4.54	3.68	3.29	3.06	2.90	2.79	2.70	2.64	2.59	2.55	2.51	2.48	2.43	2.39	2.33	2.29	2.25	2.21	2.18	2.15	2.12	2.10	2.08	2.07
	8.68	**6.36**	**5.42**	**4.89**	**4.56**	**4.32**	**4.14**	**4.00**	**3.89**	**3.80**	**3.73**	**3.67**	**3.56**	**3.48**	**3.36**	**3.29**	**3.20**	**3.12**	**3.07**	**3.00**	**2.97**	**2.92**	**2.89**	**2.87**

Critical values table (F-distribution). First column is ν_d (degrees of freedom for denominator). Each cell shows the 0.05 value (upper) and the 0.01 value (lower, bold). The numerator degree-of-freedom column headers are not printed within the visible portion of this page.

ν_d																								
16	4.49 **8.53**	3.63 **6.23**	3.24 **5.29**	3.01 **4.77**	2.85 **4.44**	2.74 **4.20**	2.66 **4.03**	2.59 **3.89**	2.54 **3.78**	2.49 **3.69**	2.45 **3.61**	2.42 **3.55**	2.37 **3.45**	2.33 **3.37**	2.28 **3.25**	2.24 **3.18**	2.20 **3.10**	2.16 **3.01**	2.13 **2.96**	2.09 **2.98**	2.07 **2.86**	2.04 **2.80**	2.02 **2.77**	2.01 **2.75**
17	4.45 **8.40**	3.59 **6.11**	3.20 **5.18**	2.96 **4.67**	2.81 **4.34**	2.70 **4.10**	2.62 **3.93**	2.55 **3.79**	2.50 **3.68**	2.45 **3.59**	2.41 **3.52**	2.38 **3.45**	2.33 **3.35**	2.29 **3.27**	2.23 **3.16**	2.19 **3.08**	2.15 **3.00**	2.11 **2.92**	2.08 **2.86**	2.04 **2.79**	2.02 **2.76**	1.99 **2.70**	1.97 **2.67**	1.96 **2.65**
18	4.41 **8.28**	3.55 **6.01**	3.16 **5.09**	2.93 **4.58**	2.77 **4.25**	2.66 **4.01**	2.58 **3.85**	2.51 **3.71**	2.46 **3.60**	2.41 **3.51**	2.37 **3.44**	2.34 **3.37**	2.29 **3.27**	2.25 **3.19**	2.19 **3.07**	2.15 **3.00**	2.11 **2.91**	2.07 **2.83**	2.04 **2.78**	2.00 **2.71**	1.98 **2.68**	1.95 **2.62**	1.93 **2.59**	1.92 **2.57**
19	4.38 **8.18**	3.52 **5.93**	3.13 **5.01**	2.90 **4.50**	2.74 **4.17**	2.63 **3.94**	2.55 **3.77**	2.48 **3.63**	2.43 **3.52**	2.38 **3.43**	2.34 **3.36**	2.31 **3.30**	2.26 **3.19**	2.21 **3.12**	2.15 **3.00**	2.11 **2.92**	2.07 **2.84**	2.02 **2.76**	2.00 **2.70**	1.96 **2.63**	1.94 **2.60**	1.91 **2.54**	1.90 **2.51**	1.88 **2.49**
20	4.35 **8.10**	3.49 **5.85**	3.10 **4.94**	2.87 **4.43**	2.71 **4.10**	2.60 **3.87**	2.52 **3.71**	2.45 **3.56**	2.40 **3.45**	2.35 **3.37**	2.31 **3.30**	2.28 **3.23**	2.23 **3.13**	2.18 **3.05**	2.12 **2.94**	2.08 **2.86**	2.04 **2.77**	1.99 **2.69**	1.96 **2.63**	1.92 **2.56**	1.90 **2.53**	1.87 **2.47**	1.85 **2.44**	1.84 **2.42**
21	4.32 **8.02**	3.47 **5.78**	3.07 **4.87**	2.84 **4.37**	2.68 **4.04**	2.57 **3.81**	2.49 **3.65**	2.42 **3.51**	2.37 **3.40**	2.32 **3.31**	2.28 **3.24**	2.25 **3.17**	2.20 **3.07**	2.15 **2.99**	2.09 **2.88**	2.05 **2.80**	2.00 **2.72**	1.96 **2.63**	1.93 **2.58**	1.89 **2.51**	1.87 **2.47**	1.84 **2.42**	1.82 **2.38**	1.81 **2.36**
22	4.30 **7.94**	3.44 **5.72**	3.05 **4.82**	2.82 **4.31**	2.66 **3.99**	2.55 **3.76**	2.47 **3.59**	2.40 **3.45**	2.35 **3.35**	2.30 **3.26**	2.26 **3.18**	2.23 **3.12**	2.18 **3.02**	2.13 **2.94**	2.07 **2.83**	2.03 **2.75**	1.98 **2.67**	1.93 **2.58**	1.91 **2.53**	1.87 **2.46**	1.84 **2.42**	1.81 **2.37**	1.80 **2.33**	1.78 **2.31**
23	4.28 **7.88**	3.42 **5.66**	3.03 **4.76**	2.80 **4.26**	2.64 **3.94**	2.53 **3.71**	2.45 **3.54**	2.38 **3.41**	2.32 **3.30**	2.28 **3.21**	2.24 **3.14**	2.20 **3.07**	2.14 **2.97**	2.10 **2.89**	2.04 **2.78**	2.00 **2.70**	1.96 **2.62**	1.91 **2.53**	1.88 **2.48**	1.84 **2.41**	1.82 **2.37**	1.79 **2.32**	1.77 **2.28**	1.76 **2.26**
24	4.26 **7.82**	3.40 **5.61**	3.01 **4.72**	2.78 **4.22**	2.62 **3.90**	2.51 **3.67**	2.43 **3.50**	2.36 **3.36**	2.30 **3.25**	2.26 **3.17**	2.22 **3.09**	2.18 **3.03**	2.13 **2.93**	2.09 **2.85**	2.02 **2.74**	1.98 **2.66**	1.94 **2.58**	1.89 **2.49**	1.86 **2.44**	1.82 **2.36**	1.80 **2.33**	1.76 **2.27**	1.74 **2.23**	1.73 **2.21**
25	4.24 **7.77**	3.38 **5.57**	2.99 **4.68**	2.76 **4.18**	2.60 **3.86**	2.49 **3.63**	2.41 **3.46**	2.34 **3.32**	2.28 **3.21**	2.24 **3.13**	2.20 **3.05**	2.16 **2.99**	2.11 **2.89**	2.06 **2.81**	2.00 **2.70**	1.96 **2.62**	1.92 **2.54**	1.87 **2.45**	1.84 **2.40**	1.80 **2.32**	1.77 **2.29**	1.74 **2.23**	1.72 **2.19**	1.71 **2.17**
26	4.22 **7.72**	3.37 **5.53**	2.98 **4.64**	2.74 **4.14**	2.59 **3.82**	2.47 **3.59**	2.39 **3.42**	2.32 **3.29**	2.27 **3.17**	2.22 **3.09**	2.18 **3.02**	2.15 **2.96**	2.10 **2.86**	2.05 **2.77**	1.99 **2.66**	1.95 **2.58**	1.90 **2.50**	1.85 **2.41**	1.82 **2.36**	1.78 **2.28**	1.76 **2.25**	1.72 **2.19**	1.70 **2.15**	1.69 **2.13**
27	4.21 **7.68**	3.35 **5.49**	2.96 **4.60**	2.73 **4.11**	2.57 **3.79**	2.46 **3.56**	2.37 **3.39**	2.30 **3.26**	2.25 **3.14**	2.20 **3.06**	2.16 **2.98**	2.13 **2.93**	2.08 **2.83**	2.03 **2.74**	1.97 **2.63**	1.93 **2.55**	1.88 **2.47**	1.84 **2.38**	1.80 **2.33**	1.76 **2.25**	1.74 **2.21**	1.71 **2.16**	1.68 **2.12**	1.67 **2.10**
28	4.20 **7.64**	3.34 **5.45**	2.95 **4.57**	2.71 **4.07**	2.56 **3.76**	2.44 **3.53**	2.36 **3.36**	2.29 **3.23**	2.24 **3.11**	2.19 **3.03**	2.15 **2.95**	2.12 **2.90**	2.06 **2.80**	2.02 **2.71**	1.96 **2.60**	1.91 **2.52**	1.87 **2.44**	1.81 **2.35**	1.78 **2.30**	1.75 **2.22**	1.72 **2.18**	1.69 **2.13**	1.67 **2.09**	1.65 **2.06**
29	4.18 **7.60**	3.33 **5.42**	2.93 **4.54**	2.70 **4.04**	2.54 **3.73**	2.43 **3.50**	2.35 **3.33**	2.28 **3.20**	2.22 **3.08**	2.18 **3.00**	2.14 **2.92**	2.10 **2.87**	2.05 **2.77**	2.00 **2.68**	1.94 **2.57**	1.90 **2.49**	1.85 **2.41**	1.80 **2.32**	1.77 **2.27**	1.73 **2.19**	1.71 **2.15**	1.68 **2.10**	1.65 **2.06**	1.64 **2.03**
30	4.17 **7.56**	3.32 **5.39**	2.92 **4.51**	2.69 **4.02**	2.53 **3.70**	2.42 **3.47**	2.34 **3.30**	2.27 **3.17**	2.21 **3.06**	2.16 **2.98**	2.12 **2.90**	2.09 **2.84**	2.04 **2.74**	1.99 **2.66**	1.93 **2.55**	1.89 **2.47**	1.84 **2.38**	1.79 **2.29**	1.76 **2.24**	1.72 **2.16**	1.69 **2.13**	1.66 **2.07**	1.64 **2.03**	1.62 **2.01**
32	4.15 **7.50**	3.30 **5.34**	2.90 **4.46**	2.67 **3.97**	2.51 **3.66**	2.40 **3.42**	2.32 **3.25**	2.25 **3.12**	2.19 **3.01**	2.14 **2.94**	2.10 **2.86**	2.07 **2.80**	2.02 **2.70**	1.97 **2.62**	1.91 **2.51**	1.86 **2.42**	1.82 **2.34**	1.76 **2.25**	1.74 **2.20**	1.69 **2.12**	1.67 **2.08**	1.64 **2.02**	1.61 **1.98**	1.59 **1.96**
34	4.13 **7.44**	3.28 **5.29**	2.88 **4.42**	2.65 **3.93**	2.49 **3.61**	2.38 **3.38**	2.30 **3.21**	2.23 **3.08**	2.17 **2.97**	2.12 **2.89**	2.08 **2.82**	2.05 **2.76**	2.00 **2.66**	1.95 **2.58**	1.89 **2.47**	1.84 **2.38**	1.80 **2.30**	1.74 **2.21**	1.71 **2.15**	1.67 **2.08**	1.64 **2.04**	1.61 **1.98**	1.59 **1.94**	1.57 **1.91**

Note: ν_n = degrees of freedom for numerator; ν_d = degrees of freedom for denominator.

Table 3-1 Critical Values of F Corresponding to P < .05 (Lightface) and P < .01 (Boldface) (Continued)

ν_n

ν_d	1	2	3	4	5	6	7	8	9	10	11	12	14	16	20	24	30	40	50	75	100	200	500	∞
36	4.11	3.26	2.86	2.63	2.48	2.36	2.28	2.21	2.15	2.10	2.06	2.03	1.98	1.93	1.87	1.82	1.78	1.72	1.69	1.65	1.62	1.59	1.56	1.55
	7.39	**5.25**	**4.38**	**3.89**	**3.58**	**3.35**	**3.18**	**3.04**	**2.94**	**2.86**	**2.78**	**2.72**	**2.62**	**2.54**	**2.43**	**2.35**	**2.26**	**2.17**	**2.12**	**2.04**	**2.00**	**1.94**	**1.90**	**1.87**
38	4.10	3.25	2.85	2.62	2.46	2.35	2.26	2.19	2.14	2.09	2.05	2.02	1.96	1.92	1.85	1.80	1.76	1.71	1.67	1.63	1.60	1.57	1.54	1.53
	7.35	**5.21**	**4.34**	**3.86**	**3.54**	**3.32**	**3.15**	**3.02**	**2.91**	**2.82**	**2.75**	**2.69**	**2.59**	**2.51**	**2.40**	**2.32**	**2.22**	**2.14**	**2.08**	**2.00**	**1.97**	**1.90**	**1.86**	**1.84**
40	4.08	3.23	2.84	2.61	2.45	2.34	2.25	2.18	2.12	2.07	2.04	2.00	1.95	1.90	1.84	1.79	1.74	1.69	1.66	1.61	1.59	1.55	1.53	1.51
	7.31	**5.18**	**4.31**	**3.83**	**3.51**	**3.29**	**3.12**	**2.99**	**2.88**	**2.80**	**2.73**	**2.66**	**2.56**	**2.49**	**2.37**	**2.29**	**2.20**	**2.11**	**2.05**	**1.97**	**1.94**	**1.88**	**1.84**	**1.81**
42	4.07	3.22	2.83	2.59	2.44	2.32	2.24	2.17	2.11	2.06	2.02	1.99	1.94	1.89	1.82	1.78	1.73	1.68	1.64	1.60	1.57	1.54	1.51	1.49
	7.27	**5.15**	**4.29**	**3.80**	**3.49**	**3.26**	**3.10**	**2.96**	**2.86**	**2.77**	**2.70**	**2.64**	**2.54**	**2.46**	**2.35**	**2.26**	**2.17**	**2.08**	**2.02**	**1.94**	**1.91**	**1.85**	**1.80**	**1.78**
44	4.06	3.21	2.82	2.58	2.43	2.31	2.23	2.16	2.10	2.05	2.01	1.98	1.92	1.88	1.81	1.76	1.72	1.66	1.63	1.58	1.56	1.52	1.50	1.48
	7.24	**5.12**	**4.26**	**3.78**	**3.46**	**3.24**	**3.07**	**2.94**	**2.84**	**2.75**	**2.68**	**2.62**	**2.52**	**2.44**	**2.32**	**2.24**	**2.15**	**2.06**	**2.00**	**1.92**	**1.88**	**1.82**	**1.78**	**1.75**
46	4.05	3.20	2.81	2.57	2.42	2.30	2.22	2.14	2.09	2.04	2.00	1.97	1.91	1.87	1.80	1.75	1.71	1.65	1.62	1.57	1.54	1.51	1.48	1.46
	7.21	**5.10**	**4.24**	**3.76**	**3.44**	**3.22**	**3.05**	**2.92**	**2.82**	**2.73**	**2.66**	**2.60**	**2.50**	**2.42**	**2.30**	**2.22**	**2.13**	**2.04**	**1.98**	**1.90**	**1.86**	**1.80**	**1.76**	**1.72**
48	4.04	3.19	2.80	2.56	2.41	2.30	2.21	2.14	2.08	2.03	1.99	1.96	1.90	1.86	1.79	1.74	1.70	1.64	1.61	1.56	1.53	1.50	1.47	1.45
	7.19	**5.08**	**4.22**	**3.74**	**3.42**	**3.20**	**3.04**	**2.90**	**2.80**	**2.71**	**2.64**	**2.58**	**2.48**	**2.40**	**2.28**	**2.20**	**2.11**	**2.02**	**1.96**	**1.88**	**1.84**	**1.78**	**1.73**	**1.70**
50	4.03	3.18	2.79	2.56	2.40	2.29	2.20	2.13	2.07	2.02	1.98	1.95	1.90	1.85	1.78	1.74	1.69	1.63	1.60	1.55	1.52	1.48	1.46	1.44
	7.17	**5.06**	**4.20**	**3.72**	**3.41**	**3.18**	**3.02**	**2.88**	**2.78**	**2.70**	**2.62**	**2.56**	**2.46**	**2.39**	**2.26**	**2.18**	**2.10**	**2.00**	**1.94**	**1.86**	**1.82**	**1.76**	**1.71**	**1.68**
60	4.00	3.15	2.76	2.52	2.37	2.25	2.17	2.10	2.04	1.99	1.95	1.92	1.86	1.81	1.75	1.70	1.65	1.59	1.56	1.50	1.48	1.44	1.41	1.39
	7.08	**4.98**	**4.13**	**3.65**	**3.34**	**3.12**	**2.95**	**2.82**	**2.72**	**2.63**	**2.56**	**2.50**	**2.40**	**2.32**	**2.20**	**2.12**	**2.03**	**1.93**	**1.87**	**1.79**	**1.74**	**1.68**	**1.63**	**1.60**
70	3.98	3.13	2.74	2.50	2.35	2.23	2.14	2.07	2.01	1.97	1.93	1.89	1.84	1.79	1.72	1.67	1.62	1.56	1.53	1.47	1.45	1.40	1.37	1.35
	7.01	**4.92**	**4.08**	**3.60**	**3.29**	**3.07**	**2.91**	**2.77**	**2.67**	**2.59**	**2.51**	**2.45**	**2.35**	**2.28**	**2.15**	**2.07**	**1.98**	**1.88**	**1.82**	**1.74**	**1.69**	**1.62**	**1.56**	**1.53**
80	3.96	3.11	2.72	2.48	2.33	2.21	2.12	2.05	1.99	1.95	1.91	1.88	1.82	1.77	1.70	1.65	1.60	1.54	1.51	1.45	1.42	1.38	1.35	1.32
	6.96	**4.88**	**4.04**	**3.56**	**3.25**	**3.04**	**2.87**	**2.74**	**2.64**	**2.55**	**2.48**	**2.41**	**2.32**	**2.24**	**2.11**	**2.03**	**1.94**	**1.84**	**1.78**	**1.70**	**1.65**	**1.57**	**1.52**	**1.49**
100	3.94	3.09	2.70	2.46	2.30	2.19	2.10	2.03	1.97	1.92	1.88	1.85	1.79	1.75	1.68	1.63	1.57	1.51	1.48	1.42	1.39	1.34	1.30	1.28
	6.90	**4.82**	**3.98**	**3.51**	**3.20**	**2.99**	**2.82**	**2.69**	**2.59**	**2.51**	**2.43**	**2.36**	**2.26**	**2.19**	**2.06**	**1.98**	**1.89**	**1.79**	**1.73**	**1.64**	**1.59**	**1.51**	**1.46**	**1.43**
120	3.92	3.07	2.68	2.45	2.29	2.18	2.09	2.02	1.96	1.91	1.87	1.84	1.78	1.73	1.66	1.61	1.56	1.50	1.46	1.39	1.37	1.32	1.28	1.25
	6.85	**4.79**	**3.95**	**3.48**	**3.17**	**2.96**	**2.79**	**2.66**	**2.56**	**2.47**	**2.40**	**2.34**	**2.23**	**2.15**	**2.03**	**1.95**	**1.86**	**1.76**	**1.70**	**1.61**	**1.56**	**1.48**	**1.42**	**1.38**
∞	3.84	2.99	2.60	2.37	2.21	2.09	2.01	1.94	1.88	1.83	1.79	1.75	1.69	1.64	1.57	1.52	1.46	1.40	1.35	1.28	1.24	1.17	1.11	1.00
	6.63	**4.60**	**3.78**	**3.32**	**3.02**	**2.80**	**2.64**	**2.51**	**2.41**	**2.32**	**2.24**	**2.18**	**2.07**	**1.99**	**1.87**	**1.79**	**1.69**	**1.59**	**1.52**	**1.41**	**1.36**	**1.25**	**1.15**	**1.00**

Note: ν_n = degrees of freedom for numerator; ν_d = degrees of freedom for denominator.

Source: Adapted from G. W. Snedecor and W. G. Cochran, Statistical Methods, Iowa State University Press, Ames, 1978, pp. 560–563.

• The variances of each population must be equal, even when the means are different, i.e., when the treatment has an effect.

When the data suggest that these assumptions do not apply, one ought not to use the procedure we just developed, the analysis of variance. Since there is one factor (the diet) that distinguishes the different experimental groups, this is known as a *single-factor* or *one-way analysis of variance*. Other forms of analysis of variance (not discussed here) can be used to analyze experiments in which there is more than one experimental factor.

Since the distribution of possible F values depends on the size of each sample and number of samples under consideration, so does the exact value of F which corresponds to the 5 percent cutoff point. For example, in our diet study, the number of samples was 4 and the size of each sample was 7. This dependence enters into the mathematical formulas used to determine the value at which F gets "big" as two parameters known as *degree-of-freedom* parameters, often denoted ν (Greek nu). For this analysis, the between-groups degrees of freedom (also called the numerator degrees of freedom because the between-groups variance is in the numerator of F) is defined to be the number of samples m minus 1, or $\nu_n = m - 1$. The within-groups (or denominator) degrees of freedom is defined to be the number of samples times 1 less than the size of each sample, $\nu_d = m(n - 1)$. For our diet example, the numerator degrees of freedom are $4 - 1 = 3$, and the denominator degrees of freedom are $4(7 - 1) = 24$. Degrees of freedom often confuse and mystify people who are trying to work with statistics. They simply represent the way *number of samples* and *sample size* enter the mathematical formulas used to construct all statistical tables.

THREE EXAMPLES

We now have the tools needed to form conclusions using statistical reasoning. We will examine examples, all based on results published in the medical literature. I have exercised some literary license with these examples for two reasons: (1) Medical and scientific authors usually summarize their raw data with descriptive statistics (like those developed in Chap. 2) rather than including the raw data. As a result, the "data from the literature" shown in this chapter—and the rest of the book—are usually my guess at what the raw data probably looked like based on the descriptive statistics in the original article.* (2) The analysis of variance as we developed it requires that each sample contain the same number of members. This is often not the case in reality, so I adjusted the sample sizes in the original studies to meet this restriction. We later generalize our statistical methods to handle experiments with different numbers of individuals in each sample or treatment group.

Relationship of Drug Prescribing to Length of Hospital Stay

Is inappropriate drug prescribing associated with a longer hospital stay? Since the daily bed rate is the single most costly item for most hospitalized patients, finding ways to reduce the length of stay without harming the quality of care would be a good way to save money without jeopardizing the patient. To investigate this question, Knapp and her colleagues† reviewed the charts of people admitted to nonprofit hospitals with a common kidney infection, uncomplicated pyelonephritis. They selected this disease because it is a well-defined condition for which there are well-established antimicrobial drug therapies.

This approach is called a *retrospective study* because it involved looking back over previous experience (here recorded in the patients' charts) to obtain data for analysis. It is an example of an *observational study* because the investigator obtains data by simply observing events without controlling them.

Such studies are prone to two potentially serious problems. First, the groups may vary in ways the investigators do not notice or choose to ignore, and these differences, rather than the treatment itself, may account for the differences the investigators find. (These factors are called *confounding effects*.) For example, smokers are more likely to develop lung cancer than nonsmokers who appear similar in all other aspects. Most people interpret this statistically demonstrated relationship as proving that smoking causes lung cancer. A few people, however,

---

*Since authors often failed to include a complete set of descriptive statistics, I had to estimate them from the results of their hypothesis tests.

†D. E. Knapp, D. A. Knapp, M. K. Speedie, D. M. Yaeger, and C. L. Baker, "Relationship of Inappropriate Drug Prescribing to Increased Length of Hospital Stay," *Am. J. Hosp. Pharm.,* **36**:1334–1337, 1979.

argue that people with a genetic predisposition to lung cancer also have a genetic predisposition to smoking cigarettes. Nothing in such an observational study can definitely distinguish between these two interpretations. Second, such studies can be subject to bias in patient recall, investigator assessment, and selection of the treatment group and, often more important, the control group. These problems are especially difficult in studies based on chart reviews when the people reading the charts often must use considerable judgment in assessing what actually happened to the patient.

Observational studies do have their advantages. First, they are relatively inexpensive, often being based on reviews of existing information or information that is already being collected for other purposes (like medical records) and requiring no direct intervention by the investigator. Second, in retrospective studies, it is possible to accumulate enough cases to perform a meaningful analysis in a relatively short time. This advantage is especially important when studying rare diseases that require years of clinical experience to accumulate even a few patients. Third, ethical considerations or prevailing medical practice can make it impossible to carry out active manipulation of the variable under study. For example, Knapp and her colleagues simply could not have divided a collection of patients into two groups at random, then instructed their physicians to treat people in one group appropriately and treat people in the other group inappropriately.

Because of the potential difficulties in all observational studies — and especially retrospective studies — it is critical that the investigators explicitly specify the criteria they used for classifying each subject in the control or treatment group. Such specifications help minimize biases when the study is done as well as help you, as a consumer of the resulting information, judge whether the classification rules made sense.

Knapp and her colleagues developed explicit criteria for including a patient in their study, including the following:

1   The primary discharge diagnosis was pyelonephritis.
2   The patient had symptons of lower back pain over the kidneys and oral temperature over $100°F$ when admitted.
3   A urine culture revealed a significant bacterial infection (over 100,000 colonies per milliliter), and the clinical laboratory had re-

ported the results of tests to determine drugs to which the bacteria responded.

4 The patient was between 18 and 44 year old (to try to exclude people with concurrent diseases and treatments).

5 The patient neither had nor was being treated for immunosuppressive, kidney, or liver disorders, nor was the patient admitted for surgery. (These conditions all complicate drug treatment.)

6 The patient did not leave the hospital against medical advice, die, or transfer to another institution, thus cutting the medical record short.

The investigators also developed explicit criteria for the appropriate use of drugs based on professional and scientific literature, in particular Food and Drug Administration–approved labeling of the drug products, the *Physicians' Desk Reference,* and the *Medical Letter.* The average practicing physician has routine access to all this material. They also considered individual differences between patients (e.g., allergies) and what laboratory information was available at the time to the physician. Using these criteria, they classified each patient as being treated appropriately or inappropriately.

Figure 3-7 shows data for 36 appropriately treated patients and 36 inappropriately treated patients. On the average, the appropriately treated patients were hospitalized for 4.51 days whereas the inappropriately treated patients were hospitalized for 6.28 days. There is, however, considerable variability in both groups of patients' lengths of stay. The standard deviation in the length of hospitalization for the appropriately treated patients was 1.98 days and for the inappropriately treated patients 2.54 days.

How consistent are these data with the hypothesis that whether or not the drugs were administered in accordance with the *Physicians' Desk Reference* and *Medical Letter* had no effect on length of hospitalization for patients with pyelonephritis? In other words, how likely are the differences between the two samples of patients shown in Fig. 3-7 to be due to random sampling rather than the differences in how they were treated?

To answer this question, we perform an analysis of variance.

We begin by estimating the within-groups variance by averaging the variances of the two patient groups

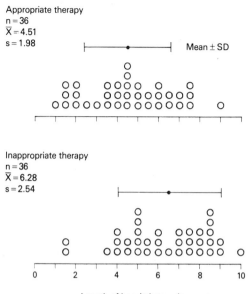

Appropriate therapy
n = 36
$\bar{X}$ = 4.51
s = 1.98

Inappropriate therapy
n = 36
$\bar{X}$ = 6.28
s = 2.54

Length of hospital stay, days

Figure 3-7 Results of a study on the lengths of stay of patients with pyelonephritis who were treated appropriately and inappropriately with drugs. Each patient's length of stay is indicated by a circle at the appropriate length of stay. The average length of stay for patients treated appropriately is below the average length of stay for patients treated inappropriately. The statistical question is to assess whether or not the difference is due simply to random-sampling effect or to an actual effect of the differences in treatment.

$$s^2_{wit} = \frac{1}{2}\left(s^2_{app} + s^2_{inap}\right)$$

$$= \frac{1}{2}(1.98^2 + 2.54^2) = 5.19 \text{ days}^2$$

We then go on to calculate the between-groups variance. This first step is to estimate the standard error of the mean by computing the standard deviation of the two sample means. The mean of the two sample means is

$$\bar{X} = \frac{1}{2}(\bar{X}_{app} + \bar{X}_{inap})$$

$$= \frac{1}{2}(4.51 + 6.28) = 5.40 \text{ days}$$

Therefore the standard deviation of the sample means is

$$s_{\bar{X}} = \sqrt{\frac{(\bar{X}_{app} - \bar{X})^2 + (\bar{X}_{inap} - \bar{X})^2}{m - 1}}$$

$$= \sqrt{\frac{(4.51 - 5.40)^2 + (6.28 - 5.40)^2}{2 - 1}} = 1.25 \text{ days}$$

Since the sample size n is 36, the estimation of the population variance from between the groups is

$$s^2_{bet} = ns^2_{\bar{X}} = 36(1.25^2) = 56.25 \text{ days}^2$$

Finally, the ratio of these two different estimates of the population variance is

$$F = \frac{s^2_{bet}}{s^2_{wit}} = \frac{56.25}{5.19} = 10.84$$

The degrees of freedom for the numerator are the number of groups minus 1, and so $\nu_n = 2 - 1 = 1$, and the degrees of freedom for the denominator are the number of groups times 1 less than the sample size, or $\nu_d = 2(36 - 1) = 70$. Look in the column headed 1 and the row headed 70 in Table 3-1. The resulting entry indicates that there is less than a 1 percent chance of F exceeding 7.01; we therefore conclude that the value of F associated with our observations is "big" and we reject the hypothesis that there is no difference in the average length of stay in the two groups of patients shown in Fig. 3-7.

Hence, this study supports the view that hospital stays could be shortened an average of about 2 days for patients with pyelonephritis if physicians could be made to use prescription drugs in closer agreement with the manufacturers' and FDA's standards.

Halothane versus Morphine for Open-Heart Anesthesia

Halothane is a popular drug to induce general anesthesia because it is potent, nonflammable, easy to use, and very safe. Since halothane can be carried with oxygen, it can be vaporized and administered to the patient with the same equipment used to ventilate the patient. The patient absorbs and releases it through the lungs, making it possible to change anesthetic states more rapidly than would be possible with drugs that have to be administered intravenously. It does, however, lessen the heart's ability to pump blood directly by depressing the myocardium itself and indirectly by increasing peripheral venous capacity. Some anesthesiologists believed that these effects could produce complications in people with cardiac problems and suggested using morphine as an anesthetic agent in these patients because it has little effect on cardiac performance in supine individuals. Conahan and his colleagues* directly compared these two anesthetic agents in a large number of patients during routine surgery for cardiac valve repair or replacement.

To obtain two similar samples of patients who differed only in the type of anesthesia used, they selected the anesthesia at random for each patient who was suitable for the study.

This procedure, called a *randomized clinical trial,* is the method of choice for evaluating therapies because it avoids the selection biases that can creep into observational studies. The randomized clinical trial is an example of what statisticans call an *experimental study* because the investigator actively manipulates the treatment under study, making it possible to draw much stronger conclusions than are possible from observational studies about whether or not a treatment produced an effect. Experimental studies are the rule in the physical sciences and animal studies in the life sciences but are less common in studies involving human subjects. Randomization reduces biases that can appear in observational studies, and since all clinical trials are *prospective,* no one knows how things will turn out at the beginning. This fact

*T. J. Conahan III, A. J. Ominsky, H. Wollman, and R. A. Stroth, "A Prospective Random Comparison of Halothane and Morphine for Open-Heart Anesthesia: One Year's Experience," *Anesthesiology,* **38**:528–535, 1973.

also reduces the opportunity for bias. Perhaps for these reasons, randomized clinical trials often show therapies to be of little or no value, even when observational studies have suggested that they were efficacious.*

Why, then, are not all therapies subjected to randomized clinical trials? Once something has become part of generally accepted medical practice—even if it did so without any objective demonstration of its value—it is extremely difficult to convince patients and their physicians to participate in a study that requires withholding it from some of the patients. Second, randomized clinical trials are always prospective; a person recruited into the study must be followed for some time, often many years. People move, lose interest, or die for reasons unrelated to the study. Simply keeping track of people in a randomized clinical trial is often a major task.

To collect enough patients to have a meaningful sample it is often necessary to have many groups at different institutions participating. While it is great fun for the people running the study, it is often just one more task for the people at the collaborating institutions. All these factors often combine to make randomized clinical trials expensive and difficult to execute. Nevertheless, when done, they provide the most definitive answers to questions regarding the relative efficacy of different treatments.

Conahan and his colleagues were not faced with many of these problems because they were studying the effects of different types of anesthesia on how a patient did during the operation and the immediate postoperative recovery in a single hospital. During the operation, they recorded many hemodynamic variables, such as blood pressures before induction of anesthesia, after anesthesia but before incision, and during other important periods during the operation. They also recorded information relating to length of stay in the postsurgical intensive care unit, total length of hospitalization, and any deaths that occurred during this period. We will analyze these latter data after we have developed the necessary statistical tools in Chap. 5. For now, we will focus on a representative pressure measurement, the lowest mean arterial blood pressure between the start of anesthesia and the time of

*For a readable and classic discussion of the place of randomized clinical trials in providing useful clinical knowledge, together with a sobering discussion of how little of commonly accepted medical practice has ever been actually shown to do any good, see A. K. Cochran, *Effectiveness and Efficiency: Random Reflections on Health Services*, Nuffield Provincial Hospitals Trust, London, 1972.

incision. This variable is thought to be a good measure of depression of the cardiovascular system before any surgical stimulation occurs. Specifically, we will investigate the hypothesis that, on the average, there was no difference in patients anesthetized with halothane or morphine.

Figure 3-8 shows the lowest mean arterial blood pressure observed from the start of anesthesia until the time of incision for 122 patients, half of whom were anesthetized with each agent. Pressures were rounded to the nearest even number, and each patient's pressure is represented by a circle. On the average, patients anesthetized with halothane had pressures 6.3 mmHg below those anesthetized with morphine. There is quite a bit of overlap in the pressures observed in the two different groups because of biological variability in how different people respond to anesthesia. The standard deviations in pressures are 12.2 and 14.4 mmHg for the people anesthetized with halothane and morphine,

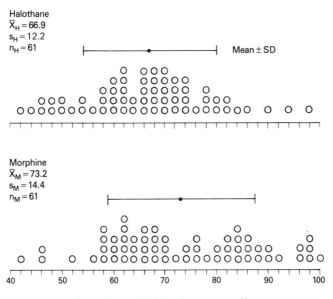

Lowest mean arterial blood pressure, mm Hg

Figure 3-8 Lowest mean arterial blood pressure between the beginning of anesthesia and the incision in patients during open-heart surgery for patients anesthetized with halothane and morphine. Are the observed differences consistent with the hypothesis that, on the average, anesthetic did not affect blood pressure?

respectively. Given this, is the 6.3-mmHg difference large enough to assert that halothane produced lower lowest mean arterial pressures?

To answer this question, we perform an analysis of variance exactly as we did to compare length of hospitalizations in the appropriately and inappropriately treated pyelonephritis patients. We estimate the within-groups variance by averaging the estimates of the variance obtained from the two samples:

$$s^2_{\text{wit}} = \tfrac{1}{2}(s^2_{\text{hlo}} + s^2_{\text{mor}}) = \tfrac{1}{2}(12.2^2 + 14.4^2) = 178.1 \text{ mmHg}^2$$

Since this estimate of the population variance is computed from the variances of the separate samples, it does not depend on whether or not the means are different.

Next, we estimate the population variance by assuming that the hypothesis that halothane and morphine produce the same effect on arterial blood pressure is true. In that case, the two groups of patients in Fig. 3-8 are simply two random samples drawn from a single population. As a result, the standard deviation of the sample means is an estimate of the standard error of the mean. The mean of the two samples means is

$$\bar{X} = \tfrac{1}{2}(\bar{X}_{\text{hlo}} + \bar{X}_{\text{mor}}) = \tfrac{1}{2}(66.9 + 73.2) = 70 \text{ mmHg}$$

The standard deviation of the $m = 2$ sample means is

$$s_{\bar{X}} = \sqrt{\frac{(\bar{X}_{\text{hlo}} - \bar{X})^2 + (\bar{X}_{\text{mor}} - \bar{X})^2}{m - 1}}$$

$$= \sqrt{\frac{(66.9 - 70.0)^2 + (73.2 - 70.0)^2}{2 - 1}} = 4.46 \text{ mmHg}$$

Since the sample size n is 61, the estimate of the population variance computed from the variability in the sample means is

$$s^2_{\text{bet}} = ns^2_{\bar{X}} = 61(4.46^2) = 1213 \text{ mmHg}^2$$

To test whether these two estimates are compatible, we compute

$$F = \frac{s^2_{bet}}{s^2_{wit}} = \frac{1213}{178.1} = 6.81$$

The degrees of freedom for the numerator are $\nu_n = m - 1 = 2 - 1 = 1$, and the degrees of freedom for the denominator are $\nu_d = m(n - 1) = 2(61 - 1) = 120$. Since $F = 6.81$ is greater than the critical value of 3.92 from (interpolating in) Table 3-1, we conclude that there is less than a 5 percent chance that our data were all drawn from a single population. In other words, we conclude that halothane produced lower lowest mean arterial blood pressures than morphine did, on the average.

Given the variability in response among patients to each drug (quantified by the standard deviations), do you expect this *statistically* significant result to be *clinically significant*? We will return to this question later.

Menstrual Dysfunction in Distance Runners

Infrequent or suspended menstruation can be a symptom of serious metabolic disorders, such as anorexia nervosa (a psychological disorder that leads people to stop eating, then waste away) or tumors of the pituitary gland. Infrequent or suspended menstruation can also frustrate a woman's wish to have children. It can also be a side effect of birth control pills or indicate that a woman is pregnant or entering menopause. Gynecologists see many women who complain about irregular menstrual cycles and must decide how to diagnose and perhaps treat this possible problem. In addition to these potential explanations, there is some evidence that strenuous exercise, perhaps by changing the percentage of body fat, may affect the ovulation cycle. Since jogging and long-distance running have become popular, Dale and his colleagues[*] decided to investigate whether there is a relationship between the frequency of menstruation and the amount of jogging young women do, as well as to look for possible effects on body weight, fat, and levels of circulating hormones that play an important role in the menstrual cycle.

[*]E. Dale, D. H. Gerlach, and A. L. Wilhite, "Menstrual Dysfunction in Distance Runners," *Obs. Gynecol,* **54**:47–53, 1979.

They did an observational study of three groups of women. The first two groups were volunteers who regularly engaged in some form of running, and the third, a control group, consisted of women who did not run but were otherwise similar to the other two groups. The runners were divided into *joggers* who jog "slow and easy" 5 to 30 miles per week, and *runners* who run more than 30 miles per week and combine long, slow distance with speed work. The investigators used a survey to show that the three groups were similar in the amount of physical activity (aside from running), distribution of ages, heights, occupations, and type of birth control methods being used.

Figure 3-9 shows the number of menstrual periods per year for the 26 women in each experimental group. The women in the control group averaged 11.5 menses per year, the joggers averaged 10.1 menses per year, and the runners averaged 9.1 menses per year. Are these differences in mean number of menses compatible with what one would expect from the variability within each group?

To answer this question, we first estimate the population variance by averaging the variance from within the groups

$$s^2_{wit} = \tfrac{1}{3}(s^2_{con} + s^2_{jog} + s^2_{run})$$

$$= \tfrac{1}{3}(1.3^2 + 2.1^2 + 2.4^2) = 3.95 \ (menses/year)^2$$

To estimate the population variance from the variability in the sample means, we must first estimate the standard error of the mean by computing the standard deviation of the means of the three samples. Since the mean of the three means is

$$\bar{X} = \tfrac{1}{3}(\bar{X}_{con} + \bar{X}_{jog} + \bar{X}_{run})$$

$$= \tfrac{1}{3}(11.5 + 10.1 + 9.1) = 10.2 \ menses/year$$

Our estimate of the standard error is

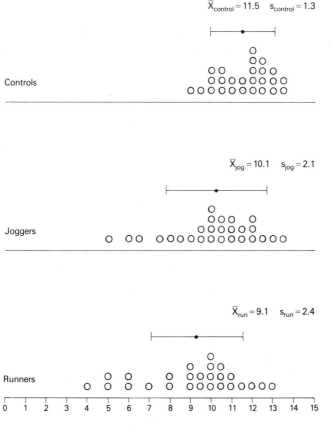

Figure 3-9 The number of menstrual cycles per year in women who were sedentary, joggers, and long-distance runners. The mean values of the three samples of women were different. Is this variation beyond what would be expected from random sampling, i.e., that the amount of running one does has no effect on the number of menstrual cycles, or is it compatible with the view that jogging affects menstruation? Furthermore, if there is an effect, is there a different effect for joggers and long-distance runners?

$$s_{\bar{X}} = \sqrt{\frac{(\bar{X}_{con} - \bar{X})^2 + (\bar{X}_{jog} - \bar{X})^2 + (\bar{X}_{run} - \bar{X})^2}{m - 1}}$$

$$= \sqrt{\frac{(11.5 - 10.2)^2 + (10.1 - 10.2)^2 + (9.1 - 10.2)^2}{3 - 1}}$$

$$= 1.2 \text{ menses/year}$$

The sample size n is 26, and so the estimate of the population variance from the variability in the means is

$$s_{bet}^2 = ns_{\bar{X}}^2 = 26(1.2^2) = 37.44 \text{ (menses/year)}^2$$

Finally,

$$F = \frac{s_{bet}^2}{s_{wit}^2} = \frac{37.44}{3.95} = 9.48$$

The numerator has $m - 1 = 3 - 1 = 2$ degrees of freedom and the denominator has $m(n - 1) = 3(26 - 1) = 75$ degrees of freedom. Interpolating in Table 3-1, we find that F will exceed 4.90 only 1 percent of the time when all the groups are drawn from a single population; we conclude that jogging or running has an effect on the frequency of menstruation.

When a woman comes to her gynecologist complaining about irregular or infrequent periods, the physician should not only look for biochemical abnormalities but also ask whether or not she jogs.

One question remains: Which of the three groups differed from the others? Does one have to be a marathon runner to expect menstrual dysfunction, or does it accompany less strenuous jogging? Or is the effect graded, becoming more pronounced with more strenuous exercise? We will have to defer answering these questions until we develop another statistical tool, the t test, in Chap. 4.

PROBLEMS

3-1 When labor has to be induced, the mother's cervix can fail to soften and enlarge, prolonging the labor and perhaps requiring delivery by cesarean section. To investigate whether the cervix can be softened and dilated by treating it with a gel containing prostaglandin E_2, C. O'Herlihy and H. MacDonald ("Influence of Preinduction Prostaglandin E_2 Vaginal Gel on Cervical Ripening and Labor," *Obstet. Gynecol.,* **54**:708–710, 1979) applied such a gel to the cervixes of 21 women who were having labor induced and a placebo gel that contained no active ingredients to 21 other women who were having labor induced. The two groups of women were of similar ages, heights, weeks of gestation, and initial extent of cervical dilation before applying the gel. The labor of women treated with prostaglandin E_2 averaged 8.5 h, and the labor of control women averaged 13.9 h. The standard deviations for these two groups were 4.7 and 4.1 h, respectively. Is there evidence that the prostaglandin gel shortens labor?

3-2 It is generally believed that infrequent and short-term exposure to pollutants in tobacco, such as carbon monoxide, nicotine, benzo-[a]pyrene, and oxides of nitrogen, will not permanently alter lung function in healthy adult nonsmokers. To investigate this hypothesis, James White and Herman Froeb ("Small-Airways Dysfunction in Nonsmokers Chronically Exposed to Tobacco Smoke," *N. Engl. J. Med.,* **302**:720–723, 1980, used by permission) measured lung function in cigarette smokers and nonsmokers during a "physical fitness profile" at the University of California, San Diego. They measured how rapidly a person could force air from the lungs (mean forced midexpiratory flow). Reduced forced mid-expiratory flow is associated with small-airways disease of the lungs. For the women they tested White and Froeb found:

Group	No. of subjects	Mean forced mid-expiratory flow, L/s^{-1}	
		Mean	SD
Nonsmokers			
Worked in clean environment	200	3.17	.74
Worked in smoky environment	200	2.72	.71
Light smokers	200	2.63	.73
Moderate smokers	200	2.29	.70
Heavy smokers	200	2.12	.72

Is there evidence that the presence of small-airways disease, as measured by this test, is any different among the different experimental groups?

3-3 Elevated levels of plasma high-density-lipoprotein (HDL) cholesterol may be associated with a lowered risk of coronary heart
disease. Several studies have suggested that vigorous exercise may
result in increased levels of HDL. To investigate whether or not
jogging is associated with an increase in the plasma HDL concentration, G. Harley Hartung and his colleagues ("Relation of Diet to
High-Density-Lipoprotein Cholesterol in Middle-Aged Marathon
Runners, Joggers, and Inactive Men," *N. Engl. J. Med.,* **302**:357–
361, 1980, used by permission) measured HDL concentrations in
middle-aged (35 to 66 years old) marathon runners, joggers, and
inactive men. The mean HDL concentration observed in the
inactive men was 43.3 mg/dL with a standard deviation of 14.2
mg/dL. The mean and standard deviation of the HDL concentration for the joggers and marathon runners were 58.0 and 17.7
mg/dL and 64.8 and 14.3 mg/dL, respectively. If there were 70
men in each group, test the hypothesis that there is no difference
in the average HDL concentration between these groups of men.

3-4 Since smoking marijuana is illegal in the United States, it is impossible to complete the kinds of epidemiological studies that
first uncovered the adverse health effects of smoking tobacco cigarettes. As a result, people who wish to investigate the health
effects of marijuana are generally limited to laboratory research,
often using animals. To explore whether or not marijuana adversely
affected the lungs' ability to cope with bacterial exposure Gary
Huber and his colleagues ("Marijuana, Tetrahydrocannabinol,
and Pulmonary Arterial Antibacterial Defenses," *Chest,* **77**:403–
410, 1980) exposed rats to an aerosol of bacteria, then placed
them in a chamber with a cigarette-smoking machine that exposed
them to the smoke of various numbers of marijuana cigarettes.
After the rats were exposed to the bacteria and smoke, Huber and
his colleagues killed them and examined their lungs to see how
effectively the bacteria had been inactivated. In addition to exposing the rats to regular marijuana cigarettes, they exposed them to
cigarettes that had the psychoactive ingredient in marijuana (tetrahydrocannabinol, THC) removed. This experiment was to see
whether any effect on bacterial inactivation was due to the smoke
per se or the psychoactive ingredient. See page 61 for findings.
(SEM = standard error of the mean.) If each group included 36
rats, is there evidence that different doses of marijuana produced
differences in the lungs' ability to cope with a bacterial insult?

Group (no. of cigarettes)	Bacterial inactivation, %	
	Mean	SEM
0 (control)	85.1	.3
15	83.5	1.0
30	80.9	.6
50	72.6	.7
75	60	1.3
75 (THC extracted)	73.5	.7
150	63.8	2.6

3-5 In a further effört to separate the effects of the THC from the
effects of the smoke, Huber and his colleagues also investigated
the effect of injected THC on the lungs' ability to inactivate bacteria. They exposed rats to the bacteria, then either injected THC
or gave a sham injection that consisted only of the ethanol used to
dissolve the THC. The 36 rats who received a 10-mg/kg injection of
THC inactivated an average of 51.4 percent of the bacteria, and the
36 rats who received the sham injection inactivated an average of
59.4 percent of the bacteria. The standard errors of the mean were
3.2 and 3.9 percent, respectively. Is there evidence that the THC
itself affects the ability of the lungs to inactivate bacteria?

3-6 *Burnout* is a term that loosely describes a condition of fatigue,
frustration, and anger manifested as a lack of enthusiasm for and
feeling of entrapment in one's job. It has been argued that professions such as teaching and nursing, which require high levels of
commitment, are most subject to burnout. Moreover, since burnout is often linked to stress, it may be that nurses who specialize
in so-called high-stress areas, such as intensive care units, experience
more burnout and experience it sooner than nurses in less-stressful
areas. Anne Keane and her associates ("Stress in ICU and Non-ICU
Nurses," *Nursing Research* **34**:231–236, 1985) studied several aspects of nursing burnout, including whether there was a difference
in burnout between nurses who worked in intensive care units
(ICU's), stepdown units (SDU's) or intermediate care units, and
general medical units. They administered a questionnaire that could
be used to construct a score called the Staff Burnout Scale for
Health Professionals (SBS-HP), in which higher scores indicate

more burnout. Do the data below suggest a difference in burnout among the units surveyed?

	ICU		SDU		General	
	Surgical	Medical	Surgical	Medical	Surgical	Medical
Mean score	49.9	51.2	57.3	46.4	43.9	65.2
Standard deviation	14.3	13.4	14.9	14.7	16.5	20.5
Sample size	16	16	16	16	16	16

3-7 Dopamine and nitroprusside are two drugs used to treat people who have had heart attacks (a blockage of one or more arteries that carry blood to the heart prevents oxygen from reaching part of the heart muscle, which then dies). Nitroprusside seems to help these people by reducing the work the heart must do and thus the demand of the heart muscle for oxygen. Dopamine seems to help by maintaining the pressure in the arteries and helping provide flow to the affected area through secondary channels (called the collateral circulation). To compare these drugs, Clayton Shatney and his colleagues ("Effects of Infusion of Dopamine and Nitroprusside on Size of Experimental Myocardial Infarction," *Chest,* 73:850–856, 1978) administered them to dogs after tying off the left anterior descending coronary artery (a major artery serving the heart). They then waited 6 h, killed the dogs, and measured the size of the damaged muscle by weighing it. The selection of drug for any given dog was made at random, and the person who measured the damaged tissue did not know which drug (if any) the animal received. They found:

		Percentage of left ventricle damaged	
Group	No. of dogs	Mean	SEM
Control	30	15	1
Dopamine			
Low dose	13	15	2
High dose	20	9	2
Nitroprusside	20	7	1

Is there sufficient evidence to conclude that any of these drugs affects the amount of damaged muscle? (The formulas for analysis of variance with unequal sample sizes are in Appendix A.)

3-8 The production of platelets (elements in blood that play a role in clotting) seems to be regulated differently in newborns and adults. As part of their study of this regulation, Hanna Bessler and her coworkers ("Thrombopoietic Activity in Newborn Infants," *Biol. Neonate* **49**:61–65, 1986) measured the platelet content of blood samples taken from adults and groups of infants of different ages:

Group	n	Platelet count (billions/liter)	
		Mean	SD
Adult	15	257	159
Infants:			
4 days	37	196	359
1 month	31	221	340
2 months	13	280	263
4 months	10	310	95

Is there any evidence that the amount of platelets differs among these groups of people?

The Special Case
of Two Groups: The *t* Test

As we have just seen in Chap. 3, many investigations require comparing only two samples. In addition, as the last example in Chap. 3 illustrated, when there are more than two samples, the analysis of variance allows you to conclude only that the data are not consistent with the hypothesis that all the samples were drawn from a single population. It does not help you decide which one or ones are most likely to differ from the others. To answer these questions, we now develop a procedure that is specifically designed to test for differences in two groups: the *t test* or *Student's t test*. While we will develop the *t* test from scratch, we will eventually show that it is just a different way of doing an analysis of variance. In particular, we will see that $F = t^2$ when there are two groups.

The *t* test is the most common statistical procedure in the medical literature; you can expect it to appear in more than half the papers you read in the general medical literature.* In addition to being used to

---

*A. R. Feinstein: "Clinical Biostatistics: A Survey of the Statistical Procedures in General Medical Journals," *Clin. Pharm. Therap.*, 15:97–107, 1974.

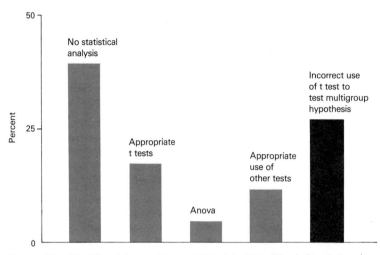

Figure 4-1 Of 142 original articles published in Vol. 56 of *Circulation* (excluding radiology, clinicopathologic, and case reports), 39 percent did not use statistics; 34 percent used a *t* test appropriately to compare two groups, analysis of variance (ANOVA), or other methods; and 27 percent used the *t* test incorrectly to compare more than two groups with each other. (*From S. A. Glantz, "How to Detect, Correct, and Prevent Errors in the Medical Literature," Circulation, 61:1–7, 1980. By permission of the American Heart Association, Inc.*)

compare two group means, it is widely applied incorrectly to compare multiple groups, by doing all the pairwise comparisons, e.g., by comparing more than one intervention with a control condition or the state of a patient at different times following an intervention. Figure 4-1 shows the results of an analysis of the use of *t* tests for the clinical journal *Circulation;* 54 percent of all the papers used the *t* test, more often than not to analyze experiments for which it is not appropriate. As we will see, this incorrect use increases the chances of rejecting the hypothesis of no effect above the nominal level, say 5 percent, used to select the cutoff value for a "big" value of the test statistic *t*. In practical terms, this boils down to increasing the chances of reporting that some therapy had an effect when the evidence does not support this conclusion.

THE GENERAL APPROACH

Suppose we wish to test a new drug that may be an effective diuretic. We assemble a group of 10 people and divide them at random into two groups, a control group that receives a placebo and a treatment group that receives the drug; then we measure their urine production for 24 h. Figure 4-2A shows the resulting data. The average urine production of the group receiving the diuretic is 240 mL higher than that of the group

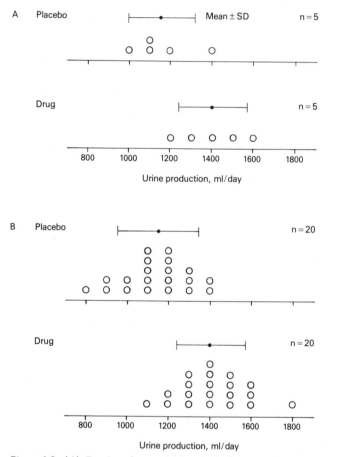

Figure 4-2 (**A**) Results of a study in which five people were treated with a placebo and five people were treated with a drug thought to increase daily urine production. On the average, the five people who received the drug produced more urine than the placebo group. Are these data convincing evidence that the drug is an effective diuretic? (**B**) Results of a similar study with 20 people in each treatment group. The means and standard deviations associated with the two groups are similar to the results in panel **A**. Are these data convincing evidence that the drug is an effective diuretic? If you changed your mind, why did you do it?

receiving the placebo. Simply looking at Fig. 4-2A, however, does not provide very convincing evidence that this difference is due to anything more than random sampling.

Nevertheless, we pursue the problem and give the placebo or drug to another 30 people to obtain the results shown in Fig. 4-2B. The mean responses of the two groups of people, as well as the standard deviations, are almost identical to those observed in the smaller samples shown in Fig. 4-2A. Even so, most observers are more confident in claiming that the diuretic increased average urine output from the data in Fig. 4-2B than the data in Fig. 4-2A, even though the samples in each case are good representatives of the underlying population. Why?

As the sample size increases, most observers become more confident in their estimates of the population means, so they can begin to discern a difference between the people taking the placebo or the drug. Recall that the standard error of the mean quantifies the uncertainty of the estimate of the true population mean based on a sample. Furthermore, as the sample size increases, the standard error of the mean decreases according to

$$\sigma_{\bar{X}} = \frac{\sigma}{\sqrt{n}}$$

where n is the sample size and σ is the standard deviation of the population from which the sample was drawn. As the sample size increases, the uncertainty in the estimate of the difference of the means between the people who received placebo and the patients who received drug decreases relative to the difference of the means. As a result, we become more confident that the drug actually has an effect. More precisely, we become less confident in the hypothesis that the drug had no effect, in which case the two samples of patients could be considered two samples drawn from a single population.

To formalize this logic, we will examine the ratio

$$t = \frac{\text{difference in sample means}}{\text{standard error of difference of sample means}}$$

When this ratio is small, we will conclude that the data are compatible with the hypothesis that both samples were drawn from a single population. When this ratio is large, we will conclude that it is unlikely that the samples were drawn from a single population and assert that the treatment (e.g., the diuretic) produced an effect.

This logic, while differing in emphasis from that used to develop the analysis of variance, is essentially the same. In both cases, we are comparing the relative magnitude of the differences in the sample means with the amount of variability that would be expected from looking within the samples.

To compute the t ratio we need to know two things: the difference of the sample means and the standard error of this difference. Computing the difference of the sample means is easy; we simply subtract. Computing an estimate for the standard error of this difference is a bit more involved. We begin with a slightly more general problem, that of finding the standard deviation of the difference of two numbers drawn at random from the same population.

THE STANDARD DEVIATION OF A DIFFERENCE OR A SUM

Figure 4-3A shows a population with 200 members. The mean is 0, and the standard deviation is 1. Now, suppose we draw two samples at random and compute their difference. Figure 4-3B shows this result for the two members indicated by solid circles in panel A. Drawing five more pairs of samples (indicated by different shadings in panel A) and computing their differences yields the corresponding shaded points in panel B. Note that there seems to be more variability in the differences of the samples than in the samples themselves. Figure 4-3C shows the results of panel B, together with the results of drawing another 50 pairs of numbers at random and computing their differences. The standard deviation of the population of differences is about 40 percent larger than the standard deviation of the population from which the samples were drawn.

In fact, it is possible to demonstrate mathematically that *the variance of the difference (or sum) of two variables selected at random equals the sum of the variances of the two populations from which the samples were drawn.* In other words, if X is drawn from a population with standard deviation σ_X and Y is drawn from a population with

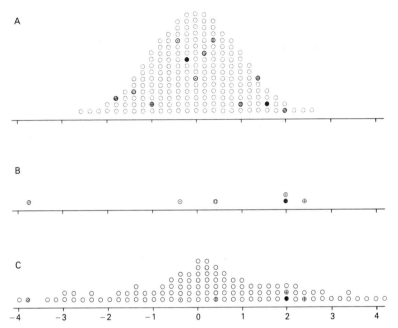

Figure 4-3 If one selects pairs of members of the population in panel *A* at random and computes the difference, the population of differences, shown in panel *B,* has a wider variance than the original population. Panel *C* shows another 100 values for differences of pairs of members selected at random from the population in *A* to make this point again.

standard deviation σ_Y, the distribution of all possible values of $X - Y$ (or $X + Y$) will have variance

$$\sigma^2_{X-Y} = \sigma^2_{X+Y} = \sigma^2_X + \sigma^2_Y$$

This result should seem reasonable to you because when you select pairs of values that are on opposite (the same) sides of the population mean and compute their difference (sum), the result will be even farther from the mean.

Returning to the example in Fig. 4-3, we can observe that both the first and second numbers were drawn from the same population, whose variance was 1, and so the variance of the difference should be

$$\sigma^2_{X-Y} = \sigma^2_X + \sigma^2_Y = 1 + 1 = 2$$

Since the standard deviation is the square root of the variance, the standard deviation of the population of differences will be $\sqrt{2}$ times the standard deviation of the original population, or about 40 percent bigger, confirming our earlier subjective impression.*

When we wish to estimate the variance in the difference or sum of members of two populations based on the observations, we simply replace the population variances σ^2 in the equation above with the estimates of the variances computed from our samples,

$$s^2_{X-Y} = s^2_X + s^2_Y$$

The standard error of the mean is just the standard deviation of the population of all possible sample means of samples of size n, and so we can find the standard error of the difference of two means using the equation above. Specifically,

$$s^2_{\bar{X}-\bar{Y}} = s^2_{\bar{X}} + s^2_{\bar{Y}}$$

*The fact that the sum of randomly selected variables has a variance equal to the sum of the variances of the individual numbers explains why the standard error of the mean equals the standard deviation divided by $\sqrt{n}$. Suppose we draw n numbers at random from a population with standard deviation σ. The mean of these numbers will be

$$\bar{X} = \frac{1}{n}(X_1 + X_2 + X_3 + \cdots + X_n)$$

so

$$n\bar{X} = X_1 + X_2 + X_3 + \cdots + X_n$$

Since the variance associated with each of the X_i's is σ^2, the variance of $n\bar{X}$ will be

$$\sigma^2_{n\bar{X}} = \sigma^2 + \sigma^2 + \sigma^2 + \cdots + \sigma^2 = n\sigma^2$$

and the standard deviation will be

$$\sigma_{n\bar{X}} = \sqrt{n}\sigma$$

But we want the standard deviation of $\bar{X}$, which is $n\bar{X}/n$, therefore

$$\sigma_{\bar{X}} = \sqrt{n}\sigma/n = \sigma/\sqrt{n}$$

which is the formula for the standard error of the mean. Note that we made no assumptions about the population from which the sample was drawn. (In particular, we did *not* assume that it had a normal distribution.)

in which case

$$s_{\bar{X}-\bar{Y}} = \sqrt{s_{\bar{X}}^2 + s_{\bar{Y}}^2}$$

Now we are ready to construct the *t* ratio from the definition in the last section.

USE OF *t* TO TEST HYPOTHESES ABOUT TWO GROUPS

Recall that we decided to examine the ratio

$$t = \frac{\text{difference of sample means}}{\text{standard error of difference of sample means}}$$

We can now use the result of the last section to translate this definition into the equation

$$t = \frac{\bar{X}_1 - \bar{X}_2}{\sqrt{s_{\bar{X}_1}^2 + s_{\bar{X}_2}^2}}$$

Alternatively, we can write *t* in terms of the sample standard deviations rather than the standard errors of the mean:

$$t = \frac{\bar{X}_1 - \bar{X}_2}{\sqrt{(s_1^2/n) + (s_2^2/n)}}$$

in which *n* is the size of each sample.

If the hypothesis that the two samples were drawn from the same population is true, the variances s_1^2 and s_2^2 computed from the two samples are both estimates of the same population variance σ^2. Therefore, we replace the two different estimates of the population variance in the equation above with a single estimate, s^2, that is obtained by averaging these two separate estimates

$$s^2 = \frac{1}{2}(s_1^2 + s_2^2)$$

This is called the *pooled-variance estimate* since it is obtained by pooling the two estimates of the population variance to obtain a single esti-mate. The t-test statistic based on the pooled-variance estimate is

$$t = \frac{\bar{X}_1 - \bar{X}_2}{\sqrt{(s^2/n) + (s^2/n)}}$$

The specific value of t one obtains from any two samples depends not only on whether or not there actually is a difference in the means of the populations from which the samples were drawn but also on which specific individuals happened to be selected for the samples. Thus, as for F, there will be a range of possible values that t can have, even when both samples are drawn from the same population. Since the means computed from the two samples will generally be close to the mean of the population from which they were drawn, the value of t will tend to be small when the two samples are drawn from the same popu-lation. Therefore, we will use the same procedure to test hypotheses with t as we did with F in the last chapter. Specifically, we will com-pute t from the data, then reject the assertion that the two samples were drawn from the same population if the resulting value of t is "big."

Let us return to the problem of assessing the value of the diuretic we were discussing earlier. Suppose the entire population of interest contains 200 people. In addition, we will assume that the diuretic had no effect, so that the two groups of people being studied can be con-sidered to represent two samples drawn from a single population. Figure 4-4A shows this population, together with two samples of 10 people each selected at random for study. The people who received the placebo are shown as dark circles, and the people who received the diuretic are shown as lighter circles. The lower part of panel A shows the data as they would appear to the investigator, together with the mean and stan-dard deviations computed from each of the two samples. Looking at these data certainly does not suggest that the diuretic had any effect. The value of t associated with these samples is -.2.

Of course, there is nothing special about these two samples, and we could just as well have selected two different groups of people to study. Figure 4-4B shows another collection of people that could have been selected at random to receive the placebo (dark circles) or diuretic (light circles). Not surprisingly, these two samples differ from each other as well as the samples selected in panel A. Given only the data in

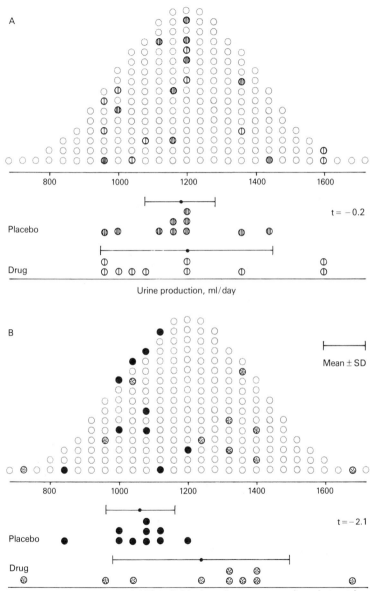

Figure 4-4 A population of 200 individuals and two groups selected at random for study of a drug designed to increase urine production but which is totally ineffective. The people shown as dark circles received the placebo and those with the lighter circles received the drug. An investigator would not see the entire

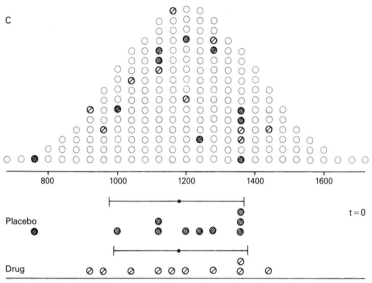

Figure 4-4 (continued)

population but just the information as reflected in the lower part of panel *A;* nevertheless, the two samples show very little difference, and it is unlikely that one would have concluded that the drug had an effect on urine production. Of course, there is nothing special about the two random samples shown in panel *A,* and an investigator could just as well have selected the two groups of people in panel *B* for study. There is more difference between these two groups than the two shown in panel *A,* and there is a chance that the investigator would think that this difference is due to the drug's effect on urine production rather than simple random sampling. Panel *C* shows yet another pair of random samples the investigator might have drawn for the study.

the lower part of panel *B*, we might think that the diuretic increases urine production. The t value associated with these data is -2.1. Panel *C* shows yet another pair of samples. They differ from each other and the other samples considered in panels *A* and *B*. The samples in panel *C* yield a value of 0 for t.

We could continue this process for quite a long time since there are more than 10^{27} different pairs of samples of 10 people each that we could draw from the population of 200 individuals shown in Fig. 4-4*A*. We can compute a value of t for each of these 10^{27} different pairs of samples. Figure 4-5 shows the values of t associated with 200 different pairs of random samples of 10 people each drawn from the original

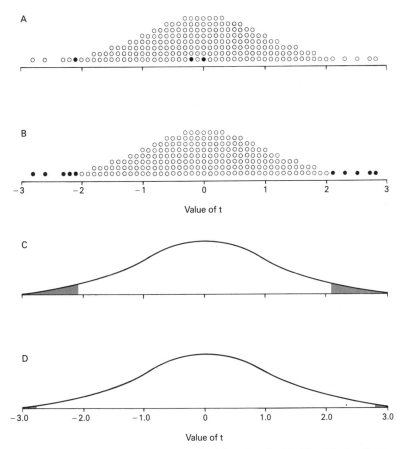

Figure 4-5 The results of 200 studies like that described in Fig. 4-4; the three specific studies from Fig. 4-4 are indicated in panel *A*. Note that most values of the *t* statistic cluster around 0, but it is possible for some values of *t* to be quite large, exceeding 1.5 or 2. Panel *B* shows that there are only 5 chances in 100 of *t* exceeding 2.1 in magnitude if the two samples were drawn from the same population. If one continues examining all possible samples drawn from the population and our pairs of samples drawn from the same population, one obtains a distribution of all possible *t* values which becomes the smooth curve in panel *C*. In this case, one defines the critical value of *t* by saying that it is unlikely that this value of *t* statistic was observed under the hypothesis that the drug had no effect by taking the 5 percent most extreme error areas under the tails of distribution and selecting the *t* value corresponding to the beginning of this region. Panel *D* shows that if one required a more stringent criterion for rejecting the hypothesis for no difference by requiring that *t* be in the most extreme 1 percent of all possible values, the cutoff value of *t* is 2.878.

population, including the three specific pairs of samples shown in Fig. 4-4. The distribution of possible t values is symmetrical about $t = 0$ because it does not matter which of the two samples we subtract from the other. As predicted, most of the resulting values of t are close to zero; t rarely is below about –2 or above +2.

Figure 4-5 allows us to determine what a big t is. Panel B shows that t will be less than –2.1 or greater than +2.1 10 out of 200, or 5 percent of the time. In other words, there is only a 5 percent chance of getting a value of t more extreme than –2.1 or +2.1 when the two samples are drawn from the same population. Just as with the F distribution, the number of possible t values rapidly increases beyond 10^{27} as the population size grows, and the distribution of possible t values approaches a smooth curve. Figure 4-5C shows the result of this limiting process. We define the cutoff values for t that are large enough to be called "big" on the basis of the total area in the two tails. Panel C shows that only 5 percent of the possible values of t will lie beyond –2.1 or +2.1 when the two samples are drawn from a single population. When the data are associated with a value of t beyond this range, it is customary to conclude that the data are inconsistent with the hypothesis of no difference between the two samples and report that there was a difference in treatment.

The extreme values of t that lead us to reject the hypothesis of no difference lie in both tails of the distribution. Therefore, the approach we are taking is sometimes called a *two-tailed t test*. Occasionally, people use a one-tailed t test, and there are indeed cases where this is appropriate. One should be suspicious of such one-tailed tests, however, because the cutoff value for calling t "big" for a given value of P is smaller. In reality, people are almost always looking for a *difference* between the control and treatment groups, and a two-tailed test is appropriate. This book always assumes a two-tailed test.

Note that the data in Fig. 4-4B are associated with a t value of –2.1, which we have decided to consider "big." If all we had were the data shown in Fig. 4-5B, we would conclude that the observations were inconsistent with the hypothesis that the diuretic had no effect and report that it *increased* urine production, and even though we did the statistical analysis correctly, *our conclusion about the drug would be wrong.*

Reporting $P < .05$ means that if the treatment had no effect, there is less than a 5 percent chance of getting a value of t from the data as far or farther from 0 as the critical value for t to be called "big." It does not mean it is impossible to get such a large value of t when the treatment has no effect. We could, of course, be more conservative and say that we will reject the hypothesis of no difference between the populations from which the samples were drawn if t is in the most extreme 1 percent of possible values. Figure 4-5D shows that this would require t to be beyond -2.88 or $+2.88$ in this case, so we would not erroneously conclude that the drug had an effect on urine output in any of the specific examples shown in Fig. 4-4. In the long run, however, we will make such errors about 1 percent of the time. The price for this conservatism is decreasing the chances of concluding that there is a difference when one really exists. Chapter 6 discusses this trade-off in more detail.

The critical values of t, like F, have been tabulated and depend not only on the level of confidence with which one rejects the hypothesis of no difference – the P value – but also on the sample size. As with the F distribution, this dependence on sample size enters the table as the *degrees of freedom v*, which is equal to $2(n - 1)$ for this t test, where n is the size of each sample. As the sample size increases, the value of t needed to reject the hypothesis of no difference decreases. In other words, as sample size increases, it becomes possible to detect smaller differences with a given level of confidence. Reflecting on Fig. 4-2 should convince you that this is reasonable.

WHAT IF THE TWO SAMPLES ARE NOT THE SAME SIZE?

It is easy to generalize the t test to handle problems in which there are different numbers of members in the two samples being studied. Recall that t is defined by

$$t = \frac{\bar{X}_1 - \bar{X}_2}{\sqrt{s_{\bar{X}_1}^2 + s_{\bar{X}_2}^2}}$$

in which $s_{\bar{X}_1}$ and $s_{\bar{X}_2}$ are the standard errors of the means of the two samples. If the first sample is of size n_1 and the second sample contains n_2 members,

$$s_{\bar{X}_1}^2 = \frac{s_1^2}{n_1} \quad \text{and} \quad s_{\bar{X}_2}^2 = \frac{s_2^2}{n_2}$$

in which s_1 and s_2 are the standard deviations of the two samples. Use these definitions to rewrite the definition of t in terms of the sample standard deviations

$$t = \frac{\bar{X}_1 - \bar{X}_2}{\sqrt{(s_1^2/n_1) + (s_2^2/n_2)}}$$

When the two samples are different sizes, the pooled estimate of the variance is given by

$$s^2 = \frac{(n_1 - 1)s_1^2 + (n_2 - 1)s_2^2}{n_1 + n_2 - 2}$$

so that

$$t = \frac{\bar{X}_1 - \bar{X}_2}{\sqrt{(s^2/n_1) + (s^2/n_2)}}$$

This is the definition of t for comparing two samples of unequal size. There are $\nu = n_1 + n_2 - 2$ degrees of freedom.

Notice that this result reduces to our earlier results when the two sample sizes are equal, i.e., when $n_1 = n_2 = n$.

THE EXAMPLES REVISITED

We can now use the t test to analyze the data from the examples we discussed to illustrate the analysis of variance. The conclusions will be no different from those obtained with analysis of variance because, as already stated, the t test is just a special case of analysis of variance.

Relationship of Drug Prescribing to Length of Hospital Stay

From Fig. 3-7, the 36 patients who were treated appropriately for pyelonephritis were hospitalized for an average of 4.51 days, and the 36 who were treated inappropriately were hospitalized an average of 6.28 days. The standard deviations of these two groups were 1.98 and 2.54 days, respectively. Since the sample sizes are equal, the pooled estimate for the variance is $s^2 = \frac{1}{2}(1.98^2 + 2.54^2) = 5.18$. Putting this information into the formula for t, we have

$$t = \frac{4.51 - 6.28}{\sqrt{(5.18/36) + (5.18/36)}} = -3.30$$

with $\nu = 2(n - 1) = 2(36 - 1) = 70$. Table 4-1 shows that, for 70 degrees of freedom, the magnitude of t will exceed 1.994 only 5 percent of the time and 2.648 only 1 percent of the time when the two samples were drawn from the same population. Since the magnitude of t associated with our data exceeds 2.648, we conclude that appropriate drug therapy led to patients having shorter hospital stays on the average ($P < .01$).

Halothane versus Morphine for Open-Heart Surgery

Figure 3-8 showed that the lowest mean arterial blood pressure between the start of anesthesia and beginning of the incision was 66.9 mmHg in the 61 patients anesthetized with halothane and 73.2 in the 61 patients anesthetized with morphine. The standard deviations of the blood pressures in the two groups of patients was 12.2 and 14.4 mmHg, respectively. Thus,

$$s^2 = \frac{1}{2}(12.2^2 + 14.4^2) = 178.1$$

and

$$t = \frac{66.9 - 73.2}{\sqrt{(178.1/61) + (178.1/61)}} = -2.607$$

with $\nu = 2(n - 1) = 2(61 - 1) = 120$ degrees of freedom. Table 4-1 shows that the magnitude of t should exceed 2.358 only 2 percent of the time when the two samples are drawn from a single population, as they would be if halothane and morphine both affected patients' blood pressure similarly. Since the value of t associated with the observations exceeds this value, we conclude that halothane is associated with a lower lowest mean arterial pressure than morphine, on the average.

Table 4-1   Critical Values of t (Two-Tailed)

v	Probability of greater value, P								
	0.50	0.20	0.10	0.05	0.02	0.01	0.005	0.002	0.001
1	1.000	3.078	6.314	12.706	31.821	63.657	127.321	318.309	636.619
2	0.816	1.886	2.920	4.303	6.965	9.925	14.089	22.327	31.599
3	0.765	1.638	2.353	3.182	4.541	5.841	7.453	10.215	12.924
4	0.741	1.533	2.132	2.776	3.747	4.604	5.598	7.173	8.610
5	0.727	1.476	2.015	2.571	3.365	4.032	4.773	5.893	6.869
6	0.718	1.440	1.943	2.447	3.143	3.707	4.317	5.208	5.959
7	0.711	1.415	1.895	2.365	2.998	3.499	4.029	4.785	5.408
8	0.706	1.397	1.860	2.306	2.896	3.355	3.833	4.501	5.041
9	0.703	1.383	1.833	2.262	2.821	3.250	3.690	4.297	4.781
10	0.700	1.372	1.812	2.228	2.764	3.169	3.581	4.144	4.587
11	0.697	1.363	1.796	2.201	2.718	3.106	3.497	4.025	4.437
12	0.695	1.356	1.782	2.179	2.681	3.055	3.428	3.930	4.318
13	0.694	1.350	1.771	2.160	2.650	3.012	3.372	3.852	4.221
14	0.692	1.345	1.761	2.145	2.624	2.977	3.326	3.787	4.140
15	0.691	1.341	1.753	2.131	2.602	2.947	3.286	3.733	4.073
16	0.690	1.337	1.746	2.120	2.583	2.921	3.252	3.686	4.015
17	0.689	1.333	1.740	2.110	2.567	2.898	3.222	3.646	3.965
18	0.688	1.330	1.734	2.101	2.552	2.878	3.197	3.610	3.922
19	0.688	1.328	1.729	2.093	2.539	2.861	3.174	3.579	3.883
20	0.687	1.325	1.725	2.086	2.528	2.845	3.153	3.552	3.850
21	0.686	1.323	1.721	2.080	2.518	2.831	3.135	3.527	3.819
22	0.686	1.321	1.717	2.074	2.508	2.819	3.119	3.505	3.792
23	0.685	1.319	1.714	2.069	2.500	2.807	3.104	3.485	3.768
24	0.685	1.318	1.711	2.064	2.492	2.797	3.091	3.467	3.745
25	0.684	1.316	1.708	2.060	2.485	2.787	3.078	3.450	3.725
26	0.684	1.315	1.706	2.056	2.479	2.779	3.067	3.435	3.707
27	0.684	1.314	1.703	2.052	2.473	2.771	3.057	3.421	3.690
28	0.683	1.313	1.701	2.048	2.467	2.763	3.047	3.408	3.674
29	0.683	1.311	1.699	2.045	2.462	2.756	3.038	3.396	3.659
30	0.683	1.310	1.697	2.042	2.457	2.750	3.030	3.385	3.646
31	0.682	1.309	1.696	2.040	2.453	2.744	3.022	3.375	3.633
32	0.682	1.309	1.694	2.037	2.449	2.738	3.015	3.365	3.622
33	0.682	1.308	1.692	2.035	2.445	2.733	3.008	3.356	3.611
34	0.682	1.307	1.691	2.032	2.441	2.728	3.002	3.348	3.601
35	0.682	1.306	1.690	2.030	2.438	2.724	2.996	3.340	3.591
36	0.681	1.306	1.688	2.028	2.434	2.719	2.990	3.333	3.582
37	0.681	1.305	1.687	2.026	2.431	2.715	2.985	3.326	3.574
38	0.681	1.304	1.686	2.024	2.429	2.712	2.980	3.319	3.566
39	0.681	1.304	1.685	2.023	2.426	2.708	2.976	3.313	3.558
40	0.681	1.303	1.684	2.021	2.423	2.704	2.971	3.307	3.551

Table 4-1   Critical Values of *t* (Two-Tailed) *(Continued)*

ν	Probability of greater value, *P*								
	0.50	0.20	0.10	0.05	0.02	0.01	0.005	0.002	0.001
42	0.680	1.302	1.682	2.018	2.418	2.698	2.963	3.296	3.538
44	0.680	1.301	1.680	2.015	2.414	2.692	2.956	3.286	3.526
46	0.680	1.300	1.679	2.013	2.410	2.687	2.949	3.277	3.515
48	0.680	1.299	1.677	2.011	2.407	2.682	2.943	3.269	3.505
50	0.679	1.299	1.676	2.009	2.403	2.678	2.937	3.261	3.496
52	0.679	1.298	1.675	2.007	2.400	2.674	2.932	3.255	3.488
54	0.679	1.297	1.674	2.005	2.397	2.670	2.927	3.248	3.480
56	0.679	1.297	1.673	2.003	2.395	2.667	2.923	3.242	3.473
58	0.679	1.296	1.672	2.002	2.392	2.663	2.918	3.237	3.466
60	0.679	1.296	1.671	2.000	2.390	2.660	2.915	3.232	3.460
62	0.678	1.295	1.670	1.999	2.388	2.657	2.911	3.227	3.454
64	0.678	1.295	1.669	1.998	2.386	2.655	2.908	3.223	3.449
66	0.678	1.295	1.668	1.997	2.384	2.652	2.904	3.218	3.444
68	0.678	1.294	1.668	1.995	2.382	2.650	2.902	3.214	3.439
70	0.678	1.294	1.667	1.994	2.381	2.648	2.899	3.211	3.435
72	0.678	1.293	1.666	1.993	2.379	2.646	2.896	3.207	3.431
74	0.678	1.293	1.666	1.993	2.378	2.644	2.894	3.204	3.427
76	0.678	1.293	1.665	1.992	2.376	2.642	2.891	3.201	3.423
78	0.678	1.292	1.665	1.991	2.375	2.640	2.889	3.198	3.420
80	0.678	1.292	1.664	1.990	2.374	2.639	2.887	3.195	3.416
90	0.677	1.291	1.662	1.987	2.368	2.632	2.878	3.183	3.402
100	0.677	1.290	1.660	1.984	2.364	2.626	2.871	3.174	3.390
120	0.677	1.289	1.658	1.980	2.358	2.617	2.860	3.160	3.373
140	0.676	1.288	1.656	1.977	2.353	2.611	2.852	3.149	3.361
160	0.676	1.287	1.654	1.975	2.350	2.607	2.846	3.142	3.352
180	0.676	1.286	1.653	1.973	2.347	2.603	2.842	3.136	3.345
200	0.676	1.286	1.653	1.972	2.345	2.601	2.839	3.131	3.340
∞	0.6745	1.2816	1.6449	1.9600	2.3263	2.5758	2.8070	3.0902	3.2905

Source: Adapted from J. H. Zar, *Biostatistical Analysis,* Prentice-Hall, Englewood Cliffs, N.J., 1974, pp. 413–414, table D.10. Used by permission.

Conahan and his colleagues also measured the amount of blood being pumped by the heart in some of the patients they anesthetized to obtain another measure of how the two anesthetic agents affected cardiac function in people having heart-valve replacement surgery. To normalize the measurements to account for the fact that patients are different sizes and hence have different sized hearts and blood flows, they computed the cardiac index, which is defined as the rate at which

Table 4-2 Comparison of Anesthetic Effects on the Cardiovascular
System

	Halothane (n = 9)		Morphine (n = 16)	
	Mean	SD	Mean	SD
Best cardiac index, induction to bypass, L/m² · min	2.08	1.05	1.75	.88
Mean arterial blood pressure at time of best cardiac index, mmHg	76.8	13.8	91.4	19.6
Total peripheral resistance associated with best cardiac index, dyn · s/cm⁵	2210	1200	2830	1130

Source: Adapted from T. J. Conahan et al., "A Prospective Random Comparison of Halothane and Morphine for Open-Heart Anesthesia," *Anesthesiology,* **38**:528–535, 1973.

the heart pumps blood (the cardiac output) divided by body surface area. Table 4-2 reproduces some of their results. Morphine seems to produce lower cardiac indexes than halothane, but is this difference large enough to reject the hypothesis that the difference reflects random sampling rather than an actual physiological difference?

From the information in Table 4-2, the pooled estimate of the variance is

$$s^2 = \frac{(9-1)(1.05^2) + (16-1)(.88^2)}{9 + 16 - 2} = .89$$

and so

$$t = \frac{2.08 - 1.75}{\sqrt{(.89/9) + (.89/16)}} = .84$$

which does not exceed the 5 percent critical value of 2.069 for $\nu = n_{hlo} + n_{mor} - 2 = 9 + 16 - 2 = 23$ degrees of freedom. Hence, we do not have strong enough evidence to assert that there is really a difference in cardiac index with the two anesthetics. Does this prove that there really was not a difference?

THE *t* TEST IS AN ANALYSIS OF VARIANCE*

The *t* test and analysis of variance we developed in Chap. 3 are really two different ways of doing the same thing. Since few people recognize this, we will prove that when comparing the means of two groups, $F = t^2$. In other words, the *t* test is simply a special case of analysis of variance applied to two groups.

We begin with two samples, each of size *n*, with means and standard deviations $\bar{X}_1$ and $\bar{X}_2$ and s_1 and s_2, respectively.

To form the *F* ratio used in analysis of variance, we first estimate the population variance as the average of the variances computed for each group

$$s^2_{\text{wit}} = \tfrac{1}{2}(s^2_1 + s^2_2)$$

Next, we estimate the population variance from the sample means by computing the standard deviation of the sample means with

$$s_{\bar{X}} = \sqrt{\frac{(\bar{X}_1 - \bar{X})^2 + (\bar{X}_2 - \bar{X})^2}{2 - 1}}$$

Therefore

$$s^2_{\bar{X}} = (\bar{X}_1 - \bar{X})^2 + (\bar{X}_2 - \bar{X})^2$$

in which $\bar{X}$ is the mean of the two sample means

$$\bar{X} = \tfrac{1}{2}(\bar{X}_1 + \bar{X}_2)$$

Eliminate $\bar{X}$ from the equation for $s^2_{\bar{X}}$ to obtain

---

*This section represents the only mathematical proof in this book and as such is a bit more technical than everything else. The reader can skip this section with no loss of continuity.

$$s_{\bar{X}}^2 = [\bar{X}_1 - \tfrac{1}{2}(\bar{X}_1 + \bar{X}_2)]^2 + [\bar{X}_2 - \tfrac{1}{2}(\bar{X}_1 + \bar{X}_2)]^2$$

$$= (\tfrac{1}{2}\bar{X}_1 - \tfrac{1}{2}\bar{X}_2)^2 + (\tfrac{1}{2}\bar{X}_2 - \tfrac{1}{2}\bar{X}_1)^2$$

Since the square of a number is always positive, $(a - b)^2 = (b - a)^2$ and the equation above becomes

$$s_{\bar{X}}^2 = (\tfrac{1}{2}\bar{X}_1 - \tfrac{1}{2}\bar{X}_2)^2 + (\tfrac{1}{2}\bar{X}_1 - \tfrac{1}{2}\bar{X}_2)^2$$

$$= 2[\tfrac{1}{2}(\bar{X}_1 - \bar{X}_2)]^2 = \tfrac{1}{2}(\bar{X}_1 - \bar{X}_2)^2$$

Therefore, the estimate of the population variance from between the groups is

$$s_{\text{bet}}^2 = ns_{\bar{X}}^2 = \tfrac{n}{2}(\bar{X}_1 - \bar{X}_2)^2$$

Finally, F is the ratio of these two estimates of the population variance

$$F = \frac{s_{\text{bet}}^2}{s_{\text{wit}}^2} = \frac{(n/2)(\bar{X}_1 - \bar{X}_2)^2}{\tfrac{1}{2}(s_1^2 + s_2^2)} = \frac{(\bar{X}_1 - \bar{X}_2)^2}{(s_1^2/n) + (s_2^2/n)}$$

$$= \left[\frac{\bar{X}_1 - \bar{X}_2}{\sqrt{(s_1^2/n) + (s_2^2/n)}}\right]^2$$

The quantity in the brackets is t, hence

$$F = t^2$$

The degrees of freedom for the numerator of F equals the number of groups minus 1, that is, $2 - 1 = 1$ for all comparisons of two groups. The degrees of freedom for the denominator equals the number of groups times 1 less than the sample size of each group, $2(n - 1)$, which is the same as the degrees of freedom associated with the *t* test.

In sum, the *t* test and analysis of variance are just two different ways of looking at the same test for two groups. Of course, if there are more than two groups, one cannot use the *t*-test form of analysis of variance but must use the more general form we developed in Chap. 3.

COMMON ERRORS IN THE USE OF THE *t* TEST AND HOW TO COMPENSATE FOR THEM

The *t* test is used to compute the probability of being wrong, the *P* value, when asserting that the mean values of *two* treatment groups are different. We have already seen (Fig. 4-1) that it is also used widely but erroneously to test for differences between more than two groups by comparing all possible pairs of means with *t* tests.

For example, suppose an investigator measured blood sugar under control conditions, in the presence of drug A, and in the presence of drug B. It is common to perform three *t* tests on these data: one to compare control versus drug A, one to compare control versus drug B, and one to compare drug A versus drug B. This practice is incorrect because the true probability of erroneously concluding that the drug affected blood sugar is actually higher than the nominal level, say 5 percent, used when looking up the "big" cutoff value of the *t* statistic in a table.

To understand why, reconsider the experiment described in the last paragraph. Suppose that if the value of the *t* statistic computed in one of the three comparisons just described is in the most extreme 5 percent of the values that would occur if the drugs really had no effect, we will reject that assumption and assert that the drugs changed blood sugar. We will be satisfied if $P < .05$; in other words, in the long run we are willing to accept the fact that 1 statement in 20 will be wrong. Therefore, when we test control versus drug A, we can expect erroneously to assert a difference 5 percent of the time. Similarly, when testing control versus drug B, we expect erroneously to assert a difference 5 percent of the time, and when testing drug A versus drug B, we expect erroneously to assert a difference 5 percent of the time. Therefore, when considering the three tests together, we expect to conclude that at least one pair of groups differs about 5 percent + 5 percent + 5 percent = 15 percent of the time, even if in reality the drugs did not affect blood sugar (P actually equals 14 percent). If there are not too many comparisons, simply adding the P values obtained in multiple tests produces a realistic and conservative estimate of the true P value for the set of comparisons.

In the example above, there were three t tests, so the effective P value was about $3(.05) = .15$, or 15 percent. When comparing four groups, there are six possible t tests (1 versus 2, 1 versus 3, 1 versus 4, 2 versus 3, 2 versus 4, 3 versus 4); so if the author concludes that there is a difference and reports $P < .05$, the effective P value is about $6(.05) = .30$; there is about a 30 percent chance of at least one incorrect statement if the author concludes that the treatments had an effect!

In Chap. 2, we discussed random samples of Martians to illustrate the fact that different samples from the same population yield different estimates of the population mean and standard deviation. Figure 2-6 showed three such samples of the heights of Martians, all drawn from a single population. Suppose we chose to study how these Martians respond to human hormones. We draw three samples at random, give one group a placebo, one group testosterone, and one group estrogen. Suppose that these hormones have no effect on the Martians' heights. Thus, the three groups shown in Fig. 2-6 represent three samples drawn at random from the same population.

Figure 4-6 shows how these data would probably appear in a typical medical journal. The large vertical bars denote the value of the mean responses, and the small vertical bars denote 1 standard error of the mean above or below the sample means. Showing 1 standard deviation would be the appropriate way to describe variability in the samples. Most authors would analyze these data by performing three t tests: placebo against testosterone, placebo against estrogen, and testosterone against estrogen. These three tests yield t values of 2.39, 0.93, and 1.34, respectively. Since each test is based on 2 samples of 10 Martians each, there are $2(10 - 1) = 18$ degrees of freedom. From Table 4-1, the critical value of t with a 5 percent chance of erroneously concluding that a difference exists is 2.101. Thus, the author would conclude that testosterone produced shorter Martians than placebo, whereas estrogen did not differ significantly from placebo, and that the two hormones did not produce significantly different results.

Think about this result for a moment. What is wrong with it?

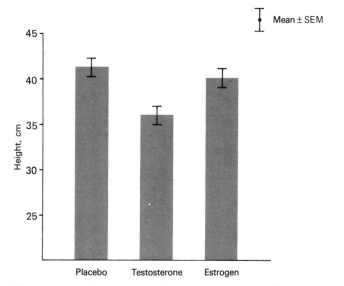

Figure 4-6 Results of a study of human hormones on Martians as it would be commonly presented in the medical literature. Each large bar has a height equal to the mean of the group; the small vertical bars indicate 1 standard error of the mean on either side of the mean (not 1 standard deviation).

If testosterone produced results no different from those of estrogen and estrogen produced results no different from those of placebo, how can testosterone have produced results different from placebo? Far from alerting medical researchers that there is something wrong with their analysis, this illogical result usually leads to a very creatively written "Discussion" section in their paper.

An analysis of variance of these data yields $F = 2.74$ [with numerator degrees of freedom = $m - 1 = 3 - 1 = 2$ and denominator degrees of freedom $m(n - 1) = 3(10 - 1) = 27$], which is below the critical value of 3.13 we have decided is required to assert that the data are incompatible with the hypothesis that all three treatments acted as placebos.

Of course, performing the analysis of variance does not ensure that we will not reach a conclusion that is actually wrong, but it will make it less likely.

We end our discussion of common errors in the use of the *t* test with three rules of thumb:

- *The t test can be used to test the hypothesis that two group means are not different.*
- *When the experimental design involves multiple groups, analysis of variance should be used.*
- *When t tests are used to test for differences between multiple groups, you can estimate the true P value by multiplying the reported P value times the number of possible t tests.*

HOW TO USE t TESTS TO ISOLATE DIFFERENCES
BETWEEN GROUPS IN ANALYSIS OF VARIANCE

The last section demonstrated that when presented with data from experiments with more than two groups of subjects, one must do an analysis of variance to determine how inconsistent the observations are with the hypothesis that all the treatments had the same effect. Doing pairwise comparisons with t tests increases the chances of erroneously reporting an effect above the nominal value, say 5 percent, used to determine the value of a "big" t. The analysis of variance, however, only tests the global hypothesis that *all* the samples were drawn from a single population. In particular, it does not provide any information on which sample or samples differed from the others.

There are a variety of methods, called *multiple-comparison procedures,* that can be used to provide information on this point. All are essentially based on the t test but include appropriate corrections for the fact that we are comparing more than one pair of means. We will develop one such approach, the *Bonferroni t test,* here. The general approach we take is first to perform an analysis of variance to see whether *anything* appears different, then use a multiple-comparison procedure to isolate the treatment or treatments producing the different results.* In the last section, we saw that if one analyzes a set of data with three t tests, each using the 5 percent critical value for concluding that there is a difference, there is about a $3(5) = 15$ percent chance of finding it. This result is a special case of a formula called the *Bonferroni inequality,* which states that if k statistical tests are per-

---

*Some statisticians believe that this approach is too conservative and that one should skip the analysis of variance and proceed directly to the multiple comparisons of interest. For an introductory treatment from this perspective, see Byron W. Brown, Jr., and Myles Hollander, *Statistics: A Biomedical Introduction,* Wiley, New York, 1977, chap. 10, "Analysis of k-Sample Problems."

formed with the cutoff value for the test statistics, for example, t or F, at the α level, the likelihood of observing a value of the test statistic exceeding the cutoff value at least once when the treatments did not produce an effect is no greater than k times α. Mathematically, the Bonferroni inequality states

$$\alpha_T < k\alpha$$

where α_T is the true probability of erroneously concluding a difference exists at least once. α_T is the error rate we want to control. From the equation above,

$$\frac{\alpha_T}{k} < \alpha$$

Thus, if we do *each* of the t tests using the critical value of t corresponding to α_T/k, the error rate for *all* the comparisons taken as a group will be at most α_T. For example, if we wish to do three comparisons with t tests while keeping the probability of making at least one mistake to less than 5 percent, we use the t value corresponding to $^5/_3 = 1.6$ percent for each of the individual comparisons. This procedure is called the Bonferroni t test because it is based on the Bonferroni inequality.

This procedure works reasonably well when there are only a few groups to compare, but as the number of comparisons k increases above 8 to 10, the value of t required to conclude that a difference exists becomes much larger than it really needs to be and the method becomes overconservative. Other multiple-comparison procedures, such as the Student-Neuman-Keuls test (discussed in the next section), are less conservative. All, however, are similar to the Bonferroni t test in that they are essentially modifications of the t test to account for the fact that we are making multiple comparisons.

One way to make the Bonferroni t test less conservative is to use the estimate of the population variance computed from within the groups in the analysis of variance. Specifically, recall that we defined t as

$$t = \frac{\bar{X}_1 - \bar{X}_2}{\sqrt{(s^2/n_1) + (s^2/n_2)}}$$

where s^2 is an estimate of the population variance. We will replace this estimate with the population variance estimated from within the groups as part of the analysis of variance, s^2_{wit}, to obtain

$$t = \frac{\bar{X}_1 - \bar{X}_2}{\sqrt{(s^2_{wit}/n_1) + (s^2_{wit}/n_2)}}$$

When the sample sizes are equal, the equation becomes

$$t = \frac{\bar{X}_1 - \bar{X}_2}{\sqrt{2s^2_{wit}/n}}$$

The degrees of freedom for this test are the same as the denominator degrees of freedom for the analysis of variance and will be higher than for a simple t test based on the two samples being compared.* Since the critical value of t decreases as the degrees of freedom increase, it will be possible to detect a difference with a given confidence with smaller absolute differences in the means.

More on Menstruation and Jogging

In the last chapter we analyzed the data in Fig. 3-9 and concluded that they were inconsistent with the hypothesis that a control group, a group of joggers, and a group of runners had on the average the same number of menstrual periods per year. At the time, however, we were unable to isolate where the difference came from. Now we can use our Bonferroni t test to compare the three groups pairwise.

Recall that our best estimate of the within-groups variance s^2_{wit} is 3.95 (menses/year)^2. There are $m = 3$ samples, each containing $n = 26$ women. Therefore, there are $m(n - 1) = 3(26 - 1) = 75$ degrees of freedom associated with the estimate of the within-groups variance. [Note that if we just used the pooled variance from the two samples, there would be only $2(n - 1) = 2(26 - 1) = 50$ degrees of freedom.] Therefore, we can compare the three different groups by computing three values of t. To compare control with the joggers, we compute

---

*The number of degrees of freedom is the same if there are only two groups.

$$t = \frac{\bar{X}_{\text{jog}} - \bar{X}_{\text{con}}}{\sqrt{2s^2_{\text{wit}}/n}} = \frac{10.1 - 11.5}{\sqrt{2(3.95)/26}} = -2.54$$

To compare the control group with the runners, we compute

$$t = \frac{\bar{X}_{\text{run}} - \bar{X}_{\text{con}}}{\sqrt{2s^2_{\text{wit}}/n}} = \frac{9.1 - 11.5}{\sqrt{2(3.95)/26}} = -4.35$$

To compare the joggers with the runners, we compute

$$t = \frac{\bar{X}_{\text{jog}} - \bar{X}_{\text{run}}}{\sqrt{2s^2_{\text{wit}}/n}} = \frac{10.1 - 9.1}{\sqrt{2(3.95)/26}} = 1.81$$

There are three comparisons, so to have an overall error rate of less than 5 percent we compare each of these values of t with the critical value of t associated with the $\frac{5}{3} = 1.6$ percent level and 75 degrees of freedom. Interpolating in Table 4-1 shows this value to be about 2.47.

Thus, we have sufficient evidence to conclude that both jogging and running decrease the frequency of menstruation, but we do not have evidence that running decreases menstruation any more than simply jogging.

A BETTER APPROACH TO MULTIPLE COMPARISON TESTING: THE STUDENT-NEWMAN-KEULS TEST*

As noted in the previous section, the Bonferroni t test is overly conservative when there are more than a few group means to compare. This section presents the *Student-Newman-Keuls (SNK) test*. The SNK test statistic q is constructed similarly to the t test statistic, but the sampling distribution used to determine the critical values reflects a more sophisticated mathematical model of the multiple-comparison problem than does the simple Bonferroni inequality. This more sophisticated model gives rise to a more realistic estimate of the total true probability

---

*This material is important for people who are using this book as a guide for analysis of their data; it can be skipped in a course on introductory biostatistics without interfering with the presentation of the rest of the material in this book.

of erroneously concluding a difference exists, α_T, than does the Bonferroni t test.

The first step in the analysis is to complete an analysis of variance on all the data to test the global hypothesis that all the samples were drawn from a single population. If this test yields a significant value of F, arrange all the means in increasing order and compute the SNK test statistic q according to

$$q = \frac{\bar{X}_A - \bar{X}_B}{\sqrt{\frac{s_{\text{wit}}^2}{2}\left(\frac{1}{n_A} + \frac{1}{n_B}\right)}}$$

where $\bar{X}_A$ and $\bar{X}_B$ are the two means being compared, s_{wit}^2 is the variance within the treatment groups estimated from the analysis of variance, and n_A and n_B are the sample sizes of the two samples being compared.

This value of q is then compared with the table of critical values (Table 4-3). This critical value depends on α_T, the total risk of erroneously asserting a difference for all comparisons combined, ν_d, the denominator degrees of freedom from the analysis of variance, and a parameter p, which is the number of means being tested. For example, when comparing the largest and smallest of four means, $p = 4$; when comparing the second smallest and smallest means, $p = 2$.

The conclusions reached by multiple-comparisons testing depend on the order that the pair-wise comparisons are made. The proper procedure is to compare first the largest mean with the smallest, then the largest with the second smallest, and so on, until the largest has been compared with the second largest. Next, compare the second largest with the smallest, the second largest with the next smallest, and so forth. For example, after ranking four means in ascending order, the sequence of comparisons should be: 4 versus 1, 4 versus 2, 4 versus 3, 3 versus 1, 3 versus 2, 2 versus 1.

Another important procedural rule is that if no significant difference exists between two means, then conclude that no difference exists between any means enclosed by the two without testing for them. Thus, in the preceding example, if we failed to find a significant difference between means 3 and 1, we would not test for a difference between means 3 and 2 or means 2 and 1.

Still More on Menstruation and Jogging

To illustrate the procedure, we once again analyze the data in Fig. 3-9, which presents the number of menses per year in women runners, joggers, and sedentary controls. The women in the control group had an average of 11.5 menses per year, the joggers had an average of 10.1 menses per year, and the runners had an average of 9.1 menses per year. We begin by ordering these means in descending order (which is how they happen to be listed). Next, we compute the change in means between the largest and smallest (control versus runners), the largest and the next smallest (control versus joggers), and the second largest and the smallest (joggers versus runners). Finally, we use the estimate of the variance from within the groups in the analysis of variance, $s_{wit}^2 = 3.95$ (menses/year)^2 with $v_d = 75$ degrees of freedom, and the fact that each test group contained 26 women to complete the computation of each value of q.

To compare the controls with the runners, we compute

$$q = \frac{\bar{X}_{con} - \bar{X}_{run}}{\sqrt{\dfrac{s_{wit}^2}{2}\left(\dfrac{1}{n_{con}} + \dfrac{1}{n_{run}}\right)}} = \frac{11.5 - 9.1}{\sqrt{\dfrac{3.95}{2}\left(\dfrac{1}{26} + \dfrac{1}{26}\right)}} = 6.157$$

This comparison spans three means, so $p = 3$. From Table 4-3, the critical value of q for $\alpha_T = .05$, $v_d = 75$ (from the analysis of variance), and $p = 3$ is 3.385. Since the value of q associated with this comparison, 6.157, exceeds this critical value, we conclude that there is a significant difference between the controls and the runners. Since this result is significant, we go on to the next comparison.

To compare the controls with the joggers, we compute

$$q = \frac{\bar{X}_{con} - \bar{X}_{jog}}{\sqrt{\dfrac{s_{wit}^2}{2}\left(\dfrac{1}{n_{con}} + \dfrac{1}{n_{jog}}\right)}} = \frac{11.5 - 10.1}{\sqrt{\dfrac{3.95}{2}\left(\dfrac{1}{26} + \dfrac{1}{26}\right)}} = 3.592$$

For this comparison, α_T and v_d are the same as before, but $p = 2$. From Table 4-3, the critical value of q is 2.822. The value of 3.592 associated

Table 4-3   Critical Values of q

				$\alpha_T = 0.05$					
ν_d	$p = 2$	3	4	5	6	7	8	9	10
1	17.97	26.98	32.82	37.08	40.41	43.12	45.40	47.36	49.0
2	6.085	8.331	9.798	10.88	11.74	12.44	13.03	13.54	13.99
3	4.501	5.910	6.825	7.502	8.037	8.478	8.853	9.177	9.4
4	3.927	5.040	5.757	6.287	6.707	7.053	7.347	7.602	7.8
5	3.635	4.602	5.218	5.673	6.033	6.330	6.582	6.802	6.9
6	3.461	4.339	4.896	5.305	5.628	5.895	6.122	6.319	6.4
7	3.344	4.165	4.681	5.060	5.359	5.606	5.815	5.998	6.1
8	3.261	4.041	4.529	4.886	5.167	5.399	5.597	5.767	5.9
9	3.199	3.949	4.415	4.756	5.024	5.244	5.432	5.595	5.7
10	3.151	3.877	4.327	4.654	4.912	5.124	5.305	5.461	5.5
11	3.113	3.820	4.256	4.574	4.823	5.028	5.202	5.353	5.4
12	3.082	3.773	4.199	4.508	4.751	4.950	5.119	5.265	5.3
13	3.055	3,735	4.151	4.453	4.690	4.885	5.049	5.192	5.3
14	3.033	3.702	4.111	4.407	4.639	4.829	4.990	5.131	5.2
15	3.014	3.674	4.076	4.367	4.595	4.782	4.940	5.077	5.1
16	2.998	3.649	4.046	4.333	4.557	4.741	4.897	5.031	5.1
17	2.984	3.628	4.020	4.303	4.524	4.705	4.858	4.991	5.1
18	2.971	3.609	3.997	4.277	4.495	4.673	4.824	4.956	5.0
19	2.960	3.593	3.977	4.253	4.469	4.645	4.794	4.924	5.0
20	2.950	3.578	3.958	4.232	4.445	4.620	4.768	4.896	5.0
24	2.919	3.532	3.901	4.166	4.373	4.541	4.684	4.807	4.9
30	2.888	3.486	3.845	4.102	4.302	4.464	4.602	4.720	4.8
40	2.858	3.442	3.791	4.039	4.232	4.389	4.521	4.635	4.7
60	2.829	3.399	3.737	3.977	4.163	4.314	4.441	4.550	4.6
120	2.800	3.356	3.685	3.917	4.096	4.241	4.363	4.468	4.5
∞	2.772	3.314	3.633	3.858	4.030	4.170	4.286	4.387	4.4

with this comparison also exceeds the critical value, so we conclude that controls are also significantly different from joggers.

To compare the joggers with the runners, we compute

$$q = \frac{\bar{X}_{\text{jog}} - \bar{X}_{\text{run}}}{\sqrt{\dfrac{s^2_{\text{wit}}}{2}\left(\dfrac{1}{n_{\text{jog}}} + \dfrac{1}{n_{\text{run}}}\right)}} = \frac{10.1 - 9.1}{\sqrt{\dfrac{3.95}{2}\left(\dfrac{1}{26} + \dfrac{1}{26}\right)}} = 2.566$$

Table 4-3   Critical Values of q (*Continued*)

ν_d	$p = 2$	3	4	5	6	7	8	9	10
				$\alpha_T = 0.01$					
1	90.03	135.0	164.3	185.6	202.2	215.8	227.2	237.0	245.6
2	14.04	19.02	22.29	24.72	26.63	28.20	29.53	30.68	31.69
3	8.261	10.62	12.17	13.33	14.24	15.00	15.64	16.20	16.69
4	6.512	8.120	9.173	9.958	10.58	11.10	11.55	11.93	12.27
5	5.702	6.976	7.804	8.421	8.913	9.321	9.669	9.972	10.24
6	5.243	6.331	7.033	7.556	7.973	8.318	8.613	8.869	9.097
7	4.949	5.919	6.543	7.005	7.373	7.679	7.939	8.166	8.368
8	4.746	5.635	6.204	6.625	6.960	7.237	7.474	7.681	7.863
9	4.596	5.428	5.957	6.348	6.658	6.915	7.134	7.325	7.495
10	4.482	5.270	5.769	6.136	6.428	6.669	6.875	7.055	7.213
11	4.392	5.146	5.621	5.970	6.247	6.476	6.672	6.842	6.992
12	4.320	5.046	5.502	5.836	6.101	6.321	6.507	6.670	6.814
13	4.260	4.964	5.404	5.727	5.981	6.192	6.372	6.528	6.667
14	4.210	4.895	5.322	5.634	5.881	6.085	6.258	6.409	6.543
15	4.168	4.836	5.252	5.556	5.796	5.994	6.162	6.309	6.439
16	4.131	4.786	5.192	5.489	5.722	5.915	6.079	6.222	6.349
17	4.099	4.742	5.140	5.430	5.659	5.847	6.007	6.147	6.270
18	4.071	4.703	5.094	5.379	5.603	5.788	5.944	6.081	6.201
19	4.046	4.670	5.054	5.334	5.554	5.735	5.889	6.022	6.141
20	4.024	4.639	5.018	5.294	5.510	5.688	5.839	5.970	6.087
24	3.956	4.546	4.907	5.168	5.374	5.542	5.685	5.809	5.919
30	3.889	4.455	4.799	5.048	5.242	5.401	5.536	5.653	5.756
40	3.825	4.367	4.696	4.931	5.114	5.265	5.392	5.502	5.559
60	3.762	4.282	4.595	4.818	4.991	5.133	5.253	5.356	5.447
120	3.702	4.200	4.497	4.709	4.872	5.005	5.118	5.214	5.299
∞	3.643	4.120	4.403	4.603	4.757	4.882	4.987	5.078	5.157

Source: H. L. Harter, *Order Statistics and Their Use in Testing and Estimation*, Vol. I: *Tests Based on Range and Studentized Range of Samples from a Normal Population*, U.S. Government Printing Office, Washington, D.C., 1970.

The value of q associated with this comparison, 2.566, is less than the critical value of 2.822 required to assert that there is a difference between joggers and runners. (The values of ν_d and p are the same as before, so the critical value of q is too.)

In sum, we conclude that runners and joggers have significantly fewer menses per year than women in the control group, but that there is not a significant difference between the runners and the joggers. Since we only did a small number of comparisons (3), this is the same conclusion we drew using the Bonferroni t test to conduct the multiple comparisons. Had we had an experiment with more test groups (and hence many more comparisons), we would see that the SNK test was capable of detecting differences that the Bonferroni t test missed because of the large values of t (i.e., small values of P) required to assert a statistically significant difference in any individual pair-wise comparison.

THE MEANING OF P

Understanding what P means requires understanding the logic of statistical hypothesis testing. For example, suppose an investigator wants to test whether or not a drug alters body temperature. The obvious experiment is to select two similar groups of people, administer a placebo to one and the drug to the other, measure body temperature in both groups, then compute the mean and standard deviation of the temperatures measured in each group. The mean responses of the two groups will probably be different, regardless of whether the drug has an effect or not for the same reason that different random samples drawn from the same population yield different estimates for the mean. Therefore, the question becomes: Is the observed difference in mean temperature of the two groups likely to be due to random variation associated with the allocation of individuals to the two experimental groups or due to the drug?

To answer this question, statisticians first quantify the observed difference between the two samples with a single number, called *a test statistic,* such as F or t. These statistics, like most test statistics, have the property that the greater the difference between the samples, the greater their value. If the drug has no effect, the test statistic will be a small number. But what is "small"?

To find the boundary between "small" and "big" values of the test statistic, statisticians assume that the drug does *not* affect temperature (the *null hypothesis*). If this assumption is correct, the two groups of people are simply random samples from a single population, all of whom received a placebo (because the drug is, in effect, a placebo). Now, in theory, the statistician repeats the experiment using all possible samples of people and computes the test statistic for each hypothetical experiment. Just as random variation produced different values for means of different samples, this procedure will yield a range of values for the test statistic. Most of these values will be relatively small, but sheer bad luck requires that there be a few samples that are not representative of the entire population. These samples will yield relatively large values of the test statistic *even if the drug had no effect.* This exercise produces only a few of the possible values of the test statistic, say 5 percent of them, above some cutoff point. The test statistic is "big" if it is larger than this cutoff point.

Having determined this cutoff point, we execute an experiment on a drug with unknown properties and compute the test statistic. It is "big." Therefore, we conclude that *there is less than a 5 percent chance of observing data which led to the computed value of the test statistic if the assumption that the drug had had no effect was true.* Traditionally, if the chances of observing the computed test statistic when the intervention has no effect are below 5 percent, one rejects the working assumption that the drug has no effect and asserts that the drug *does* have an effect. There is, of course, a chance that this assertion is wrong: about 5 percent. This 5 percent is known as the *P value* or *significance level.*

Precisely,

> *The P value is the probability of obtaining a value of the test statistic as large as or larger than the one computed from the data when in reality there is no difference between the different treatments.*

Or, in other words,

> *The P value is the probability of being wrong when asserting that a true difference exists.*

If we are willing to assert a difference when $P < .05$, we are tacitly agreeing to accept the fact that, over the long run, we expect 1 assertion of a difference in 20 to be wrong.

It is commonly believed that the *P* value is the probability of making a mistake. There are obviously two ways an investigator can reach a mistaken conclusion based on the data, reporting that the treatment had an effect when in reality it did not or reporting that the treatment did not have an effect when in reality it did. As noted above, the *P* value only quantifies the probability of making the first kind of error (called a *Type I* or α *error*), that of erroneously concluding that the treatment had an effect when in reality it did not. It gives no information about the probability of making the second kind of error (called a *Type II* or β *error*), that of concluding that the treatment had no effect when in reality it did. Chapter 6 discusses how to estimate the probability of making Type II errors.

PROBLEMS

4-1 Conahan and his associates also measured the mean arterial pressure and total peripheral resistance (a measure of how hard it is to produce a given flow through the arterial bed) in 9 patients who were anesthetized with halothane and 16 patients who were anesthetized with morphine. The results are summarized in Table 4-2. Is there evidence that these two anesthetic agents are associated with differences in either of these two variables?

4-2 People with some abnormalities of their retinas show increased permeability of the retinal blood vessels. This permeability is measured by injecting a fluorescent dye into the blood and measuring how much penetrates into the eye. Gerald Fishman and his coworkers ("Blood-Retinal Barrier Function in Patients with Cone or Cone-Rod Dystrophy," *Arch. Ophthalmol.* **104**:545–548, 1986) studied a group of people with normal retinas and a group of people with obvious abnormalities of only the foveal part of the retina. The dye-penetration ratios of these two groups are

Penetration ratios, 10^{-6}/min

Normal retina	Foveal abnormality
0.5	1.2
0.7	1.4
0.7	1.6
1.0	1.7
1.0	1.7
1.2	1.8
1.4	2.2
1.4	2.3
1.6	2.4
1.6	6.4
1.7	19.0
1.2	23.6

Do these data support the hypothesis that there is a difference in retinal permeability between people with normal retinas and ones with foveal abnormalities?

4-3 Atrial natriuretic factor (ANF) is a recently discovered hormone synthesized by the heart that affects sodium and water loss by the kidneys. Wladimiro Jimenez and his coworkers ("Atrial Natriuretic Factor: Reduced Cardiac Content in Cirrhotic Rats with Ascites," *Am. J. Physiol.* **250**:F749–F752, 1986) investigated its role as a possible cause of sodium-water retention in cirrhosis of the liver. To determine if ANF was decreased with cirrhosis, they measured the percent increase in sodium loss through the kidneys caused by giving equal amounts of a crude ANF extract to two different groups of rats. The first group received an extract from normal rats and the second group received an extract from rats with cirrhosis of the liver. The results are given below. What do these data indicate?

Percent change in sodium extraction

Control	Cirrhotic
760	80
1000	80
1370	80
1680	210
1970	210
2420	320
3260	500
5000	610
5400	760
7370	760
	890
	890
	1870
	1950

4-4 Rework Probs. 3-1 and 3-5 using the *t* test. What is the relationship between the value of *t* computed here and the value of *F* computed for these data in Chap. 3?

4-5 Problem 3-2 presented the data that White and Froeb collected on the lung function of nonsmokers working in smoke-free environments, nonsmokers working in smoky environments, and smokers of various intensity. Analysis of variance revealed that these data were inconsistent with the hypothesis that the lung function was the same in all these groups. Isolate the various subgroups with similar lung function. What does this result mean in terms of the original question they posed: Does chronic exposure to other people's smoke affect the health of healthy adult nonsmokers?

4-6 Problem 3-3 led to the conclusion that HDL concentration is not the same in inactive men, joggers, and marathon runners. Use Bonferroni t tests to compare each of these groups pairwise.

4-7 Use the data from Probs. 3-4 and 3-5 to determine what doses of marijuana seem to affect the ability of the lungs to inactivate bacteria. Does the presence or absence of THC seem to be a factor in how marijuana smoke affects the lungs' defenses against infection?

4-8 Use Bonferroni t tests to isolate which of the drugs discussed in Prob. 3-7 affected the amount of damaged heart muscle after the left anterior descending coronary artery was tied off.

4-9 Repeat Prob. 4-8 using the SNK test. Compare the results with those of Prob. 4-8 and explain any differences.

4-10 In Prob. 3-6 you determined there was a difference in burnout among nursing staffs of different patient care units. Isolate these differences and discuss them.

4-11 In a test of significance, the P value of the test statistic is .063. Are the data statistically significant at

   a both the $\alpha = .05$ and $\alpha = .01$ levels?

   b the $\alpha = .05$ level but not at the $\alpha = .01$ level?

   c the $\alpha = .01$ level but not at the $\alpha = .05$ level?

   d neither the $\alpha = .05$ nor the $\alpha = .01$ levels?

How to Analyze Rates
and Proportions

The statistical procedures developed in Chaps. 2 to 4 are appropriate for analyzing the results of experiments in which the variable of interest takes on a continuous range of values, such as blood pressure, urine production, or length of hospital stay. These, and similar variables, are measured on an *interval scale* because they are measured on a scale with constant intervals, e.g., millimeters of mercury, milliliters, or days. Much of the information physicians, nurses, and medical scientists use cannot be measured on interval scales. For example, an individual may be male or female, dead or alive, or Caucasian, Negro, Mexican American, or Asian. These variables are measured on a *nominal scale,* in which there is no arithmetic relationship between the different classifications. We now develop the statistical tools necessary to describe and analyze such information.*

*There is a third class of variables in which responses can be *ordered* without an arithmetic relationship between the different possible states. Ordinal scales often appear in clinical practice; Chaps. 8 and 10 develop statistical procedures to analyze variables measured on ordinal scales.

It is easy to describe things measured on a nominal scale; simply count the number of patients or experimental subjects with each condition and (perhaps) compute the corresponding percentages.

Let us continue our discussion of the use of halothane versus morphine in open-heart surgery.* We have already seen that these two anesthetic agents produce differences in blood pressure that are unlikely to be due to random-sampling effects. This finding is interesting, but the important clinical question is: Was there any difference in mortality? Of the patients anesthetized with halothane 8 of 61, or 13.1 percent, died compared with 10 of the 67 anesthetized with morphine (14.9 percent). This study showed that halothane was associated with a 2 percent lower mortality rate *in the 128 patients who were studied.* Is this difference due to a real clinical effect or simply to random variation?

To answer this and other questions about nominal data we must first invent a way to estimate the precision with which percentages based on limited samples approximate the true rates that would be observed if we could examine the entire population, in this case *all* people who will be anesthetized for open-heart surgery. We will use these estimates to construct statistical procedures to test hypotheses.

BACK TO MARS

Before we can quantify the certainty of our descriptions of a population on the basis of a limited sample, we need to know how to describe the population itself. Since we have already visited Mars and met all 200 Martians (in Chap. 2), we will continue to use them to develop ways to describe populations. In addition to measuring the Martians' heights, we noted that 50 of them were left-footed and the remaining 150 were right-footed. Figure 5-1 shows the entire population of Mars divided according to footedness. The first way in which we can describe this population is by giving the *proportion p* of Martians who are in each class. In this case $p_{\text{left}} = {}^{50}\!/_{200} = .25$ and $p_{\text{rt}} = {}^{150}\!/_{250} = .75$. Since there are only two possible classes, notice that $p_{\text{rt}} = 1 - p_{\text{left}}$. Thus, whenever there are only two possible classes and they are mutually exclusive, we can completely describe the division in the population

---

*When this study was discussed in Chap. 4, we assumed the same number of patients in each treatment group to simplify the computation. In this chapter we use the actual number of patients in the study.

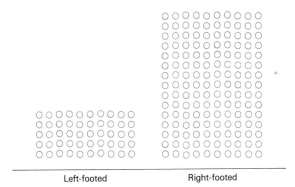

Left-footed   Right-footed

Figure 5-1 Of the 200 Martians 50 are left-footed, and the remaining 150 are right-footed. Therefore, if we select one Martian at random from this population, there is a $p_{left} = {}^{50}/_{200} = .25 = 25$ percent chance it will be left-footed.

with the single parameter p, the proportion of members with one of the attributes. The proportion of the population with the other attribute is *always* $1 - p$.

Note that p also is the *probability* of drawing a left-footed Martian if one selects one member of the population at random.

Thus p plays a role exactly analogous to that played by the population mean μ in Chap. 2. To see why, suppose we associate the value $X = 1$ with each left-footed Martian and a value of $X = 0$ with each right-footed Martian. The mean value of X for the population is

$$\mu = \frac{\Sigma X}{N} = \frac{1 + 1 + \cdots + 1 + 0 + 0 + \cdots + 0}{200} = \frac{50(1) + 150(0)}{200} = \frac{50}{200} = .25$$

which is p_{left}.

This idea can be generalized quite easily using a few equations. Suppose M members of a population of N individuals have some attribute and the remaining $N - M$ members of the population do not. Associate a value of $X = 1$ with the population members having the attribute and a value of $X = 0$ with the others. The mean of the resulting collection of numbers is

$$\mu = \frac{\Sigma X}{N} = \frac{M(1) + (N - M)(0)}{N} = \frac{M}{N} = p$$

the proportion of the population having the attribute.

Since we can compute a mean in this manner, why not compute a standard deviation in order to describe variability in the population? Even though there are only two possibilities, $X = 1$, and $X = 0$, the amount of variability will differ, depending on the value of p. Figure 5-2 shows three more populations of 200 individuals each. In Fig. 5-2*A* only 10 of the individuals are left-footed; it exhibits less variability than the population shown in Fig. 5-1. Figure 5-2*B* shows the extreme case in which half the members of the population fall into each of the two classes; the variability is greatest. Figure 5-2*C* shows the other extreme; all the members fall into one of the two classes, and there is no variability at all.

To quantify this subjective impression, we compute the standard deviation of the 1s and 0s associated with each member of the population when we computed the mean. By definition, the population standard deviation is

$$\sigma = \sqrt{\frac{\Sigma(X - \mu)^2}{N}}$$

$X = 1$ for M members of the population and 0 for the remaining $N - M$ members, and $\mu = p$; therefore

$$\sigma = \sqrt{\frac{(1-p)^2 + (1-p)^2 + \cdots + (1-p)^2 + (0-p)^2 + (0-p)^2 + \cdots + (0-p)^2}{N}}$$

$$= \sqrt{\frac{M(1-p)^2 + (N-M)p^2}{N}} = \sqrt{\frac{M}{N}(1-p)^2 + \left(1 - \frac{M}{N}\right)p^2}$$

Figure 5-2   This figure illustrates three different populations, each containing 200 members but with different proportions of left-footed members. The standard deviation, $\sigma = \sqrt{p(1-p)}$ quantifies the variability in the population. (*A*) When most of the members fall in one class, σ is a small value, 0.2, indicating relatively little variability. (*B*) In contrast, if half the members fall into each class, σ reaches its maximum value of .5, indicating the maximum possible variability. (*C*) At the other extreme, if all members fall into the same class, there is no variability at all and $\sigma = 0$.

p = 0.05
σ = 0.2

A

p = 0.50
σ = 0.50

B

p = 0
σ = 0

C

Left-footed   Right-footed

But since $M/N = p$ is the proportion of population members with the attribute,

$$\sigma = \sqrt{p(1-p)^2 + (1-p)p^2} = \sqrt{[p(1-p)+p^2](1-p)}$$

which simplifies to

$$\sigma = \sqrt{p(1-p)}$$

This equation for the population standard deviation produces quantitative results that agree with the qualitative impressions we developed from Figs. 5-1 and 5-2. As Fig. 5-3 shows, $\sigma = 0$ when $p = 0$ or $p = 1$, that is, when all members of the population either do or do not have the attribute, and σ is maximized when $p = .5$, that is, when any given member of the population is as likely to have the attribute as not.

Since σ depends only on p, it really does not contain any additional information (in contrast to the mean and standard deviation of a normally distributed variable, where μ and σ provide two independent pieces of information). It will be most useful in computing a standard error associated with estimates of p based on samples drawn at random from populations like those shown in Figs. 5-1 or 5-2.

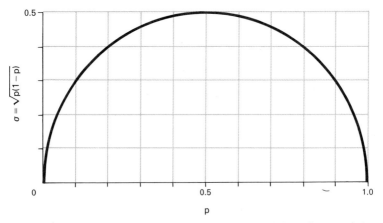

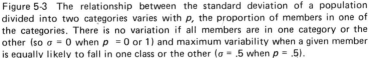

Figure 5-3 The relationship between the standard deviation of a population divided into two categories varies with p, the proportion of members in one of the categories. There is no variation if all members are in one category or the other (so $\sigma = 0$ when $p = 0$ or 1) and maximum variability when a given member is equally likely to fall in one class or the other ($\sigma = .5$ when $p = .5$).

ESTIMATING PROPORTIONS FROM SAMPLES

Of course, if we could observe all members of a population, there would not be any statistical question. In fact, all we ever see is a limited, hopefully representative, sample drawn from that population. How accurately does the proportion of members of a sample with an attribute reflect the proportion of individuals in the population with that attribute? To answer this question, we do a sampling experiment, just as we did in Chap. 2 when we asked how well the sample mean estimated the population mean.

Suppose we select 10 Martians at random from the entire population of 200 Martians. Figure 5-4 (top) shows which Martians were drawn; Fig. 5-4 (bottom) shows all the information the investigators who drew the sample would have. Half the Martians in the sample are left-footed and half are right-footed. Given only this information, one would probably report that the proportion of left-footed Martians is .5 or 50 percent.

Of course, there is nothing special about this sample, and one of

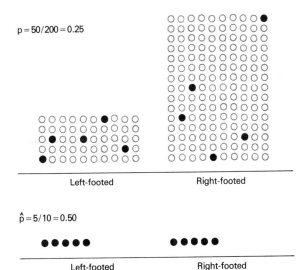

Figure 5-4 The top panel shows one random sample of 10 Martians selected from the population in Fig. 5-1; the bottom panel shows what the investigator would see. Since this sample included 5 left-footed Martians and 5 right-footed Martians, the investigator would estimate the proportion of left-footed Martians to be $\hat{p}_{\text{left}} = \frac{5}{10} = .5$, where the circumflex denotes an estimate.

the four other random samples shown in Fig. 5-5 could just as well have been drawn, in which case the investigator would have reported that the proportion of left-footed Martians was 30, 30, 10, or 20 percent, depending on which random sample happened to be drawn. In each case we have computed an estimate of the population proportion p based on a sample. Denote this estimate $\hat{p}$. Like the sample mean, the possible values of $\hat{p}$ depend on both the nature of the underlying population and the specific sample that is drawn. Figure 5-6 shows the five values of $\hat{p}$ computed from the specific samples in Figs. 5-4 and 5-5 together with the results of drawing another 20 random samples of 10

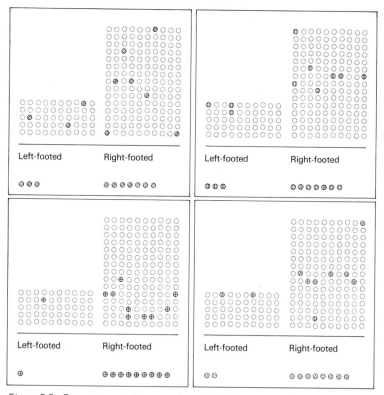

Figure 5-5 Four more random samples of 10 Martians each, together with the sample as it would appear to the investigator. Depending which sample happened to be drawn, the investigator would estimate the proportion of left-footed Martians to be 30, 30, 10, or 20 percent.

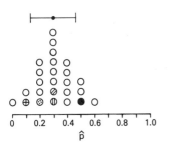

Figure 5-6 There will be a distribution of estimates of the proportion of left-footed Martians $\hat{p}_{\text{left}}$ depending on which random sample the investigator happens to draw. This figure shows the 5 specific random samples drawn in Figs. 5-4 and 5-5 together with 20 more random samples of 10 Martians each. The mean of the 25 estimates of p and the standard deviation of these estimates are also shown. The standard deviation of this distribution is the standard error of the estimate of the proportion $\sigma_{\hat{p}}$; it quantifies the precision with which $\hat{p}$ estimates p.

Martians each. Now we change our focus from the population of Martians to the population of all values of $\hat{p}$ computed from random samples of 10 Martians each. There are more than 10^{16} such samples with their corresponding estimates $\hat{p}$ of the value of p for the population of Martians.

The mean estimate of p for the 25 samples of 10 Martians each shown in Fig. 5-6 is 30 percent, which is remarkably close to the true proportion of left-footed Martians in the population (25 percent or .25). There is some variation in the estimates. To quantify the variability in the possible values of $\hat{p}$, we compute the *standard deviation* of values of $\hat{p}$ computed from random samples of 10 Martians each. In this case, it is about 14 percent or .14. This number describes the variability in the population of all possible values of the proportion of left-footed Martians computed from random samples of 10 Martians each.

Does this sound familiar? It should. It is just like the standard error of the mean. Therefore, we define the *standard error of the estimate of a proportion* to be the standard deviation of the population of all possible values of the proportion computed from samples of a given size. Just as with the standard error of the mean

$$\sigma_{\hat{p}} = \frac{\sigma}{\sqrt{n}}$$

in which $\sigma_{\hat{p}}$ is the standard error of the proportion, σ is the standard deviation of the population from which the sample was drawn, and n is the sample size. Since $\sigma = \sqrt{p(1-p)}$,

$$\sigma_{\hat{p}} = \sqrt{\frac{p(1-p)}{n}}$$

We estimate the true standard error by replacing the true value of p in this equation with our estimate $\hat{p}$ obtained from the random sample. Thus,

$$s_{\hat{p}} = \sqrt{\frac{\hat{p}(1-\hat{p})}{n}}$$

The standard error is a very useful way to describe the uncertainty in the estimate of the proportion of a population with a given attribute because the central-limit theorem (Chap. 2) also leads to the conclusion that the distribution of $\hat{p}$ is approximately normal, with mean p and standard deviation $\sigma_{\hat{p}}$ for large enough sample sizes. On the other hand, this approximation fails for values of p near 0 or 1 or when the sample size n is small. When can you use the normal distribution? Statisticians have shown that it is adequate when $n\hat{p}$ and $n(1-\hat{p})$ both exceed about 5.* Recall that about 95 percent of all members of a normally distributed population fall within 2 standard deviations of the mean. When the distribution of $\hat{p}$ approximates the normal distribution, we can assert, with about 95 percent confidence, that the true proportion of population members with the attribute of interest p lies within $2s_{\hat{p}}$ of $\hat{p}$.

These results provide a framework within which to consider the question we posed earlier in the chapter regarding the mortality rates associated with halothane and morphine anesthesia; 13.1 percent of 61 patients anesthetized with halothane and 14.9 percent of 67 patients anesthetized with morphine died following open-heart surgery. The standard errors of the estimates of these percentages are

$$s_{\hat{p}_{hlo}} = \sqrt{\frac{.131(1-.131)}{61}} = .043 = 4.3\%$$

---

*When the sample size is too small to use the normal approximation, you need to solve the problem exactly using the binomial distribution. For a discussion of the binomial distribution, see J. H. Zar, *Biostatistical Analysis,* Prentice-Hall, Englewood Cliffs, N.J., 1974, chap. 20, "The Binomial Distribution."

for halothane and

$$s_{\hat{p}_{\text{mor}}} = \sqrt{\frac{.149(1 - .149)}{67}} = .044 = 4.4\%$$

for morphine. Given that there was only a 2 percent difference in the observed mortality rate, it does not seem likely that the difference in observed mortality rate is due to anything beyond random sampling.

Before moving on, we should pause to list explicitly the assumptions that underlie this approach. We have been analyzing what statisticians call *independent Bernoulli trials,* in which

- *Each individual trial has two mutually exclusive outcomes.*
- *The probability p of a given outcome remains constant.*
- *All the trials are independent.*

In terms of a population, we can phrase these assumptions as follows:

- *Each member of the population belongs to one of two classes.*
- *The proportion of members of the population in one of the classes p remains constant.*
- *Each member of the sample is selected independently of all other members.*

HYPOTHESIS TESTS FOR PROPORTIONS

In Chap. 4 the sample mean and standard error of the mean provided the basis for constructing the t test to quantify how compatible observations were with the null hypothesis. We defined the t statistic as

$$t = \frac{\text{difference of sample means}}{\text{standard error of difference of sample means}}$$

The role of $\hat{p}$ is analogous to that of the sample mean in Chaps. 2 and 4, and we have also derived an expression for the standard error of $\hat{p}$. We now use the observed proportion of individuals with a given attribute and its standard error to construct a test statistic analogous to t to test the hypothesis that the two samples were drawn from populations containing the same proportion of individuals with a given attribute.

The test statistic analogous to t is

$$z = \frac{\text{difference of sample proportions}}{\text{standard error of difference of sample proportions}}$$

Let $\hat{p}_1$ and $\hat{p}_2$ be the observed proportions of individuals with the attribute of interest in the two samples. The standard error is the standard deviation of the population of all possible values of $\hat{p}$ associated with samples of a given size, and since variances of differences add, the standard error of the difference in proportions is

$$s_{\hat{p}_1 - \hat{p}_2} = \sqrt{s_{\hat{p}_1}^2 + s_{\hat{p}_2}^2}$$

Therefore

$$z = \frac{\hat{p}_1 - \hat{p}_2}{s_{\hat{p}_1 - \hat{p}_2}} = \frac{\hat{p}_1 - \hat{p}_2}{\sqrt{s_{\hat{p}_1}^2 + s_{\hat{p}_1}^2}}$$

If n_1 and n_2 are the sizes of the two samples,

$$s_{\hat{p}_1} = \sqrt{\frac{\hat{p}_1(1 - \hat{p}_1)}{n_1}} \quad \text{and} \quad s_{\hat{p}_2} = \sqrt{\frac{\hat{p}_2(1 - \hat{p}_2)}{n_2}}$$

then

$$z = \frac{\hat{p}_1 - \hat{p}_2}{\sqrt{[\hat{p}_1(1 - \hat{p}_1)/n_1] + [\hat{p}_2(1 - \hat{p}_2)/n_2]}}$$

is our test statistic.

z replaces t because this ratio is approximately normally distributed for large enough sample sizes,* and it is customary to denote a normally distributed variable with the letter z.

Just as it was possible to improve the sensitivity of the t test by

---

*The criterion for a large sample is the same as in the last section, namely that $n\hat{p}$ and $n(1 - \hat{p})$ both exceed about 5 for both samples. When this is not the case, one should use the *Fisher exact test*. For a discussion of it see ibid.

pooling the observations in the two sample groups to estimate the population variance, it is possible to increase the sensitivity of the z test for proportions by pooling the information from the two samples to obtain a single estimate of the population standard deviation $s_{\hat{p}}$. Specifically, if the hypothesis that the two samples were drawn from the same population is true, $\hat{p}_1 = m_1/n_1$ and $\hat{p}_2 = m_2/n_2$, in which m_1 and m_2 are the number of individuals in each sample with the attribute of interest, are both estimates of the same population proportion p. In this case, we could consider all the individuals drawn as a single sample of size $n_1 + n_2$ containing a total of $m_1 + m_2$ individuals with the attribute and use this single pooled sample to estimate p:

$$\hat{p} = \frac{m_1 + m_2}{n_1 + n_2}$$

in which case

$$s_{\hat{p}} = \sqrt{\hat{p}(1 - \hat{p})}$$

and we can estimate

$$s_{\hat{p}_1 - \hat{p}_2} = \sqrt{\frac{s_{\hat{p}}^2}{n_1} + \frac{s_{\hat{p}}^2}{n_2}} = \sqrt{\hat{p}(1 - \hat{p})\left(\frac{1}{n_1} + \frac{1}{n_2}\right)}$$

Therefore, our test statistic, based on a pooled estimate of the uncertainty in the population proportion, is

$$z = \frac{\hat{p}_1 - \hat{p}_2}{\sqrt{\hat{p}(1 - \hat{p})(1/n_1 + 1/n_2)}}$$

Like the t statistic, z will have a range of possible values depending on which random samples happen to be drawn to compute $\hat{p}_1$ and $\hat{p}_2$, even if both samples were drawn from the same population. If z is sufficiently "big," however, we will conclude that the data are inconsistent with this hypothesis and assert that there is a difference in the proportions. This argument is exactly analogous to that used to define the critical values of the t for rejecting the hypothesis of no difference. The only change is that in this case we use the standard normal distribution (Fig. 2-5) to define the cutoff values. In fact, the standard normal distribution and the t distribution with an infinite number of degrees of freedom are identical, so we can get the critical values for 5 or 1 percent confidence levels from Table 4-1. This table shows that there is less than a 5 percent chance of z being beyond -1.96 or $+1.96$ and less than a 1 percent chance of z being beyond -2.58 or $+2.58$ when, in fact, the two samples were drawn from the same population.

The Yates Correction for Continuity

The standard normal distribution only approximates the actual distribution of the z test statistic in a way that yields P values that are always smaller than they should be. Thus the results are biased toward concluding that the treatment had an effect when the evidence does not support such a conclusion. The mathematical reason for this problem has to do with the fact that the z test statistic can only take on discrete values, whereas the theoretical standard normal distribution is continuous. To obtain values of the z test statistic which are more compatible with the theoretical standard normal distribution, statisticians have introduced the *Yates correction* (or *continuity correction*), in which the expression for z is modified to become

$$z = \frac{|\hat{p}_1 - \hat{p}_2| - \frac{1}{2}(1/n_1 + 1/n_2)}{\sqrt{\hat{p}(1 - \hat{p})(1/n_1 + 1/n_2)}}$$

This adjustment slightly reduces the value of z associated with the data and compensates for the mathematical problem just described.

Mortality Associated with Anesthesia for Open-Heart Surgery with Halothane or Morphine

We can now formally test the hypothesis that halothane and morphine are associated with the same mortality rate when used as anesthetic agents in open-heart surgery. Recall that the logic of the experiment was that halothane depressed cardiac function whereas morphine did not, so in patients with cardiac problems it ought to be better to use morphine anesthesia. Indeed, Chaps. 3 and 4 showed that halothane produces lower mean arterial blood pressures during the operation than morphine; so the supposed physiological effect is present.

Nevertheless, the important question is: Does either anesthetic agent lead to a detectable improvement in mortality associated with this operation in the period immediately following the operation? Since 8 of the 61 patients anesthetized with halothane (13.1 percent) and 10 of the 67 patients anesthetized with morphine (14.9 percent) died, $n\hat{p}$ for the two samples is $.131(61) = 8$ and $.149(67) = 10$. Since both exceed 5, we can use the test described in the last section.*

The proportion of *all* patients, regardless of anesthesia, who died is

$$\hat{p} = \frac{8 + 10}{61 + 67} = .141$$

Our test statistic is therefore

$$z = \frac{|\hat{p}_{\text{hlo}} - \hat{p}_{\text{mor}}| - \frac{1}{2}(1/n_{\text{hlo}} + 1/n_{\text{mor}})}{\sqrt{\hat{p}(1 - \hat{p})(1/n_{\text{hlo}} + 1/n_{\text{mor}})}}$$

$$= \frac{|.131 - .149| - \frac{1}{2}(\frac{1}{61} + \frac{1}{67})}{\sqrt{(.141)(1 - .141)(\frac{1}{61} + \frac{1}{67})}} = .04$$

which is quite small. Specifically, it comes nowhere near 1.96, the z value that defines the most extreme 5 percent of all possible values of z when the two samples were drawn from the same population. Hence, we do not have evidence that there is any difference in the mortality associated with these two anesthetic agents, despite the fact that they do seem to have different physiological effects on the patient during surgery.

This study illustrates the importance of looking at *outcomes* in clinical trials. The human body has tremendous capacity to adapt not only to trauma but also to medical manipulation. Therefore, simply showing that some intervention (like a difference in anesthesia) changed a patient's physiological state (by producing different blood pressure) does not mean that in the long run it will make any difference in the clinical outcome. Focusing on these intermediate variables, often called *process variables,* rather than the more important outcome variables may lead you to think something made a clinical difference when it did not. For example, in this study there was the expected change in the process variable, i.e., blood pressure, but not the outcome variable, i.e., mortality. If we had stopped with the process variables, we

---

*$n(1 - \hat{p})$ also exceeds 5 in both cases. We did not need to check this because $\hat{p} < .5$, so $n\hat{p} < n(1 - \hat{p})$.

might have concluded that morphine anesthesia was superior to halo-thane in patients with cardiac problems, even though the choice of anesthesia does not appear to have affected the most important vari-able, whether or not the patient survived.

Keep this distinction in mind when reading medical journals and listening to proponents argue for their tests, procedures, and thera-pies. It is much easier to show that something affects process variables than the more important outcome variables. In addition to being easier to produce a demonstrable change in process variables than outcome variables, process variables are generally easier to measure. Observing outcomes may require following the patients for some time and often present difficult subjective problems of measurement, especially when one tries to measure "quality of life" variables. Nevertheless, when assessing whether or not some new procedure deserves to be adopted in an era of limited medical resources, you should seek evidence that something affects the patient's outcome. The patient and the patient's family care about outcome, not process.

Prevention of Thrombosis in People Receiving Hemodialysis

People with chronic kidney disease can be kept alive by dialysis; their blood is passed through a machine that does the work of their kidneys and removes metabolic products and other chemicals from their blood. The dialysis machine must be connected to one of the patient's arteries and veins to allow the blood to pass through the machine. Since pa-tients must be connected to the dialysis machine on a regular basis, it is necessary to create surgically a more or less permanent connection that can be used to attach the person's body to the machine. One way of doing this is to attach a small Teflon tube containing a coupling fitting, called a *shunt,* between an artery and vein in the wrist or arm. When the patient is to be connected to the dialysis machine, the tubing is connected to these fittings on the Teflon tube; otherwise, the two fittings are simply connected together so that the blood just flows directly from the small artery to the vein. For a variety of reasons, including the surgical technique used to place the shunt, disease of the artery or vein, local infection, or a reaction to the Teflon adapter, blood clots (thromboses) tend to form in these shunts. These clots have to be removed regularly to permit dialysis and can be severe enough to require tying off the shunt and creating a new one. The clots can spread down the artery or vein, making it necessary to pass a catheter into the artery or vein to remove the clot. In addition, these clots may break loose and lodge elsewhere in the body, where they may cause problems. Harter and his colleagues* knew that aspirin tends to inhibit blood clotting and wondered whether thrombosis could be reduced in people who were receiving chronic dialysis by giving them a low dose of aspirin (160 mg, one-half a common aspirin tablet) every day to inhibit the blood's tendency to clot.

They completed a randomized clinical trial in which all people being dialyzed at their institution who agreed to participate in the study and who had no reason for not taking aspirin (like an allergy) were randomly assigned to a group that received either a placebo or aspirin. To avoid bias on either the investigators' or patients' parts, the study was *double-blind.* Neither the physician administering the drug nor the patient receiving it knew whether the tablet was placebo or aspirin. This procedure adjusts for the placebo effect in the patients and prevents the investigators from looking harder for clots in one group or the other. The double-blind randomized clinical trial is the best way to test a new therapy.

They continued the study until 24 patients developed thrombi, because they assumed that with a total of 24 patients with thrombi any differences between the placebo and aspirin-treated groups would be detectable. Once they reached this point, they broke the code on the bottles of the pills and analyzed their results: 19 people had received aspirin and 25 people had received placebo. There did not seem to be any clinically important difference in these two groups in terms of age distribution, sex, time on dialysis at entry into the study, or other variables.

Of the 19 people receiving aspirin, 6 developed thrombi; of the 25 people receiving placebo 18 developed thrombi. Is this difference beyond what we would expect if aspirin had no effect and acted like a placebo, so the two groups of patients could be considered as having been drawn from the same population in which a constant proportion p of patients were destined to develop thrombi?

*H. R. Harter, J. W. Burch, P. W. Majerus, N. Stanford, J. A. Delmez, C. B. Anderson, and C. A. Weerts, "Prevention of Thrombosis in Patients on Hemodialysis by Low-Dose Aspirin," *N. Engl. J. Med.,* **301**:577–579, 1979.

We first estimate p for the two groups:

$$\hat{p}_{asp} = {}^{6}/_{19} = .32$$

for the people who received aspirin and

$$\hat{p}_{pla} = {}^{18}/_{25} = .72$$

for the people who received placebo.

Next, we make sure that $n\hat{p}$ and $n(1 - \hat{p})$ are greater than about 5 for both groups, to be certain that the sample sizes are large enough for the normal distribution to reasonably approximate the distribution of our test statistic z if the hypothesis that aspirin had no effect is true. For the people who received aspirin

$$n_{asp}\hat{p}_{asp} = 6$$
$$n_{asp}(1 - \hat{p}_{asp}) = 13$$

and for the people who received placebo

$$n_{pla}\hat{p}_{pla} = 18$$
$$n_{pla}(1 - \hat{p}_{pla}) = 7$$

We can use the methods we have developed.

The proportion of all patients who developed thromboses was

$$\hat{p} = \frac{6 + 18}{19 + 25} = .55$$

and so

$$s_{\hat{p}_{asp} - \hat{p}_{pla}} = \sqrt{\hat{p}(1 - \hat{p})\left(\frac{1}{n_{asp}} + \frac{1}{n_{pla}}\right)} = \sqrt{.55(1 - .55)\left(\frac{1}{19} + \frac{1}{25}\right)} = .15$$

Finally, we compute z according to

$$z = \frac{|\hat{p}_{asp} - \hat{p}_{pla}| - \frac{1}{2}(\frac{1}{19} + \frac{1}{25})}{s_{\hat{p}_{asp} - \hat{p}_{pla}}} = \frac{|.32 - .72| - .05}{-.15} = 2.33$$

Table 4-1 indicates that z will exceed 2.3263 in magnitude less than 2 percent of the time if the two samples are drawn from the same population. Since the value of z associated with our experiment is more extreme than 2.3263, it is very unlikely that the two samples were drawn from a single population. Therefore, we conclude that they were not, with $P < .02$.* In other words, we will conclude that giving patients low doses of aspirin while they are receiving chronic kidney dialysis decreases the likelihood that they will develop thrombosis in the shunt used to connect them to the dialysis machine.

ANOTHER APPROACH TO TESTING NOMINAL DATA: ANALYSIS OF CONTINGENCY TABLES

The methods we just developed based on the z statistic are perfectly adequate for testing hypotheses when there are only two possible attributes or outcomes of interest. The z statistic plays a role analogous to the t test for data measured on an interval scale. There are many situations, however, where there are more than two samples to be compared or more than two possible outcomes. To do this, we need to develop a testing procedure, analogous to analysis of variance, that is more flexible than the z test just described. While the following approach may seem quite different from the one we just used to design the z test for proportions, it is essentially the same.

To keep things simple, we begin with the problem we just solved, assessing the efficacy of low-dose aspirin in preventing thrombosis. In the last section we analyzed the *proportion* of people in each of the two treatment groups (aspirin and placebo) who developed thromboses.

---

*The value of z associated with these data, 2.33, is so close to the critical value of 2.3263 associated with p less than .02 that it would be prudent to report $p < .05$ (corresponding to a critical value of 1.960) because the mathematical models that are used to compute the table of critical values are only approximations of reality.

Now we change our emphasis slightly and analyze the *number* of people in each group who developed thrombi. Since the procedure we will develop does not require assuming anything about the nature or parameters of the population from which the samples were drawn, it is called a *nonparametric* method.

Table 5-1 shows the results of placebo and aspirin in the experiment, with the number of people in each treatment group who did and did not develop thromboses. This table is called a *2 × 2 contingency table.* Most of the patients in the study fell along the diagonal in this table, suggesting an association between the presence of thrombi and the absence of aspirin treatment. Table 5-2 shows what the experimental results might have looked like *if the aspirin had no effect on thrombus formation.* It also shows the total number of patients who received each treatment as well as the total number who did and did not develop thrombi. These numbers are obtained by summing the rows and col-

Table 5-1 Thrombus Formation in People Receiving Dialysis and Treated with Placebo or Aspirin

Sample group	Number of patients	
	Developed thrombi	Free of thrombi
Placebo	18	7
Aspirin	6	13

Source: H. R. Harter, J. W. Burch, P. W. Majerus, N. Stanford, J. A. Delmez, C. B. Anderson, and C. A. Weerts, "Prevention of Thrombosis in Patients on Hemodialysis by Low-Dose Aspirin," *N. Engl. J. Med.,* **301:**577–579, 1979. Reprinted by permission of the *New England Journal of Medicine.*

Table 5-2 Expected Thrombus Formation If Aspirin Had No Effect

Sample group	Number of patients		
	Developed thrombi	Free of thrombi	Treated
Placebo	13.64	11.36	25
Aspirin	10.36	8.64	19
Total	24	20	44

umns, respectively, in the table; these sums are the same as Table 5-1. More patients developed thrombi under each treatment; the differences in absolute numbers of patients are due to the fact that more patients received the placebo than aspirin. In contrast to Table 5-1, there does not seem to be a pattern relating treatment to thrombus formation.

To understand better why most people have this subjective impression, let us examine where the numbers in Table 5-2 came from. Of the 44 people in the study 25, or $^{25}/_{44}$ = 57 percent, received placebo and 19, or $^{19}/_{44}$ = 43 percent, received aspirin. Of the people in the study 24, or $^{24}/_{44}$ = 55 percent, developed thrombi and 20, or $^{20}/_{44}$ = 45 percent, did not. Now, let us hypothesize that the treatment did *not* affect the likelihood that someone would develop a thrombus. In this case, we would expect 55 percent of the 25 patients treated with placebo (13.64 patients) to develop thrombi and 55 percent of the 19 patients treated with aspirin (10.36 patients) to develop thrombi. The remaining patients should be free of thrombi. Note that we compute the expected frequencies to two decimal places (i.e., to the hundredth of a patient); this procedure is necessary to ensure accurate results in the computation of the χ^2 test below. Thus, Table 5-2 shows how we would *expect* the data to look if 25 patients were given placebo and 19 patients were given aspirin and 24 of them were destined to develop thrombi *regardless of how they were treated*. Compare Tables 5-1 and 5-2. Do they seem similar? Not really; the actual pattern of observations seems quite different from what we expected if the treatment had no effect.

The next step in designing a statistical procedure to test the hypothesis that the pattern of observations is due to random sampling rather than a treatment effect is to reduce this subjective impression to a single number, a test statistic, like F, t, or z, so that we can reject the hypothesis of no effect when this statistic is "big."

Before constructing this test statistic, however, let us return to another example, the relationship between type of anesthesia and mortality following open-heart surgery. Table 5-3 shows the results of our investigation, presented in the same format as Table 5-1. Table 5-4 presents what the table might look like if the type of anesthesia had no effect on mortality. Out of 128 people, 110, or $^{110}/_{128}$ = 86 percent, lived. If the type of anesthesia had no effect on mortality rate, 86 percent of the 61 people anesthetized with halothane (52.42 people) and 86 percent of the 67 people anesthetized with morphine (57.58 people)

Table 5-3 Mortality Associated with Open-Heart Surgery

Anesthesia	Lived	Died	Total no. of cases
Halothane	53	8	61
Morphine	57	10	67
Total	110	18	128

Table 5-4 Expected Mortality with Open-Heart Surgery If Anesthesia Did Not Matter

Anesthesia	Lived	Died	Total no. of cases
Halothane	52.42	8.58	61
Morphine	57.58	9.42	67
Total	110	18	128

would be expected to live, the rest dying in each case. Compare Tables 5-3 and 5-4; there is little difference between the expected and observed frequencies in each cell in the table. The observations are compatible with the assumption that there is no relationship between type of anesthesia and mortality.

The Chi-Square Test Statistic

Now we are ready to design our test statistic. It should describe, with a single number, how much the observed frequencies in each cell in the table differ from the frequencies we would expect if there is no relationship between the treatments and the outcomes that define the rows and columns of the table. In addition, it should allow for the fact that if we expect a large number of people to fall in a given cell, a difference of one person between the expected and observed frequencies is less important than in cases where we expect only a few people to fall in the cell.

We define the test statistic χ^2 (the square of the Greek letter chi) as

$$\chi^2 = \text{sum of } \frac{(\text{observed} - \text{expected number of individuals in cell})^2}{\text{expected number of individuals in cell}}$$

The sum is calculated by adding the results for all cells in the contingency table. The equivalent mathematical statement is

$$\chi^2 = \Sigma \frac{(O - E)^2}{E}$$

in which O is the observed number of individuals (frequency) in a given cell, E is the expected number of individuals (frequency) in that cell, and the sum is over all the cells in the contingency table. Note that if the observed frequencies are similar to the expected frequencies, χ^2 will be a small number and if the observed and expected frequencies differ, χ^2 will be a big number.

We can now use the information in Tables 5-1 and 5-2 to compute the χ^2 statistic associated with the data on the use of low-dose aspirin to prevent thrombosis in people undergoing chronic dialysis. Table 5-1 gives the observed frequencies, and Table 5-2 gives the expected frequencies. Thus,

$$\chi^2 = \Sigma \frac{(O - E)^2}{E} = \frac{(18 - 13.64)^2}{13.64} + \frac{(7 - 11.36)^2}{11.36}$$
$$+ \frac{(6 - 10.36)^2}{10.36} + \frac{(13 - 8.64)^2}{8.64} = 7.10$$

To begin getting a feeling for whether or not 7.10 is "big," let us compute χ^2 for the data on mortality associated with halothane and morphine anesthesia given in Table 5-3. Table 5-4 gives the expected frequencies, so

$$\chi^2 = \frac{(53 - 52.42)^2}{52.42} + \frac{(8 - 8.58)^2}{8.58} + \frac{(57 - 57.58)^2}{57.58} + \frac{(10 - 9.42)^2}{9.42}$$
$$= .09$$

which is pretty small, in agreement with our intuitive impression that the observed and expected frequencies were quite similar. (Of course, it is also in agreement with our earlier analysis of the same data using the z statistic in the last section.) In fact, it is possible to show that $\chi^2 = z^2$ when there are only two samples and two possible outcomes.

Like all test statistics, χ^2 can take on a range of values even when there is no relationship between the treatments and outcomes because of the effects of random sampling. Figure 5-7 shows the distribution of possible values for χ^2 computed from data in 2 × 2 contingency tables like those in Tables 5-1 or 5-3. It shows that when the hypothesis of no relationship between the rows and columns of the table is true, χ^2 would be expected to exceed 6.635 only 1 percent of the time. Because the observed value of χ^2, 7.10 exceeds this critical value of 6.635, we can conclude that the data in Table 5-1 are unlikely to occur when the hypothesis that aspirin and placebo have the same effect on thrombus formation is true. We report that aspirin is associated with lower rates of thrombus formation ($P < .01$).

In contrast, the data in Table 5-3 seem very compatible with the hypothesis that halothane and morphine produce the same mortality rates in patients being operated on for repair of heart valves.

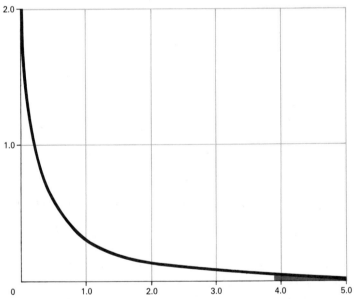

Figure 5-7 The chi-square distribution with 1 degree of freedom. The shaded area denotes the biggest 5 percent of possible values of the χ^2 test statistic when there is no relationship between the treatments and observations.

Of course, neither of these cases *proves* that aspirin did or did not have an effect, or that halothane and morphine did or did not produce the same mortality rates. What they show is that in one case the pattern of the observations is unlikely to arise if the aspirin acts like a placebo, whereas on the other hand the pattern of observations are very likely to arise if halothane and morphine produce similar mortality rates. Like all the other procedures we have been using to test hypotheses, however, when we reject the hypothesis of no association at the 5 percent level, we are implicitly willing to accept the fact that, in the long run, about 1 reported effect in 20 will be due to random variation rather than a real treatment effect.

As with all theoretical distributions of test statistics used for testing hypotheses, there·are assumptions built into the use of χ^2. For the resulting theoretical distribution to be reasonably accurate, *the expected number of individuals in all the cells must be at least 5.** (This is essentially the same as the restriction on the z test in the last section.)

Like most test statistics, the distribution of χ^2 depends on the number of treatments being compared. It also depends on the number of possible outcomes. This dependency is quantified in a *degrees of freedom* parameter ν equal to the number of rows in the table minus 1 times the number of columns in the table minus 1

$$\nu = (r - 1)(c - 1)$$

where r is the number of rows and c is the number of columns in the table. For the 2×2 tables we have been dealing with so far, $\nu = (2 - 1)(2 - 1) = 1$.

As with the z test statistic discussed earlier in this chapter, when analyzing 2×2 contingency tables ($\nu = 1$), the value of χ^2 computed using the formula above and the theoretical χ^2 distribution leads to P values that are smaller than they ought to be. Thus, the results are biased toward concluding that the treatment had an effect when the evidence does not support such a conclusion. The mathematical reason for this problem has to do with the fact that the theoretical χ^2 distribution is continuous whereas the set of all possible values that the χ^2 test statis-

---

*When the data do not meet this requirement, one should use the Fisher exact probability test.

tic can take on is not. To obtain values of the test statistic that are more compatible with the critical values computed from the theoretical χ^2 distribution when $\nu = 1$, apply the *Yates correction* (or *continuity correction*) to compute a corrected χ^2 test statistic according to

$$\chi^2 = \Sigma \frac{(|O - E| - \frac{1}{2})^2}{E}$$

This correction slightly reduces the value of χ^2 associated with the contingency table and compensates for the mathematical problem just described. The Yates correction is used only when $\nu = 1$, that is, for 2 × 2 tables.

To illustrate the use and effect of the continuity correction, let us recompute the value of χ^2 associated with the data on the use of low-dose aspirin to prevent thrombosis in people undergoing chronic dialysis. From the observed and expected frequencies in Tables 5-1 and 5-2, respectively,

$$\chi^2 = \frac{(|18 - 13.64| - \frac{1}{2})^2}{13.64} + \frac{(|7 - 11.36| - \frac{1}{2})^2}{11.36}$$

$$+ \frac{(|6 - 10.36| - \frac{1}{2})^2}{10.36} + \frac{(|13 - 8.64| - \frac{1}{2})^2}{8.64} = 5.57$$

Note that this value of χ^2, 5.57, is smaller than the uncorrected value of χ^2, 7.10, we obtained before. The corrected value of χ^2 no longer exceeds the critical value of 6.635 associated with the greatest 1 percent of possible χ^2 values (i.e., for $P < .01$). After applying the continuity correction, χ^2 now only exceeds 5.024, the critical value that defines the greatest 2.5 percent of possible values (i.e., for $P < .025$).

CHI-SQUARE APPLICATIONS TO EXPERIMENTS WITH MORE THAN TWO TREATMENTS OR OUTCOMES

It is easy to generalize what we have just done to analyze the results of experiments with more than two treatments or outcomes. The z test we developed earlier in this chapter will not work for such experiments.

Recall that in Chap. 3 we demonstrated that women who jog

regularly or engage in long-distance running have fewer menstrual periods on the average than women who do not participate in this sport.* Does this physiological change lead women to consult their physician about menstrual problems? Table 5-5 shows the results of a survey of the same women discussed in conjunction with Fig. 3-9. Are these data consistent with the hypothesis that running does not increase the likelihood that a woman will consult her physician for a menstrual problem?

Of the 165 women in the study 69, or $^{69}/_{165}$ = 42 percent, consulted their physicians for a menstrual problem, while the remaining 96, or $^{96}/_{165}$ = 58 percent, did not. If the extent of running did not affect the likelihood that a woman would consult her physician, we would expect 42 percent of the 54 controls (22.58 women) to have visited their physicians, 42 percent of the 23 joggers (9.62 women) to have consulted their physicians, and 42 percent of the 88 distance runners (36.80 women) to have consulted their physicians. Table 5-6 shows these expected frequencies, together with the expected frequencies of women who did not consult their physicians. Are the differences between the observed and expected frequencies "big?"

To answer this question, we compute the χ^2 statistic

$$\chi^2 = \frac{(14 - 22.58)^2}{22.58} + \frac{(40 - 31.42)^2}{31.42} + \frac{(9 - 9.62)^2}{9.62} + \frac{(14 - 13.38)^2}{13.38}$$

$$+ \frac{(46 - 36.80)^2}{36.80} + \frac{(42 - 51.20)^2}{51.20} = 9.63$$

The contingency table in Table 5-5 has three rows and two columns, so the χ^2 statistic has $\nu = (r - 1)(c - 1) = (3 - 1)(2 - 1) = 2$ degrees of freedom associated with it. Table 5-7 shows that χ^2 will exceed 9.21 less than 1 percent of the time when the difference between the observed and expected frequencies is due to random variation rather than an effect of the treatment (in this case, running). Thus, we conclude that there is a relationship between running and the chances that

---

*When this study was discussed in Chap. 3, we assumed the same number of patients in each treatment group to simplify the computation. In this chapter we use the actual number of patients in the study.

Table 5-5   Consult Physician for Menstrual Problem

Group	Yes	No	Total
Controls	14	40	54
Joggers	9	14	23
Runners	46	42	88
Total	69	96	165

Source: E. Dale, D. H. Gerlach, and A. L. Wilhite, "Menstrual Dysfunction in Distance Runners," *Obstet. Gynecol.,* **54**:47–53, 1979.

Table 5-6   Expected Frequencies of Physician Consultation If Running Did Not Matter

Group	Yes	No	Total
Controls	22.58	31.42	54
Joggers	9.62	13.38	23
Runners	36.80	51.20	88
Total	69	96	165

Table 5-7   Critical Values for the χ^2 Distribution

	Probability of greater value *P*							
ν	.50	.25	.10	.05	.025	.01	.005	.001
1	.455	1.323	2.706	3.841	5.024	6.635	7.879	10.828
2	1.386	2.773	4.605	5.991	7.378	9.210	10.597	13.816
3	2.366	4.108	6.251	7.815	9.348	11.345	12.838	16.266
4	3.357	5.385	7.779	9.488	11.143	13.277	14.860	18.467
5	4.351	6.626	9.236	11.070	12.833	15.086	16.750	20.515
6	5.348	7.841	10.645	12.592	14.449	16.812	18.548	22.458
7	6.346	9.037	12.017	14.067	16.013	18.475	20.278	24.322
8	7.344	10.219	13.362	15.507	17.535	20.090	21.955	26.124
9	8.343	11.389	14.684	16.919	19.023	21.666	23.589	27.877
10	9.342	12.549	15.987	18.307	20.483	23.209	25.188	29.588
11	10.341	13.701	17.275	19.675	21.920	24.725	26.757	31.264
12	11.340	14.845	18.549	21.026	23.337	26.217	28.300	32.909
13	12.340	15.984	19.812	22.362	24.736	27.688	29.819	34.528

Table 5-7 Critical Values for the χ^2 Distribution *(Continued)*

	Probability of greater value *P*							
v	.50	.25	.10	.05	.025	.01	.005	.001
14	13.339	17.117	21.064	23.685	26.119	29.141	31.319	36.123
15	14.339	18.245	22.307	24.996	27.488	30.578	32.801	37.697
16	15.338	19.369	23.542	26.296	28.845	32.000	34.267	39.252
17	16.338	20.489	24.769	27.587	30.191	33.409	35.718	40.790
18	17.338	21.605	25.989	28.869	31.526	34.805	37.156	42.312
19	18.338	22.718	27.204	30.144	32.852	36.191	38.582	43.820
20	19.337	23.828	28.412	31.410	34.170	37.566	39.997	45.315
21	20.337	24.935	29.615	32.671	35.479	38.932	41.401	46.797
22	21.337	26.039	30.813	33.924	36.781	40.289	42.796	48.268
23	22.337	27.141	32.007	35.172	38.076	41.638	44.181	49.728
24	23.337	28.241	33.196	36.415	39.364	42.980	45.559	51.179
25	24.337	29.339	34.382	37.652	40.646	44.314	46.928	52.620
26	25.336	30.435	35.563	38.885	41.923	45.642	48.290	54.052
27	26.336	31.528	36.741	40.113	43.195	46.963	49.645	55.476
28	27.336	32.020	37.916	41.337	44.461	48.278	50.993	56.892
29	28.336	33.711	39.087	42.557	45.722	49.588	52.336	58.301
30	29.336	34.800	40.256	43.773	46.979	50.892	53.672	59.703
31	30.336	35.887	41.422	44.985	48.232	52.191	55.003	61.098
32	31.336	36.973	42.585	46.194	49.480	53.486	56.328	62.487
33	32.336	38.058	43.745	47.400	50.725	54.776	57.648	63.870
34	33.336	39.141	44.903	48.602	51.966	56.061	58.964	65.247
35	34.336	40.223	46.059	49.802	53.203	57.342	60.275	66.619
36	35.336	41.304	47.212	50.998	54.437	58.619	61.581	67.985
37	36.336	42.383	48.363	52.192	55.668	59.893	62.883	69.346
38	37.335	43.462	49.513	53.384	56.896	61.162	64.181	70.703
39	38.335	44.539	50.660	54.572	58.120	62.428	65.476	72.055
40	39.335	45.616	51.805	55.758	59.342	63.691	66.766	73.402
41	40.335	46.692	52.949	56.942	60.561	64.950	68.053	74.745
42	41.335	47.766	54.090	58.124	61.777	66.206	69.336	76.084
43	42.335	48.840	55.230	59.304	62.990	67.459	70.616	77.419
44	43.335	49.913	56.369	60.481	64.201	68.710	71.893	78.750
45	44.335	50.985	57.505	61.656	65.410	69.957	73.166	80.077
46	45.335	52.056	58.641	62.830	66.617	71.201	74.437	81.400
47	46.335	53.127	59.774	64.001	67.821	72.443	75.704	82.720
48	47.335	54.196	60.907	65.171	69.023	73.683	76.969	84.037
49	48.335	55.265	62.038	66.339	70.222	74.919	78.231	85.351
50	49.335	56.334	63.167	67.505	71.420	76.154	79.490	86.661

Source: Adapted from J. H. Zar, *Biostatistical Analysis,* Prentice-Hall, Englewood Cliffs, N.J., 1974, p. 408, table D.8. Used by permission.

a woman will consult her physician about a menstrual problem ($P <$ .01). Note, however, that we do not yet know which group or groups of women account for this difference.

Let us now sum up how to use the χ^2 statistic.

- *Tabulate the data in a contingency table.*
- *Sum the number of individuals in each row and each column and figure the percentage of all individuals who fall in each row and column, independent of the column or row in which they fall.*
- *Use these percentages to compute the number of people that would be expected in each cell of the table if the treatment had no effect.*
- *Summarize the differences between these expected frequencies and the observed frequencies by computing χ^2. If the data form a 2 X 2 table, include the Yates correction.*
- *Compute the number of degrees of freedom associated with the contingency table and use Table 5-7 to see whether the observed value of χ^2 exceeds what would be expected from random variation.*

Recall that when the data fell into a 2 X 2 contingency table, all the expected frequencies had to exceed about 5 for the χ^2 test to be accurate. In larger tables, most statisticians recommend that the expected number of individuals in each cell never be less than 1 and that no more than 20 percent of them be less than 5. When this is the case, the χ^2 test can be quite inaccurate. The problem can be remedied by collecting more data to increase the cell numbers or by reducing the number of categories to increase the numbers in each cell of the table.

Subdividing Contingency Tables

Our analysis of Table 5-6 revealed that there is probably a difference in the likelihood that the different groups of women will consult their physicians regarding a menstrual problem, but our analysis did not isolate *which* groups of women accounted for this effect. This situation is analogous to the multiple-comparison problem in analysis of variance. The analysis of variance will help decide whether *something* is different, but you need to go on to the multiple-comparison procedure to define *which group it was.* You can do the same thing with a contingency table.

Looking at the numbers in Table 5-5 suggests that joggers and runners are more likely to consult their physicians than women in the control group, but they seem similar to each other.

To test this latter hypothesis, we *subdivide* the contingency table to look only at the joggers and runners. Table 5-8 shows the data for the joggers and runners. The numbers in parentheses are the expected number of women in each cell. The observed and expected number of women in each cell appear quite similar; since it is a 2 × 2 contingency table, we compute χ^2 with the Yates correction

$$
\begin{aligned}
\chi^2 &= \Sigma \frac{(|O - E| - \frac{1}{2})^2}{E} \\
&= \frac{(|9 - 11.40| - \frac{1}{2})^2}{11.40} + \frac{(|14 - 11.60| - \frac{1}{2})^2}{11.60} \\
&\quad + \frac{(|46 - 43.60| - \frac{1}{2})^2}{43.60} + \frac{(|42 - 44.40| - \frac{1}{2})^2}{44.40} = .79
\end{aligned}
$$

which is small enough for us to conclude that the joggers and runners are equally likely to visit their physicians. Since they are so similar, we combine the two groups and compare this combined group with the control group. Table 5-9 shows the resulting 2 × 2 contingency table, together with the expected frequencies in parentheses. χ^2 for this contingency table is 7.39, which exceeds 6.63, the critical value that defines the upper 1 percent of probable values of χ^2 when there is no relationship between the rows and columns in a 2 × 2 table.

Note, however, that because we have done *two* tests on the same data, we must use the Bonferroni inequality to adjust the P values to

Table 5-8 Physician Consultation among Women Joggers and Runners[*]

Group	Yes	No	Total
Joggers	9 (11.40)	14 (11.60)	23
Runners	46 (43.60)	42 (44.40)	88
Total	55	56	111

[*]Numbers in parentheses are expected frequencies if the amount of running does not affect physician consultation.

Table 5-9 Physician Consultation among Women Who Did and Did Not Run*

Group	Yes	No	Total
Controls	14 (22.58)	40 (31.42)	54
Joggers and runners	55 (46.42)	56 (64.58)	111
Total	69	96	165

*Numbers in parentheses are expected frequencies of physician consultation if whether a woman ran or not did not affect the likelihood of her consulting a physician for a menstrual problem.

account for the fact that we are doing multiple tests. Since we did two tests, we multiply the nominal 1 percent P value obtained from Table 5-7 by 2 to obtain $2(1) = 2$ percent. Therefore, we conclude that the joggers and runners did not differ in their medical consultations from each other but did differ from the women in the control group $(P < .02)$.

We now have the tools to analyze data measured on a nominal scale as long as the sample sizes are large enough. So far we have been focusing on how to demonstrate a difference and quantify the certainty with which we can assert this difference or effect with the P value. Now we turn to the other side of the coin: What does it mean if the test statistic is *not* big enough to reject the hypothesis of no difference?

PROBLEMS

5-1 Because local dental anesthetic administration is often accompanied by patient anxiety and other adverse sequelae, Timothy Bishop ("High Frequency Neural Modulation in Dentistry," *J. Am. Dental Assoc.* **112**:176–177, 1986) studied the effectiveness of high-frequency neural modulation (similar to that used in physical therapy to control chronic pain) to prevent pain during a variety of dental procedures, including restorations and tooth extractions. People were given either the electrical stimulation or simply had the inactive device attached as though it were being used (a placebo control). Neither the dentist nor the patient knew whether or not the neural modulator was turned on. Do the following data suggest that high-frequency neural modulation is an effective analgesic? Use both χ^2 and z statistics.

	Treatment Received	
	Active	Placebo
Effective analgesia	24	3
Ineffective analgesia	6	17

5-2 In sudden infant death syndrome (SIDS) apparently normal infants die without warning while sleeping. SIDS is said to occur more commonly in infants who are premature, black, or in lower socioeconomic groups. In an effort to identify the characteristics of infants who will develop SIDS when they are born, Normal Lewak and his colleagues ("Sudden Infant Death Syndrome Risk Factors: Prospective Data Review," *Clin. Pediatr.*, **18**:404–411, 1979) collected data on 19,047 infants born at a health maintenance organization in Oakland, California, between 1960 and 1967. Using hospital, Department of Motor Vehicles, and vital statistics records, the investigators were able to follow all but 48 of the infants until they were 1 year old and past risk of SIDS. Table 5-10 summarizes some of their findings. Use these data to identify the characteristics of infants who develop SIDS. Are these factors specific enough to be of predictive value in a specific infant? Why or why not?

5-3 Discuss the potential problems, if any, associated with the 48 infants lost to follow-up in the study discussed in Prob. 5-2.

5-4 Recurrent urinary tract infections can be prevented by giving preventative (prophylactic) doses of antibiotics. R. Fennell and his colleagues ("Urinary Tract Infections in Children: Effect of Short Course Antibiotic Therapy on Recurrence Rate in Children with Previous Infections," *Clin. Pediatr.*, **19**:121–124, 1980) tested three different antibiotics in girls between 3 and 16 years old who had a history of recurrent urinary tract infections. They randomly assigned girls who met the study criteria to the three drugs, then monitored their urine for the presence of bacteria. They found:

Antibiotic	Infection recurred	Nonrecurrence
Ampicillin	20	7
Trimethoprim-sulfamethoxazole	24	19
Cephalexin	14	1

Table 5-10

Factor	No. in SIDS group*	No. not in SIDS group*
Mother's age:		
Below 25 years	29	7,301
Over 25 years	15	11,241
Time from end of last pregnancy to start of this one:		
Less than 1 year	23	4,694
More than 1 year	11	7,339
Pregnancy planned:		
No	23	7,654
Yes	5	4,253
Previous pregnancy(ies):		
Yes	36	12,987
No	8	4,999
Smoked during pregnancy:		
Yes	24	5,228
No	10	9,595
Prenatal visits:		
Under 11	31	10,512
11 or more	11	8,154
Lowest hemoglobin during pregnancy:		
Below 12 mg/dL	26	12,613
12 mg/dL or higher	7	2,678
Race:		
Caucasian	31	12,240
Negro	9	4,323
Other	4	2,153

*In some cases, the numbers do not add up to 44 or 18,716 because the relevant information was not available for all the infants and their parents.

Is there any evidence that these drugs produce different responses? If so, which one seems to work best?

5-5 Public health officials often investigate the source of widespread outbreaks of disease. Agnes O'Neil and her coworkers ("A Waterborn Epidemic of Acute Infectious Non-Bacterial Gastroenteritis in Alberta, Canada," *Can. J. Public Health* **76**:199–203, 1985) recently reported on an outbreak of gastroenteritis in a small Canadian town. They hypothesized that the source of contamination was the municipal water supply. They examined the association between amount of water consumed and the rate at which people got sick. What do these data suggest?

Water consumption, glasses per day	Number ill	Number not ill
Less than 1	39	121
1 to 4	265	258
5 or more	265	146

5-6 In general, the quality of a research project is higher and the applicability of data to a specific question is higher if the data are collected *after* the research is planned. Robert Fletcher and Suzanne Fletcher ("Clinical Research in General Medical Journals: A 30-Year Perspective," *N. Engl. J. Med.,* **301**:180–183, 1979, used by permission) studied 612 articles randomly selected from the *Journal of the American Medical Association, Lancet,* and *New England Journal of Medicine* to see whether the authors collected their data before or after planning the research. They found:

	1946	1956	1966	1976
No. of articles examined	151	149	157	155
Data collection, %:				
After research planned	76	71	49	44
Before research planned	24	29	51	56

Estimate the certainty with which these percentages estimate the true percentage of articles in which the data were collected before the research was planned. Have things changed over time? If so, when? Was the change (if any) for the better or the worse?

5-7 Narrowing of the carotid arteries, which carry blood through the neck to the head, can reduce flow to the brain and starve the brain of oxygen, a condition called cerebral ischemia. To study whether medical or surgical treatment of this problem produced better results, W. Fields and his colleagues ("Joint Study of Extracranial Arterial Occlusion, V: Progress Report of Prognosis Following Surgery or Nonsurgical Treatment for Transient Ischemic Attacks and Cervical Carotid Artery Lesions, *JAMA,* **211**:1993–2003, 1970, copyright 1970–1973, American Medical Association) compared the outcomes among patients available for follow-up who received surgical and medical therapy and found:

Therapy	Recurrent ischemia, stroke, or death, no. of patients	
	Yes	No
Surgical	43	36
Medical	53	19

Is there sufficient evidence to conclude that one treatment is better than the other?

5-8 David Sackett and Michael Gent ("Controversy in Counting and Attributing Events in Clinical Trials," *N. Engl. J. Med.*, **301**:1410–1412, 1979, used by permission) took note of two important points with regard to the study described in Prob. 5-5: (1) "available for follow-up" patients had to be discharged alive and free of stroke after their hospitalization; (2) this procedure excluded 15 surgically treated patients (5 who died and 10 who had strokes during or shortly after their operations) but only 1 medically treated patient. Including these 16 patients in the data from the previous problem yields the following result:

Therapy	Recurrent ischemia, stroke, or death, no. of patients	
	Yes	No
Surgical	58	36
Medical	54	19

Does including these patients change the conclusions of the trial? If so, should the trial be analyzed excluding them (as in Prob. 5-5) or including them (as in this problem)? Why?

5-9 The chance of contracting disease X is 10 percent, regardless of whether or not a given individual has disease A or disease B. Assume that you can diagnose all three diseases with perfect accuracy and that in the entire population 1000 people have disease A and 1000 have disease B. People with X, A, and B have different chances of being hospitalized. Specifically, 50 percent of the people with A, 20 percent of the people with B, and 40 percent of the people with X are hospitalized. Then:

- Out of the 1000 people with A 10 percent (100 people) also have X; 50 percent (50 people) are hospitalized because they have A. Of the remaining 50 (who also have X), 40 percent (20 people) are hospitalized because of X. Therefore, 70 people will be hospitalized with both A and X.
- Out of the 900 people with A but not X, 50 percent are hospitalized for disease A (450 people).
- Out of the 1000 with B 10 percent (100 people) also have X; 20 percent (20 people) are hospitalized because of B, and of the remaining 80, 40 percent (32 patients) are hospitalized because they have X. Thus, 52 people with B and X are in the hospital.
- Of the 900 with B but not X, 20 percent (180 people) are hospitalized because they have disease B.

A hospital-based investigator will encounter these patients in the hospital and observe the following relationship:

	Disease X	No disease X
Disease A	70	450
Disease B	52	180

Is there a statistically significant difference in the chances that an individual has X depending on whether or not he has A or B in the sample of patients the hospital-based investigator will encounter? Would the investigator reach the same conclusion if she could observe the entire population? If not, explain why. (This example is from D. Mainland, "The Risk of Fallacious Conclusions from Autopsy Data on the Incidence of Diseases with Applications to Heart Disease," *Am. Heart J.*, **45**:644–654, 1953.)

What Does
"Not Significant"
Really Mean?

Thus far, we have used statistical methods to reach conclusions by seeing how compatible the observations were with the hypothesis that the treatment had no effect (the null hypothesis). When the data were unlikely to occur if this hypothesis were true, we rejected it and concluded that the treatment had an effect. We used a test statistic (F, t, z, or χ^2) to quantify the difference between the actual observations and those we would expect if the hypothesis of no effect were true. We concluded that the treatment had an effect if the value of this test statistic was bigger than 95 percent of the values that would occur if the treatment had no effect. When this is so, it is common for medical investigators to report a *statistically significant* effect. On the other hand, when the test statistic is not big enough to reject the hypothesis of no treatment effect, these investigators often report *no statistically significant difference* and then discuss their results as if they had proved that the treatment had no effect. All they really did was fail to demonstrate that it did have an effect. The distinction between positively demonstrating that a treatment had no effect and failing to demonstrate that it does have an effect is subtle but very important, especially in the light of the small numbers of subjects included in most clinical studies.

As already mentioned in our discussion of the t test, the ability to detect a treatment effect with a given level of confidence depends on the size of the treatment effect, the variability within the population, and the size of the samples used in the study. Just as bigger samples make it more likely that you will be able to detect an effect, smaller sample sizes make it harder. In practical terms, this means that studies of therapies that involve only a few subjects and fail to reject the hypothesis of no treatment effect may arrive at this result because the statistical procedures lacked the *power* to detect the effect because of a too small sample size, even though the treatment did have an effect. Conversely, considerations of the power of a test permit you to compute the sample size needed to detect a treatment effect of a given size that you believe is present.

AN EFFECTIVE DIURETIC

Now, we make a radical departure from everything that has preceded: we assume that the treatment *does* have an effect.

Figure 6-1 shows the same population of people we studied in Fig. 4-4 except that this time the drug given to increase daily urine production works. It increases the average urine production for members of this population from 1200 to 1400 mL/day. Figure 6-1*A* shows the distribution of values of daily urine production for all 200 members of the population under control conditions, and Fig. 6-1*B* shows how much urine every member of the population on the diuretic would produce.

Of course, an investigator cannot observe all members of the population, so she selects two groups of 10 people at random, gives one group the diuretic and the other placebo, and measures their daily urine production. Figure 6-1*C* shows what she would see. The people receiving placebo produced an average of 1180 mL/day, and those receiving the drug produced an average of 1400 mL/day. The standard deviations of these two samples are 159 and 245 mL/day, respectively. The pooled estimate of the population variance is

$$s^2 = \tfrac{1}{2}(s_{\text{drug}}^2 + s_{\text{pla}}^2) = \tfrac{1}{2}(245^2 + 144^2) = 40{,}381 = 201^2$$

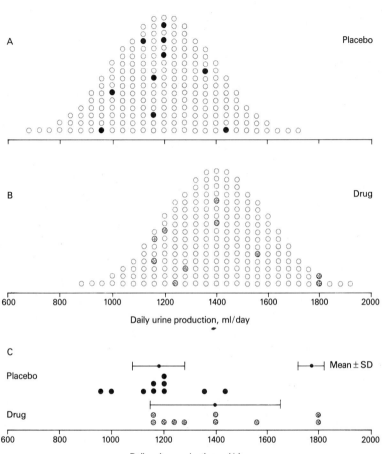

Figure 6-1   Daily urine production in a population of 200 people while they are taking a placebo and while they are taking an effective diuretic that increases urine production by 200 mL/day on the average. Panels *A* and *B* show the specific individuals selected at random for study. Panel *C* shows the results as they would appear to the investigator. *t* = 2.447 for these observations. Since the critical value of *t* for *P* < .05 with 2(10 − 1) = 18 degrees of freedom is 2.101, the investigator would probably report that the diuretic was effective.

The value of t associated with these observations is

$$t = \frac{\bar{X}_{dr} - \bar{X}_{pla}}{\sqrt{(s^2/n_{dr}) + (s^2/n_{pla})}} = \frac{1400 - 1180}{\sqrt{(201^2/10) + (201^2/10)}} = 2.447$$

which exceeds 2.101, the value that defines the most extreme 5 percent of possible values of the t statistic when the two samples are drawn from the same population. [There are $2(n - 1) = 18$ degrees of freedom.] The investigator would conclude that the observations are not consistent with the assumption that two samples came from the same population and report that the drug increased urine production. And she would be right.

Of course, there is nothing special about the two random samples of people selected for the experiment. Figure 6-2 shows two more groups of people selected at random to test the drug, together with the results as they would appear to the investigator. In this case, the mean urine production was 1216 mL/day for the people given the placebo and 1368 mL/day for the people taking the drug. The standard deviation of urine production in the two groups was 97 and 263 mL/day, respectively, so the pooled estimate of the variance is $\frac{1}{2}(97^2 + 263^2)$ $= 198^2$. The value of t associated with these observations is

$$t = \frac{1368 - 1216}{\sqrt{(198^2/10) + (198^2/10)}} = 1.71$$

which is less than 2.101. Had the investigator selected these two groups of people for testing, she would not have obtained a value of t large enough to reject the hypothesis that the drug had no effect; she would probably report "no significant difference." If she went on to conclude that the drug had no effect, she would be wrong.

Notice that this is a different type of error from that discussed in Chaps. 3 to 5. In the earlier chapters we were concerned with *rejecting* the hypothesis of no effect when it was true. Now we are concerned with *not rejecting it when it is not true.*

What are the chances of making this second kind of error?

Just as we could repeat this experiment more than 10^{27} times when the drug had no effect to obtain the distribution of possible values of t (compare the discussion of Fig. 4-5), we can do the same thing

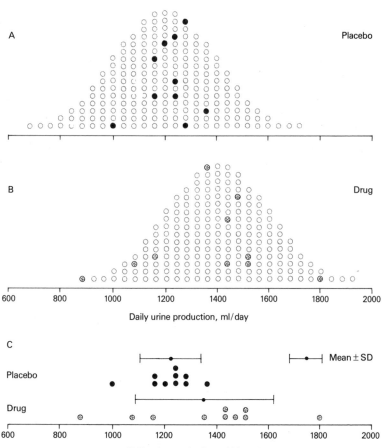

Figure 6-2 There is nothing special about the two random samples shown in Fig. 6-1. This illustration shows another random sample of two groups of 10 people each selected at random to test the diuretic and the results as they would appear to the investigator. The value of t associated with these observations is only 1.71, not great enough to reject the hypothesis of no drug effect with $P < .05$, that is, $\alpha = .05$. If the investigator reported the drug had no effect, she would be wrong.

when the drug does have an effect. Figure 6-3 shows the results of 200 such experiments; 111 out of the resulting values of t fall at or above 2.101, the value we are using to define a "big" t. Put another way, if we wish to keep the P value at or below 5 percent, there is a $^{111}/_{200} = 55$

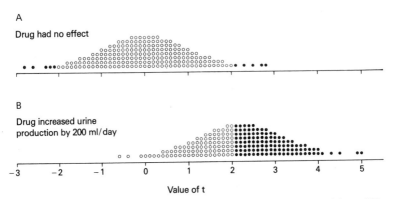

Figure 6-3 (A) The distribution of values of the *t* statistic computed from 200 experiments that consisted of drawing two samples of size 10 each from a single population; this is the distribution we would expect if the diuretic had no effect on urine production. (Compare with Fig. 4-5A.) (B) The distribution of *t* values from 200 experiments in which the drug increased average urine production by 200 mL/day. $t = 2.1$ defines the most extreme 5 percent of the possible values of *t* when the drug has no effect; 111 of the 200 values of *t* we would expect to observe from our data fall above this point when the drug increases urine production by 200 mL/day. Therefore, there is a 55 percent chance that we will conclude that the drug actually increases urine production from our experiment.

percent chance of concluding that the diuretic increases urine output when average urine output actually increases by 200 mL/day. We say the *power* of the test is .55. The power quantifies the chances of detecting a real difference of a given size.

Alternatively, we could concentrate on the 89 of the 200 experiments that produced *t* values below 2.101, in which case we would fail to reject the hypothesis that the treatment had no effect and be wrong. Thus, there is a $^{89}/_{200}$ = 45 percent = .45, chance of continuing to accept the hypothesis of no effect when the drug really increased urine production by 200 mL/day on the average.

TWO TYPES OF ERRORS

Now we have isolated the two different ways the random-sampling process can lead to erroneous conclusions. These two types of errors are analogous to the false positive and false negative results one obtains from diagnostic tests. Before this chapter we concentrated on controlling the likelihood of making a false positive error, i.e., concluding that a treatment has an effect when it really does not. In keeping with tradition, we have generally sought to keep the chances of making such an error below 5 percent; of course, we could arbitrarily select any cut-off value we wanted at which to declare the test statistic "big." Statisticians denote the maximum acceptable risk of this error by α, the Greek letter alpha. If we reject the hypothesis of no effect whenever $P < .05$, $\alpha = .05$ or 5 percent. If we actually obtain data that lead us to reject the hypothesis of no effect when this hypothesis is true, statisticians say that we have made a *Type I error*. They denote the chances of making such an error with α. All this logic is relatively straightforward because we have specified how much we believe the treatment affects the variable of interest, i.e., not at all.

What about the other side of the coin, the chances of making a false negative conclusion and not reporting an effect when one exists? Statisticians denote the chance of erroneously accepting the hypothesis of no effect by β, the Greek letter beta. The chance of detecting a true positive, i.e., reporting a statistically significant difference when the treatment really produces an effect, is $1 - \beta$. The *power* of the test that we discussed earlier is equal to $1 - \beta$. For example, if a test has power equal to .55, there is a 55 percent chance of actually reporting a statistically significant effect when one is really present. Table 6-1 summarizes these definitions.

WHAT DETERMINES A TEST'S POWER?

So far we have developed procedures for estimating and controlling the Type I, or α, error; now we turn our attention to keeping the Type II, or β, error as small as possible. In other words, we want the power to be as high as possible. In theory, this problem is not very different from the one we already solved with one important exception. Since the treatment has an effect, *the size of this effect influences how easy it is to detect.* Large effects are easier to detect than small ones. To estimate the power of a test, you need to specify how small an effect is worth detecting.

Just as with false positives and false negatives in diagnostic testing, the Type I and Type II errors are intertwined. As you require stronger evidence before reporting that a treatment has an effect, i.e., make α smaller, you also increase the chance of missing a true effect, i.e., make β bigger or power smaller. The only way to reduce both α and β simul-

Table 6-1   Types of Erroneous Conclusions in Statistical Hypothesis Testing

Conclude from observations	Actual situation	
	Treatment has an effect	Treatment has no effect
Treatment has an effect	True positive, correct conclusion $1 - \beta$	False positive, Type I error α
Treatment has no effect	False negative, Type II error β	True negative correct conclusion $1 - \alpha$

taneously is to increase the sample size, because with a larger sample you can be more confident in your decision, whatever it is.

In other words, the power of a given statistical test depends on three interacting factors:

- *The risk of error you will tolerate when rejecting the hypothesis of no treatment effect*
- *The size of the difference you wish to detect relative to the amount of variability in the populations*
- *The sample size*

To keep things simple, we will examine each of these factors separately.

The Size of the Type I Error α

Figure 6-3 showed the complementary nature of the maximum size of the Type I error α and the power of the test. The acceptable risk of erroneously rejecting the hypothesis of no effect, α, determines the critical value of the test statistic above which you will report that the treatment had an effect, $P < \alpha$. (We have usually taken $\alpha = .05$.) This critical value is defined from the distribution of the test statistic for all possible experiments with a specific sample size *given that the treatment had no effect*. The power is the proportion of possible values of the test statistic that fall above this cutoff value *given that the treat-*

ment had a specified effect (here a 200 mL/day increase in urine production). Changing α, or the P value required to reject the hypothesis of no difference, moves this cutoff point, affecting the power of the test.

Figure 6-4 illustrates this point further. Figure 6-4*A* essentially reproduces Fig. 6-3 except that it depicts the distribution of t values for all 10^{27} possible experiments involving two groups of 10 people as a continuous distribution. The top part, copied from Fig. 4-5*D*, shows the distribution of possible t values that would occur if the drug did not affect urine production. Suppose we require $P < .05$ before we are willing to assert that the observations were unlikely to have arisen from random sampling rather than the effect of the drug. In other words, we make $\alpha = .05$, in which case -2.101 and +2.101 delimit the most extreme 5 percent of all possible t values we would expect to observe if the diuretic did not affect urine production.

We know, however, that the drug actually increased average urine production by 200 mL/day. Therefore, we do not expect the distribution of possible t values associated with our experiment to be given by the distribution at the top of the figure. It will be centered not on zero but above zero (because we expect $\bar{X}_{dr} - \bar{X}_{pla}$ to average around 200 mL/day). The lower distribution in Fig. 6-4*A* shows the actual distribution of possible t values associated with our experiment; 55 percent of these possible values of t, that is, 55 percent of the area under the curve, fall above the 2.101 cutoff, so we say the power of the test is .55. In other words, if the drug increases average urine production by 200 mL/ day in this population and we do an experiment using two samples of 10 people each to test the drug, there is a 55 percent chance that we will conclude that the drug is effective ($P < .05$). Conversely, we can say that β, the likelihood that we will make the false negative, or Type II, error and accept the hypothesis of no effect when it is not true, is $1 - .55 = .45 = 45$ percent.

Now look at Fig. 6-4*B*. The two distributions of t values are identical to those in Fig. 6-4*A*. (After all, the drug's true effect is still the same.) This time, however, we will insist on stronger evidence before concluding that the drug actually increased urine production. We will require that the test statistic fall in the most extreme 1 percent of possible values before concluding that the data are inconsistent with the hypothesis that the drug has no effect. Thus, $\alpha = .01$ and t must exceed -2.878 or +2.878 to fall in the most extreme 1 percent of values. The top part of panel *B* shows this cutoff point. From the actual distribu-

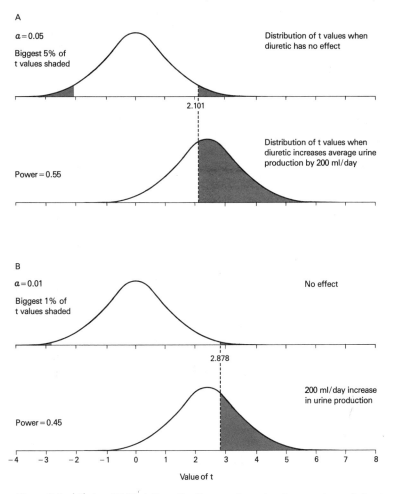

A

$\alpha = 0.05$

Biggest 5% of t values shaded

Distribution of t values when diuretic has no effect

2.101

Power = 0.55

Distribution of t values when diuretic increases average urine production by 200 ml/day

B

$\alpha = 0.01$

Biggest 1% of t values shaded

No effect

2.878

Power = 0.45

200 ml/day increase in urine production

Value of t

Figure 6-4 (A) t = 2.101 defines the 5 percent most extreme values of the t statistic we would expect to be associated with our experiment if the drug did not increase urine production. Of the possible values of the t statistic that will actually be associated with our experiment, 55 percent fall above this point because the drug increased urine production by 200 mL/day on the average. (B) If we increase the confidence with which we wish to reject the hypothesis that the drug had no effect (make α smaller), the proportion of possible t values that will actually arise from the experiment also goes down, so the power of the test to detect an effect of a given size decreases. For example, if we change α from .05 to .01, the power of the test drops from 55 to 45 percent because the cutoff for a "big" t increases from 2.101 to 2.878.

tion of t values in the lower part of Fig. 6-4B we see that only 45 percent of them fall above 2.878, so the power of the test has fallen to .45. In other words, there is less than an even chance that we will report that the drug is effective even though it actually is.

By requiring stronger evidence that there be a treatment effect before reporting it we have decreased the chances of erroneously reporting an effect (the Type I error), but we have increased the chances of failing to detect a difference when one actually exists (the Type II error) because we decreased the power of the test. This trade-off always exists.

The Size of the Treatment Effect

We just demonstrated that the power of a test decreases as we reduce the acceptable risk of making a Type I error, α. The entire discussion was based on the fact that the drug increased average urine production by 200 mL/day, from 1200 to 1400 mL/day. Had this change been different, the actual distribution of t values connected with the experiment also would have been different. In other words, the power of a test depends on the size of the difference to be detected.

Let us consider three specific examples. Figure 6-5A shows the t distribution (the distribution of possible values of the t statistic) for a sample size of 10 if the diuretic had no effect and the two treatment groups could be considered two random samples drawn from the same population. The most extreme 5 percent of the values are shaded, just as in Fig. 6-4. Figure 6-5B shows the distribution of t values we would expect if the drug increased urine production an average of 200 mL/day over the placebo; 55 percent of the possible values are beyond -2.101 or $+2.101$, so the power of the test is .55. (So far we are just recapitulating the results in Fig. 6-4.) Figure 6-5C shows the distribution of t values that would occur if the drug increased urine production only by 100 mL/day on the average. Now only 17 percent of the possible values (corresponding to 17 percent of the area under the curve) fall above 2.101, that is, the power of the test to detect a difference of only 100 mL/day is only 0.17. In other words, there is less than 1 chance in 5 that doing a study of two groups of 10 people would detect a change in urine production of 100 mL/day if we required that $P < .05$ before reporting an effect. Finally, Fig. 6-5D shows the distribution of t values that would occur if the drug increased urine production by an average of 400 mL/day. Now, 99 percent of all possible t values fall above

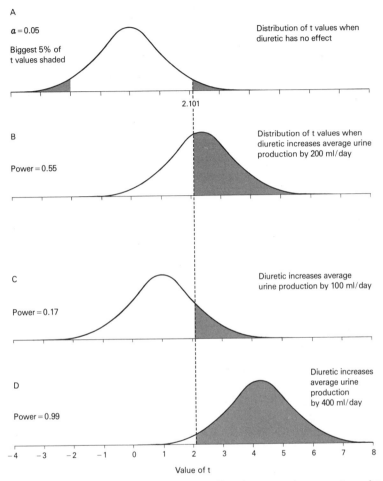

Figure 6-5 As the size of the treatment effect increases, the proportion of *t* values that will actually arise from the experiment increases, so the power of the test increases.

2.101; the power of the test to detect a difference this large is 0.99. The chances are quite good that our experiment will produce accurate results. Figure 6-5 illustrates the general rule: *It is easier to detect big differences than small ones.*

We could repeat this process for all possible sizes of the treatment effect, from no effect at all up to very large effects, then plot the power of the test as it varies with the change in urine production actually produced by the drug. Figure 6-6 shows a plot of the results, called a *power function,* of the test. It quantifies how much easier it is to detect a change (when we require a value of t corresponding to $P < .05$ and two samples of 10 people each) in urine production as the actual drug effect gets larger and larger. This plot shows that if the drug increases urine production by 200 mL/day, there is a 55 percent chance that we will detect this change with the experiment designed as we have it; if urine production increases by 350 mL/day, the chance of our detecting this effect improves to 95 percent.

The Population Variability

The power of a test increases as the size of the treatment effect increases, but the variability in the population under study also affects the likelihood with which we can detect a treatment effect of a given size. In particular, recall that the t-test statistic is defined as

$$ t = \frac{\bar{X}_1 - \bar{X}_2}{\sqrt{(s^2/n_1) + (s^2/n_2)}} $$

in which $\bar{X}_1$ and $\bar{X}_2$ are the means, s is the pooled estimate of the population standard deviation σ, and n_1 and n_2 are the sizes of the two samples. $\bar{X}_1$ and $\bar{X}_2$ are estimates of μ_1 and μ_2, the two (different) population means. In the interest of simplicity, let us assume that the two samples are the same size; that is, $n_1 = n_2 = n$. Then t computed from our observations is an estimate of

$$ t' = \frac{\mu_1 - \mu_2}{\sqrt{(\sigma^2/n) + (\sigma^2/n)}} = \frac{\mu_1 - \mu_2}{\sigma\sqrt{2/n}} $$

Denote the change in population mean value with the treatment by δ, Greek delta; then $\mu_1 - \mu_2 = \delta$, and

$$ t' = \frac{\delta/\sigma}{\sqrt{2/n}} = \frac{\delta}{\sigma}\sqrt{\frac{n}{2}} $$

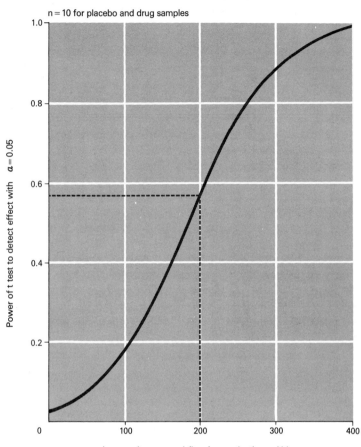

Figure 6-6 The power of a *t* test to detect a change in urine production based on experiments with two groups of people, each containing 10 individuals. The dashed line indicates how to read the graph. A *t* test has a power of .55 for detecting a 200 mL per day change in urine production.

Therefore, t' depends on the change in the mean response normalized by the population standard deviation.

For example, the standard deviation in urine production in the population we are studying is 200 mL/day (from Fig. 6-1). In this context, an increase in urine production of 200 or 400 mL/day can be seen to be 1 or 2 standard deviations, a fairly substantial change. These same absolute changes in urine production would be even more striking if the population standard deviation were only 50 mL/day, in which case a 200 mL/day absolute change would be 4 standard deviations. On the other hand, these changes in urine production would be hard to detect—indeed one wonders if you would want to detect them—if the population standard deviation were 500 mL/day. In this case 200 mL/day would be only .4 standard deviation of the normal population.

As the variability in the population σ decreases, the power of the test for detecting a fixed absolute size of treatment effects δ increases and vice versa. In fact, we can combine the influence of these two factors by considering the dimensionless ratio δ/σ rather than each one separately.

Bigger Samples Mean More Powerful Tests

So far we have seen two things: (1) The power of a test to correctly reject the hypothesis that a treatment has no effect decreases as the confidence with which you wish to reject that hypothesis increases; (2) the power increases as the size of the treatment effect, measured with respect to the population standard deviation, increases. In most cases, investigators cannot control either of these factors and for a given sample size are stuck with whatever the power of the test is. However, the situation is not totally beyond their control. They can increase the power of the test without sacrificing the confidence with which they reject the hypothesis of no treatment effect (α) by *increasing the sample size.*

Increasing the sample size generally increases the power, for two reasons. First, as the sample size grows, the number of degrees of freedom increases, and the value of the test statistic that defines the "biggest" 100α percent of possible values under the assumption of no treatment effect generally decreases. Second, as the equation for t' above shows, the value of t (and many other test statistics) increases as sample size n increases. As a result, the distribution of t values that occur when the treatment has an effect of a given size δ/σ is located at higher t values as sample size increases.

For example, Fig. 6-7A shows the same information as Fig. 6-4A, with the sample size equal to 10 in each of the two groups. Figure 6-7B shows the distribution of possible t values if the hypothesis of no effect

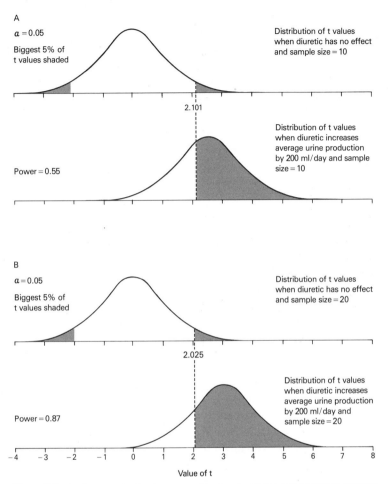

Figure 6-7 As the sample size increases, the power of the test increases for two reasons: (1) the critical value of t for a given confidence level in concluding that the treatment had an effect decreases, and (2) the values of the t statistic associated with the experiment increase.

were true as well as the distribution of t values that would appear if the drug still increased urine production by 200 mL/day but now based on an experiment with 20 people in each group. Since there are 20 people in each group, the experiment has $\nu = 2(20 - 1) = 38$ degrees of freedom. From Table 4-1 the critical value of t defining the most extreme 5 percent of possible values is 2.025 (compared with 2.101 when there were 10 people in each group). The larger sample size also produces larger values of t, on the average, when the treatment increases urine production by 200 mL/day (with a population standard deviation of 200 mL/day, as before) than it did with the smaller sample size. These two factors combine to make 87 percent of the possible values of t fall above 2.025. Therefore, there is an 87 percent chance of concluding that the drug has an effect; the power of the test under these circumstances is .87, up substantially from the value of .55 associated with the smaller sample size.

We could repeat this analysis over and over again to compute the power of this test to detect a 200 mL/day increase in urine production for a variety of sample sizes. Figure 6-8 shows the results of such computations. As the sample size increases, so does the test's power. In fact, estimating the sample size required to detect an effect large enough to be clinically significant is probably the major practical use to which power computations are put. Such computations are especially important in planning randomized clinical trials to estimate how many patients will have to be recruited and how many centers will have to be involved to accumulate enough patients to obtain a large enough sample to complete a meaningful analysis.

What Determines Power?   A Summary

Figure 6-9 shows a general power curve for the t test, allowing for a variety of sample sizes and differences of interest. All these curves assume that we will reject the hypothesis of no treatment effect whenever we compute a value of t from the data that corresponds to $P < .05$ (so $\alpha = .05$). If we were more or less stringent in our requirement concerning the size of t necessary to report a difference, we would obtain a family of curves different from those in Fig. 6-9.

There is one curve for each value of the sample size n in Fig. 6-9. This value of n represents the size of *each* of the two sample groups being compared with the t test. Most power charts (and tables) present the results assuming that each of the experimental groups is of the same size, because, for a given total sample size, power is greatest when there are equal numbers of subjects in each treatment group. Thus, when using power analysis to estimate the sample size for an experiment, the result actually yields the size of each of the sample groups. Power anal-

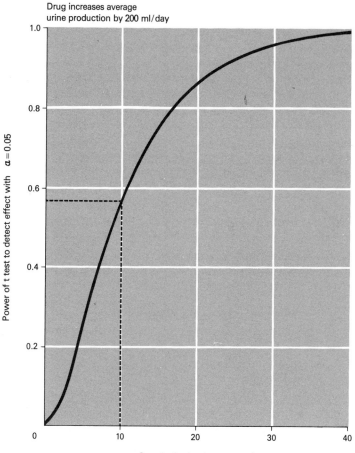

Figure 6-8 The effect of sample size on the power of a *t* test to detect a 200 mL per day increase in urine production with $\alpha = .05$ and a population standard deviation in urine production of 200 mL per day. The dashed line illustrates how to read the graph. A sample size of 10 yields a power of .55 for a *t* test to detect a 200 mL per day change in urine production.

ysis also can be used to estimate the power of a test that yielded a negative finding; in the case of unequal sample sizes, use the size of the smaller sample in the power analysis. This procedure will give you a conservative (low) estimate for the power of the test.

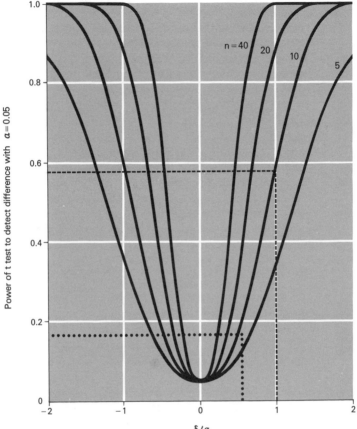

δ/σ

Figure 6-9 The power function for a test for comparing two experimental groups, each of size n, with α = .05. δ is the size of the change we wish to detect, σ is the population standard deviation. If we had taken α = .01 or any other value, we would have obtained a different set of curves. The dashed line indicates how to read the power of a test to detect a δ = 200 mL per day change in urine production with a σ = 200 mL per day standard deviation in the underlying population with a sample size of n = 10 in each test group; the power of this test is .55. The dotted line indicates how to find the power of an experiment designed to study the effects of anesthesia on the cardiovascular system in which δ/σ = .55 with a sample size of 9; the power of this test is only .16.

To illustrate the use of Fig. 6-9, again consider the effects of diuretic presented in Fig. 6-1. We wish to compute the power of a t test (with a 5 percent risk of a type I error, $\alpha = .05$) to detect a mean change in urine production of 200 mL per day when the population has a standard deviation of 200 mL per day. Hence

$$\frac{\delta}{\sigma} = \frac{200 \text{ mL per day}}{200 \text{ mL per day}} = 1$$

Since the sample size is $n = 10$ (in both the placebo and drug groups), we use the "$n = 10$" line in Fig. 6-9 to find that this test will have a power of .55.

All the examples in this chapter deal with estimating the power of an experiment that is analyzed with a t test. It is also possible to compute the power for all the other statistical procedures described in this book. Although the details of the computations are different, the same variables are important and play the same general roles in the computation. We will not discuss the details of these computations, however.*

We summarize our discussion of the power of hypothesis-testing procedures with these five statements:

• *The power of a test tells the likelihood that the hypothesis of no treatment effect will be rejected when the treatment has an effect.*
• *The more stringent our requirement for reporting that the treatment produced an effect (i.e., the smaller the chances of erroneously reporting that the treatment was effective), the lower the power of the test.*
• *The smaller the size of the treatment effect (with respect to the population standard deviation), the harder it is to detect.*
• *The larger the sample size, the greater the power of the test.*
• *The exact procedure to compute the power of a test depends on the test itself.*

---

*For a discussion of how to compute the power for tests on rates and proportions, together with a good supplementary discussion of the issues raised in this chapter, see A. F. Feinstein, *Clinical Biostatistics,* Mosby, St. Louis, 1977, chap. 22, "Sample Size and the Other Side of Statistical Significance." For a discussion of power computations for all the statistical procedures covered in this book, see W. J. Dixon and F. J. Massey, Jr., *Introduction to Statistical Analysis,* McGraw-Hill, New York, 1969, chap. 14, "Probability of Accepting a False Hypothesis."

PRACTICAL PROBLEMS IN USING POWER

If you know the size of the treatment effect, population standard deviation, α, and sample size, you can use graphs like Fig. 6-9 to estimate the power of a t test after the fact. Unfortunately, in practice, one does not know how large an effect a given treatment will have (finding that out is usually the reason for the study in the first place); so you must specify how large a change is *worth detecting* to compute the power of the test.

This requirement to go on record about how small a change is worth detecting may be one reason that very few people report the power of the tests they use. While such information is not especially important when investigators report that they detected a difference, it can be quite important when they report that they failed to detect one. If the power of the test to detect a clinically significant effect is small, say 25 percent, this report will mean something quite different than if the test was powerful enough to detect a clinically significant difference 85 percent of the time.

These difficulties are even more acute when using power computations to decide on the sample size for a study in advance. Completing this computation requires that investigators estimate not only the size of the effect they think is worth detecting and the confidence with which they hope to accept (β) or reject (α) the hypothesis that the treatment is effective but also the standard deviation of the population being studied. Sometimes existing information can be used to estimate these numbers; sometimes investigators do a pilot study to estimate them; sometimes they simply guess.

Another Look at Halothane versus Morphine for Open-Heart Surgery

Table 4-2 presented data on the effects of anesthesia on the cardiovascular system. When we analyzed these data with a t test, we did not conclude that halothane and morphine anesthesia produced significantly different values of cardiac index, which is defined as the rate at which the heart pumps blood (the cardiac output) divided by body surface area. This conclusion, however, was based on relatively small samples ($n = 9$ for the halothane group and $n = 16$ for the morphine group), and there was a 15 percent change in mean cardiac index (from 2.08

L/m^2 for halothane to 1.75 L/m^2 for morphine) between these two anesthetic regimes. While a 15 percent change in cardiac index may not be clinically important, a 25 percent change could be. The question then becomes: What is the power of this experiment to detect a 25 percent change in cardiac index?

We have already decided that a 25 percent change in cardiac index, .52 L/m^2 (25 percent of 2.08 L/m^2), is the size of the treatment effect worth detecting. From the data in Table 4-2, the pooled estimate of the variance in the underlying population is $s_{wit}^2 = .89$ $(L/m^2)^2$; take the square root of this number to obtain the estimate of the population standard deviation of .94 L/m^2. Hence

$$\frac{\delta}{\sigma} = \frac{.52 \, L/m^2}{.94 \, L/m^2} = .55$$

Since the two sample groups have different sizes, we estimate the power of the test based on the size of the smaller group, 9. From Fig. 6-9, the power is only .16! Thus it is very unlikely that this experiment would be able to detect a 25 percent change in cardiac index.

WHAT DIFFERENCE DOES IT MAKE?

In Chap. 4 we discussed the most common error in the use of statistical methods in the medical literature, inappropriate use of the t test. Repeated use of t tests increases the chances of reporting a "statistically significant" difference above the nominal levels one obtains from the t distribution. In the language of this chapter, it increases the Type I error. In practical terms, this increases the chances that an investigator will report some procedure or therapy capable of producing an effect beyond what one would expect from chance variation when the evidence does not actually support this conclusion.

This chapter examined the other side of the coin, the fact that perfectly correctly designed studies employing statistical methods correctly may fail to detect real, perhaps clinically important, differences simply because the sample sizes are too small to give the procedure enough power to detect the effect. This chapter shows how you can estimate the power of a given test after the results are reported in the literature and also how investigators can estimate the number of subjects they need to study to detect a specified difference with a given level of confidence (say, 95 percent; that is, $\alpha = .05$). Such computations are often quite distressing because they often reveal the need for a large number of experimental subjects, especially compared with the relatively few patients who typically form the basis for clinical studies.* Sometimes the investigators increase the size of the difference they say they wish to detect, decrease the power they find acceptable, or ignore the whole problem in an effort to reduce the necessary sample size. Most medical investigators never confront these problems because they have never heard of power.

Freiman and her colleagues[†] examined 71 randomized clinical trials published in journals such as *Lancet,* the *New England Journal of Medicine*, and the *Journal of the American Medical Association* reporting that the treatment studied did not produce a "statistically significant" ($P < .05$) improvement in clinical outcome. Only 20 percent of these studies included enough subjects to detect a 25 percent improvement in clinical outcome with a power of .50 or better. In other words, if the treatment produced a 25 percent reduction in mortality rate or other clinically important endpoint, there was less than a 50:50 chance that the clinical trial would be able to detect it with $P < .05$. Moreover, Freiman and her colleagues found that *only one* of the 71 papers stated that α and β were considered at the start of the study; 18 recognized a trend in the results, whereas 14 commented on the need for a larger sample size. They also pointed out that this problem has been around for a long time. Thus, in this area, like the rest of statistical applications in the medical literature, it is up to responsible readers to interpret what they read rather than take it at face value.

Other than throwing your hands up when a study with low power fails to detect a statistically significant effect, is there anything an investigator or clinician reading the literature can learn from the results? Yes. Instead of focusing on the accept-reject logic of statistical hypothe-

*R. A. Fletcher and S. W. Fletcher ("Clinical Research in General Medical Journals: A 30-Year Perspective," *N. Engl. J. Med.,* 301:180–183, 1979) report the median number of subjects included in clinical studies published in the *Journal of the American Medical Association*, *Lancet*, and the *New England Journal of Medicine* in 1946 to 1976 ranged from 16 to 36 people.
†J. A. Freiman, T. C. Chalmers, H. Smith, Jr., and R. R. Kuebler, "The Importance of Beta, the Type II Error and Sample Size in the Design and Interpretation of the Randomized Controlled Trial," *N. Engl. J. Med.,* 299:690–694, 1978.

sis testing,* one can try to estimate how strongly the observations *suggest* an effect by estimating the size of the hypothesized effect together with the uncertainty of this estimate. We laid the groundwork for this procedure in Chaps. 2, 4, and 5 when we discussed the standard error and the *t* distribution. The next chapter builds on this base to develop the idea of confidence limits.

PROBLEMS

6-1 Use the data in Table 4-2 to find the power of a *t* test to detect a 50 percent difference in cardiac index between halothane and morphine anesthesia.

6-2 How large a sample size would be necessary to have an 80 percent chance of detecting a 25 percent difference in cardiac index between halothane and morphine anesthesia?

6-3 Use the data in Table 4-2 to find the power of the experiments reported there to detect a 25 percent change in mean arterial blood pressure and total peripheral resistance.

6-4 In Prob. 3-5 (and again in Prob. 4-4), we decided that there was insufficient evidence to conclude that the psychoactive agent in marijuana (THC) was responsible for the fact that rats who breathed marijuana smoke had an impaired ability to inactivate inhaled bacteria in their lungs. What are the chances of concluding (with $\alpha = .05$) that THC actually decreases the ability of lungs to inactivate bacteria by 20 percent? In other words, what is the power of this experiment to detect a 20 percent change in ability to inactivate bacteria?

*There is another approach that can be used in some clinical trials to avoid this accept-reject problem. In a *sequential trial* the data are analyzed after each new individual is added to the study and the decision made to (1) accept the hypothesis of no treatment effect, (2) reject the hypothesis, or (3) study another individual. Sequential tests generally allow one to achieve the same levels of α and β for a given size treatment effect with a smaller sample size than the methods discussed in this book. This smaller sample size is purchased at the cost of increased complexity of the statistical procedures. Sequential analyses are often performed by repeated use of the statistical procedures presented in this book, such as the *t* test. This procedure is incorrect because it produces overoptimistic *P* values, just as the repeated use of *t* tests (without the Bonferroni correction) produces erroneous results when one should do an analysis of variance. K. McPherson ("Statistics: The Problem of Examining Accumulating Data More than Once," *N. Engl. J. Med.*, 290:501–502, 1974) presents a succinct discussion of this problem. See Dixon and Massey, op. cit., chap. 18, "Sequential Analysis," for an introduction to sequential analysis.

6-5 How large a sample would be necessary to be 90 percent confident that THC affected the lungs' ability to inactivate bacteria by at least 20 percent when you wished to be 95 percent confident in any conclusion that THC did not reduce bacterial inactivation by at least 20 percent?

6-6 How large a sample would be needed to have a 90 percent chance of detecting a change in cure rate from 30 to 90 percent with $P < .05$? The following information about the normal distribution will be helpful in solving this problem:

Number of SD from mean, z	Area under curve to right of z, %	Number of SD from mean, z	Area under curve to right of z, %
−2.5	.999	.5	.309
−2.0	.977	1.0	.159
−1.7	.955	1.3	.097
−1.5	.933	1.5	.067
−1.3	.903	1.7	.045
−1.0	.841	2.0	.023
− .5	.691	2.5	.001
.0	.500		

Confidence Intervals

All the statistical procedures developed so far were designed to help decide whether or not a set of observations is compatible with some hypothesis. These procedures yielded P values to estimate the chance of reporting that a treatment has an effect when it really does not and the power to estimate the chance that the test would detect a treatment effect of some specified size. This decision-making paradigm does not characterize the size of the difference or illuminate results that may not be statistically significant (i.e., not associated with a value of P below .05) but does nevertheless suggest an effect. In addition, since P depends not only on the magnitude of the treatment effect but also the sample size, it is common for experiments to yield very small values of P (what investigators often call "highly significant" results) when the magnitude of the treatment effect is so small that it is clinically or scientifically unimportant. As Chap. 6 noted, it can be more informative to think not only in terms of the accept-reject approach of statistical hypothesis testing but also to estimate the size of the treatment effect together with some measure of the uncertainty in that estimate.

This approach is not new; we used it in Chap. 2 when we defined the standard error of the mean to quantify the certainty with which we could estimate the population mean from a sample. We observed that since the population of all sample means at least approximately follows a normal distribution, the true (and unobserved) population mean will lie within about 2 standard errors of the mean of the sample mean 95 percent of the time. We now develop the tools to make this statement more precise and generalize it to apply to other estimation problems, such as the size of the effect a treatment produces. The resulting estimates, called *confidence intervals,* can also be used to test hypotheses.*
This approach yields exactly the same conclusions as the procedures we discussed earlier because it simply represents a different perspective on how to use concepts like the standard error, t, and normal distributions. Confidence intervals are also used to estimate the range of values that include a specified proportion of all members of a population, such as the "normal range" of values for a laboratory test.

THE SIZE OF THE TREATMENT EFFECT MEASURED AS THE DIFFERENCE OF TWO MEANS

In Chap. 4, we defined the t statistic to be

$$t = \frac{\text{difference of sample means}}{\text{standard error of difference of sample means}}$$

then computed its value for the data observed in an experiment. Next, we compared the result with the value t_α that defined the most extreme 100α percent of the possible values of t that would occur (in both tails) if the two samples were drawn from a single population. If the observed value of t exceeded t_α, we reported a "statistically significant" difference, with $P < \alpha$. As Fig. 4-5 showed, the distribution of possible values of t has a mean of zero and is symmetric about zero when the two samples are drawn from the *same* population.

*Some statisticians believe that confidence intervals provide a better way to think about the results of experiments than traditional hypothesis testing. For a brief exposition from this perspective, see K. J. Rothman, "A Show of Confidence," *N. Engl. J. Med.,* **299**:1362–1363, 1978.

On the other hand, if the two samples are drawn from populations with *different* means, the distribution of values of t associated with all possible experiments involving two samples of a given size is *not* centered on zero; it does not follow the t distribution. As Figs. 6-3 and 6-5 showed, the actual distribution of possible values of t has a nonzero mean that depends on the size of the treatment effect. It is possible to revise the definition of t so that it will be distributed according to the t distribution in Fig. 4-5 *regardless of whether or not the treatment actually has an effect.* This modified definition of t is

$$t = \frac{\begin{array}{c}\text{difference of sample means} - \\ \text{true difference in population means}\end{array}}{\text{standard error of difference of sample means}}$$

Notice that if the hypothesis of no treatment effect is correct, the difference in population means is zero and this definition of t reduces to the one we used before.

The equivalent mathematical statement is

$$t = \frac{(\bar{X}_1 - \bar{X}_2) - (\mu_1 - \mu_2)}{s_{\bar{X}_1 - \bar{X}_2}}$$

In Chap. 4 we computed t from the observations, then compared it with the critical value for a "big" value of t with $\nu = n_1 + n_2 - 2$ degrees of freedom to obtain a P value. Now, however, we cannot follow this approach since we do not know all the terms on the right side of the equation. Specifically, *we do not know the true difference in mean values of the two populations* from which the samples were drawn, $\mu_1 - \mu_2$. We can, however, use this equation to estimate the size of the treatment effect, $\mu_1 - \mu_2$.

Instead of using the equation to determine t, we will select an appropriate value of t and use the equation to estimate $\mu_1 - \mu_2$. The only problem is that of selecting an appropriate value for t.

By definition, 100α percent of all possible values of t are more negative than $-t_\alpha$ or more positive than $+t_\alpha$. For example, only 5 percent of all possible t values will fall outside the interval between $-t_{.05}$ and $+t_{.05}$, where $t_{.05}$ is the critical value of t that defines the most extreme 5 percent of the t distribution (tabulated in Table 4-1).

Therefore, $100(1 - \alpha)$ percent of all possible values of t fall between $-t_\alpha$ and $+t_\alpha$. For example, 95 percent of all possible values of t will fall between $-t_{.05}$ and $+t_{.05}$.

Every different pair of random samples we draw in our experiment will be associated with different values of $\bar{X}_1$, $\bar{X}_2$, and $s_{\bar{X}_1 - \bar{X}_2}$; and $100(1 - \alpha)$ percent of all possible experiments involving samples of a given size will yield values of t that fall between $-t_\alpha$ and $+t_\alpha$. Therefore, for $100(1 - \alpha)$ percent of all possible experiments

$$-t_\alpha < \frac{(\bar{X}_1 - \bar{X}_2) - (\mu_1 - \mu_2)}{s_{\bar{X}_1 - \bar{X}_2}} < +t_\alpha$$

Solve this equation for the true difference in sample means:

$$(\bar{X}_1 - \bar{X}_2) - t_\alpha s_{\bar{X}_1 - \bar{X}_2} < \mu_1 - \mu_2 < (\bar{X}_1 - \bar{X}_2) + t_\alpha s_{\bar{X}_1 - \bar{X}_2}$$

In other words, the actual difference of the means of the two populations from which the samples were drawn will fall within t_α standard errors of the difference of the sample means of the observed difference in the sample means (t_α has $\nu = n_1 + n - 2$ degrees of freedom, just as when we used the t distribution in hypothesis testing.) This range is called the $100(1 - \alpha)$ percent *confidence interval for the difference of the means*. For example, the 95 percent confidence interval for the true difference of the sample means is

$$(\bar{X}_1 - \bar{X}_2) - t_{.05} s_{\bar{X}_1 - \bar{X}_2} < \mu_1 - \mu_2 < (\bar{X}_1 - \bar{X}_2) + t_{.05} s_{\bar{X}_1 - \bar{X}_2}$$

This equation defines the range that will include the true difference in the means for 95 percent of all possible experiments that involve drawing samples from the two populations under study.

Since this procedure to compute the confidence interval for the difference of two means uses the t distribution, it is subject to the same limitations as the t test. In particular, the samples must be drawn from populations that follow a normal distribution at least approximately.

THE EFFECTIVE DIURETIC

Figure 6-1 showed the distributions of daily urine production for a population of 200 individuals when they are taking a placebo or a drug that is an effective diuretic. The mean urine production of the entire population when all members are taking the placebo is μ_{pla} = 1200 mL/day. The mean urine production for the population when all members are taking the drug is μ_{dr} = 1400 mL/day. Therefore, the drug increases urine production by an average of $\mu_{dr} - \mu_{pla}$ = 1400 - 1200 = 200 mL/day. An investigator, however, cannot observe every member of the population and must estimate the size of this effect from samples of people observed when they are taking the placebo or the drug. Figure 6-1 shows one pair of such samples, each of 10 individuals. The people who received the placebo had a mean urine output of 1150 mL/day, and the people receiving the drug had a mean urine output of 1400 mL/day. Thus, these two samples suggest that the drug increased urine production by $\bar{X}_{dr} - \bar{X}_{pla}$ = 1400 - 1150 = 250 mL/day. The random variation associated with the sampling procedure led to a different estimate of the size of the treatment effect from that really present. Simply presenting this single estimate of 250 mL/day increase in urine output ignores the fact that there is some uncertainty in the estimates of the true mean urine output in the two populations, so there will be some uncertainty in the estimate of the true difference in urine output. We now use the confidence interval to present an alternative description of how large a change in urine output accompanies the drug. This interval describes the average change seen in the people included in the experiment and also reflects the uncertainty introduced by the random-sampling process.

To estimate the standard error of the difference of the means $s_{\bar{X}_{dr} - \bar{X}_{pla}}$ we first compute a pooled estimate of the population variance. The standard deviations of observed urine production were 245 and 159 mL/day for people taking the drug and the placebo, respectively. Both samples included 10 people; therefore,

$$s^2 = \frac{1}{2}(s_{dr}^2 + s_{pl}^2) = \frac{1}{2}(245^2 + 159^2) = 206^2$$

and

$$s_{\bar{X}_{dr} - \bar{X}_{pla}} = \sqrt{\frac{s^2}{n_{dr}} + \frac{s^2}{n_{pla}}} = \sqrt{\frac{206^2}{10} + \frac{206^2}{10}} = 92.1 \text{ mL/day}$$

To compute the 95 percent confidence interval, we need the value of $t_{.05}$ from Table 4-1. Since each sample contains $n = 10$ individuals, we use the value of $t_{.05}$ corresponding to $\nu = 2(n - 1) = 2(10 - 1) = 18$ degrees of freedom. From Table 4-1, $t_{.05} = 2.101$.

Now we are ready to compute the 95 percent confidence interval for the mean change in urine production that accompanies use of the drug

$$(\bar{X}_{dr} - \bar{X}_{pla}) - t_{.05} s_{\bar{X}_{dr} - \bar{X}_{pla}} < \mu_{dr} - \mu_{pla} < (\bar{X}_{dr} - \bar{X}_{pla}) + t_{.05} s_{\bar{X}_{dr} - \bar{X}_{pla}}$$
$$250 - 2.101(92.1) < \mu_{dr} - \mu_{pla} < 250 + 2.101(92.1)$$
$$57 \text{ mL/day} < \mu_{dr} - \mu_{pla} < 444 \text{ mL/day}$$

Thus, on the basis of this particular experiment, we can be 95 percent confident that the drug increases average urine production somewhere between 57 and 444 mL/day. The *range* of values from 57 to 444 *is* the 95 percent *confidence interval* corresponding to this experiment. As Fig. 7-1*A* shows, this interval includes the actual change in mean urine production, $\mu_{dr} - \mu_{pla}$, 200 mL/day.

More Experiments

Of course, there is nothing special about the two samples of 10 people each selected in the study we just analyzed. Just as the values of the

---

Figure 7-1 (*A*) The 95 percent confidence interval for the change in urine production produced by the drug using the random samples shown in Fig. 6-1. The interval contains the true change in urine production, 200 mL/day (indicated by the dashed line). Since the interval does not include zero (indicated by the solid line), we can conclude that the drug increases urine output ($P < .05$). (*B*) The 95 percent confidence interval for change in urine production computed for the random samples shown in Fig. 6-2. The interval includes the actual change in urine production (200 mL/day), but it also includes zero, so that it is not possible to reject the hypothesis of no drug effect (at the 5 percent level). (*C*) The 95 percent confidence intervals for 48 more sets of random samples, e.g., experiments, drawn from the two populations in Fig. 6-1*A*. All but 3 of the 50 intervals shown in this figure include the actual change in urine production; 5 percent of *all* possible 95 percent confidence intervals will not include the 200 mL/day. Of the 50 confidence intervals, 22 include zero, meaning that the data do not permit rejecting the hypothesis of no difference at the 5 percent level. In these cases, we would make a Type II error. Since 45 percent of *all* possible 95 percent confidence intervals include zero, the probability of detecting a change in urine production is $1 - \beta = .55$.

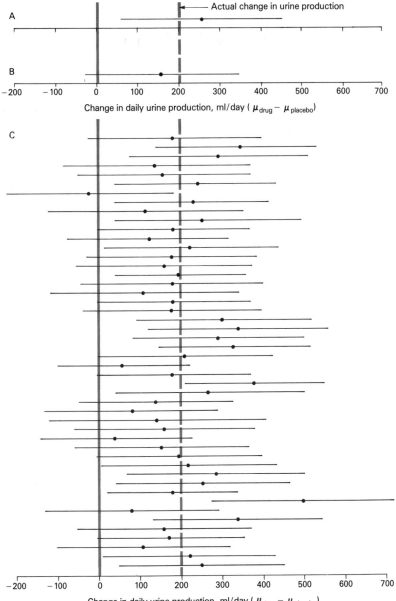

Change in daily urine production, ml/day ($\mu_{drug} - \mu_{placebo}$)

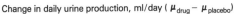

Change in daily urine production, ml/day ($\mu_{drug} - \mu_{placebo}$)

sample mean and standard deviation vary with the specific random sample of people we happen to draw, so will the confidence interval we compute from the resulting observations. (This should not be surprising, since the confidence interval is computed from the sample means and standard deviations.) The confidence interval we just computed corresponds to the specific random sample of individuals shown in Fig. 6-1. Had we selected a *different random sample* of people, say those in Fig. 6-2, we would have obtained a *different 95 percent confidence interval* for the size of the treatment effect.

The individuals selected at random for the experiment in Fig. 6-2 show a mean urine production of 1216 mL/day for the people taking the placebo and 1368 mL/day for the people taking the drug. The standard deviations of the two samples are 97 and 263 mL/day, respectively. In these two samples, the drug increased average urine production by $\bar{X}_{dr} - \bar{X}_{pla} = 1368 - 1216 = 152$ mL/day. The pooled estimate of the population variance is

$$s^2 = \tfrac{1}{2}(97^2 + 263^2) = 198^2$$

in which case,

$$s_{\bar{X}_{dr} - \bar{X}_{pla}} = \sqrt{\frac{198^2}{10} + \frac{198^2}{10}} = 89 \text{ mL/day}$$

So the 95 percent confidence interval for the mean change in urine production associated with the sample shown in Fig. 6-2 is

$$152 - 2.101(89) < \mu_{dr} - \mu_{pla} < 152 + 2.101(89)$$
$$-35 \text{ mL/day} < \mu_{dr} - \mu_{pla} < 339 \text{ mL/day}$$

This interval, while different from the first one we computed, also includes the actual mean increase in urine production, 200 mL/day (Fig. 7-1B). Had we drawn this sample rather than the one in Fig. 6-1, we would have been 95 percent confident that the drug increased average urine production somewhere between −35 and 339 mL/day. (Note that this interval includes negative values, indicating that the data do not permit us to exclude the possibility that the drug decreased as well as increased average urine production. This observation is the basis for using confidence intervals to test hypotheses later in this chapter.)

In sum, *the specific 95 percent confidence interval we obtain depends on the specific random sample we happen to select for observation.*

So far, we have seen two such intervals that could arise from random sampling of the populations in Fig. 6-1; there are more than 10^{27} possible samples of 10 people each, so there are more than 10^{27} possible 95 percent confidence intervals. Figure 7-1C shows 48 more of them, computed by selecting two samples of 10 people each from the populations of placebo and drug takers. Of the 50 intervals shown in Fig. 7-1, all but 3 (about 5 percent) include the value of 200 mL/day, the actual change in average urine production associated with the drug.

WHAT DOES "CONFIDENCE" MEAN?

We are now ready to attach a precise meaning to the term *95 percent confident.* The specific 95 percent confidence interval associated with a given set of data will or will not actually include the true size of the treatment effect, but in the long run 95 percent of *all possible 95 percent confidence intervals* will include the true difference of mean values associated with the treatment. As such, it describes not only the size of the effect but quantifies the certainty with which one can estimate the size of the treatment effect.

The size of the interval depends on the level of confidence you want to have that it will actually include the true treatment effect. Since t_α increases as α decreases, requiring a greater and greater fraction of all possible confidence intervals to cover the true effect will make the intervals larger. To see this, let us compute the 90 percent, 95 percent, and 99 percent confidence intervals associated with the data in Fig. 6-1. To do so, we need only substitute the values of $t_{.10}$ and $t_{.01}$ corresponding to $\nu = 18$ from Table 4-1 for t_α in the formula derived above. (We have already solved the problem for $t_{.05}$.)

For the 90 percent confidence interval, $t_{.10} = 1.734$, so the interval associated with the samples in Fig. 6-1 is

$$250 - 1.734(92.1) < \mu_{dr} - \mu_{pla} < 250 + 1.734(92.1)$$
$$90 \text{ mL/day} < \mu_{dr} - \mu_{pla} < 410 \text{ mL/day}$$

which, as Fig. 7-2 shows, is narrower than the 95 percent interval. Does this mean the data now magically yield a more precise estimate of

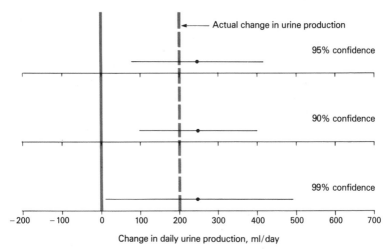

Figure 7-2 Increasing the level of confidence you wish to have that a confidence interval includes the true treatment effect makes the interval wider. All the confidence intervals in this figure were computed from the two random samples shown in Fig. 6-1. The 90 percent confidence interval is narrower than the 95 percent confidence interval, and the 99 percent confidence interval is wider. The actual change in urine production, 200 mL/day, is indicated with the dashed line.

the treatment effect? No. If you are willing to accept the risk that 10 percent of all possible confidence intervals will not include the true change in mean values, you can get by with a narrower interval.

On the other hand, if you want to specify an interval selected from a population of confidence intervals 99 percent of which include the true change in population means, you compute the confidence interval with $t_{.01}$ = 2.552. The 99 percent confidence interval associated with the samples in Fig. 6-1 is

$$250 - 2.552(92.1) < \mu_{dr} - \mu_{pla} < 250 + 2.552(92.1)$$
$$15 \text{ mL/day} < \mu_{dr} - \mu_{pla} < 485 \text{ mL/day}$$

This interval is wider than the other two in Fig. 7-2.

In sum, the confidence interval gives a range that is computed in the hope that it will include the parameter of interest (in this case, the difference of two population means). The confidence level associated with the interval (say 95, 90, or 99 percent) gives the percentage of all such possible intervals that will actually include the true value of the parameter. A *particular* interval will or will not include the true value of the parameter. Unfortunately, you can never know whether or not that interval does. All you can say is that the chances of selecting an interval that does not include the true value is small (say 5, 10, or 1 percent). The more confidence you wish to have that the interval will cover the true value, the wider the interval.

CONFIDENCE INTERVALS CAN BE USED TO TEST HYPOTHESES

As already noted, confidence intervals can provide another route to testing statistical hypotheses. This fact should not be surprising because we use all the same ingredients, the difference of the sample means, the standard error of the difference of sample means, and the value of t that corresponds to the biggest α fraction of the possible values defined by the t distribution with ν degrees of freedom.

Given a confidence interval, one cannot say where within the interval the true difference in population means lies. If the confidence interval contains zero, the evidence represented by the experimental observations is not sufficient to rule out the possibility that $\mu_1 - \mu_2 = 0$, that is, that $\mu_1 = \mu_2$, the hypothesis that the t test tests. Hence, we can state the following rule:

If the $100(1 - \alpha)$ percent confidence interval associated with a set of data includes zero, there is not sufficient evidence to reject the hypothesis of no effect with $P < \alpha$. If the confidence interval does not include zero, there is sufficient evidence to reject the hypothesis of no effect with $P < \alpha$.

Apply this rule to the two examples just discussed. The 95 percent confidence interval in Fig. 7-1*A* does not include zero, so we can report that the drug produced a statistically significant change in urine production ($P < .05$), just as we did using the t test. The 95 percent confidence interval in Fig. 7-1*B* includes zero, so the random sample (shown in Fig. 6-2) used to compute it does not provide sufficient evidence to reject the hypothesis that the drug has no effect. This, too, is the same conclusion we reached before.

Of the fifty 95 percent confidence intervals shown in Fig. 7-1, twenty-two include zero. Hence $^{22}/_{50}$ = 44 percent of these random samples do not permit reporting a difference with 95 percent confidence, i.e., with $P < .05$. If we looked at all possible 95 percent confidence intervals computed for these two populations with two samples of 10 people each, we would find that 45 percent of them include zero, meaning that we would fail to report a true difference, i.e., would make a Type II error, 45 percent of the time. Hence, $\beta = .45$, and the power of the test is .55, just as before (compare Fig. 6-4).

The confidence-interval approach to hypothesis testing offers two potential advantages. In addition to permitting you to reject the hypothesis of no effect when the interval does not include zero, it also gives information about the size of the effect. Thus, if a result reaches statistical significance more because of a large sample size than because of a large treatment effect, the confidence interval will show it. In other words, it will make it easier to recognize effects that can be detected with confidence but are too small to be of clinical or scientific significance.

For example, suppose we wish to study the potential value of a proposed antihypertensive drug. We select two samples of 100 people each and administer a placebo to one group and the drug to the other. The treated group has a mean diastolic pressure of 81 mmHg and a standard deviation of 11 mmHg; the control (placebo) group has a mean blood pressure of 85 mmHg and a standard deviation of 9 mmHg. Are these data consistent with the hypothesis that the diastolic blood pressure among people taking the drug and placebo were actually no different? To answer this question, we use the data to complete a t test. The pooled-variance estimate is

$$s^2 = \tfrac{1}{2}(11^2 + 9^2) = 10^2$$

so

$$t = \frac{\bar{X}_{dr} - \bar{X}_{pla}}{s_{\bar{X}_{dr} - \bar{X}_{pla}}} = \frac{81 - 85}{\sqrt{(10^2/100) + (10^2/100)}} = -2.83$$

This value is more negative than -2.61, the critical value of t that defines the 1 percent most extreme of the t distribution with $\nu =$

$2(n - 1) = 198$ degrees of freedom (from Table 4-1). Thus, we can assert that the drug lowers diastolic blood pressure $(P < .01)$.

But is this result clinically significant? To gain a feeling for this, compute the 95 percent confidence interval for the mean difference in diastolic blood pressure for people taking placebo versus the drug. Since $t_{.05}$ for 198 degrees of freedom is (from Table 4-1) 1.973, the confidence interval is

$$-4 - 1.973(1.42) < \mu_{dr} - \mu_{pla} < -4 + 1.973(1.42)$$
$$-6.8 \text{ mmHg} < \mu_{dr} - \mu_{pla} < -1.2 \text{ mmHg}$$

In other words, we can be 95 percent confident that the drug lowers blood pressure between 1.2 and 6.8 mmHg. This is not a very large effect, especially when compared with standard deviations of the blood pressures observed within each of the samples, which are around 10 mmHg. Thus, while the drug does seem to lower blood pressure on the average, examining the confidence interval permitted us to see that the size of the effect is not very impressive. The small value of P was more a reflection of the sample size than the size of the effect on blood pressure.

This example also points up the importance of examining not only the P values reported in a study but also the *size* of the treatment effect compared with the variability within each of the treatment groups. Usually this requires converting the standard errors of the mean reported in the paper to standard deviations by multiplying them by the square root of the sample size. This simple step often shows clinical studies to be of potential interest in illuminating physiological mechanisms but of little value in diagnosing or managing a specific patient because of person-to-person variability.

CONFIDENCE INTERVAL FOR THE POPULATION MEAN

The procedure we developed above can be used to compute a confidence interval for the mean of population from which a sample was drawn. The resulting confidence interval is the origin of the rule, stated in Chap. 2, that the true (and unobserved) mean of the original population will lie within 2 standard errors of the mean of the sample mean for about 95 percent of all possible samples.

The confidence intervals we computed up to this point are based on the fact that

$$t = \frac{\text{difference of sample means} - \text{difference in population means}}{\text{standard error of difference of sample means}}$$

follows the t distribution. It is also possible to show that

$$t = \frac{\text{sample mean} - \text{population mean}}{\text{standard error of mean}}$$

follows the t distribution. The equivalent mathematical statement is

$$t = \frac{\bar{X} - \mu}{s_{\bar{X}}}$$

We can compute the $100(1 - \alpha)$ percent confidence interval for the population mean by obtaining the value of t_α corresponding to $\nu = n - 1$ degrees of freedom, in which n is the sample size. Substitute this value for t in the equation and solve for μ (just as we did for $\mu_1 - \mu_2$ earlier):

$$\bar{X} - t_\alpha s_{\bar{X}} < \mu < \bar{X} + t_\alpha s_{\bar{X}}$$

The interpretation of the confidence interval for the mean is analogous to the interpretation of the confidence interval for the difference of two means: every possible random sample of a given size can be used to compute a, say, 95 percent confidence interval for the population mean, and this same percentage (95 percent) of all such intervals will include the true population mean.

It is common to approximate the 95 percent confidence interval with the sample mean plus or minus twice the standard error of the mean because the values of $t_{.05}$ are approximately 2 for sample sizes above about 20 (see Table 4-1). This approximate rule of thumb does underestimate the size of the confidence interval for the mean, however, especially for the small sample sizes common in biomedical research.

THE SIZE OF THE TREATMENT EFFECT MEASURED AS THE DIFFERENCE OF TWO RATES OR PROPORTIONS

It is easy to generalize the procedures we just developed to permit us to compute confidence intervals for rates and proportions. In Chap. 5 we used the statistic

$$z = \frac{\text{difference of sample proportions}}{\text{standard error of difference of proportions}}$$

to test the hypothesis that the observed proportions of events in two samples were consistent with the hypothesis that the event occurred at the same rate in the two populations. It is possible to show that even when the two populations have different proportions of members with the attribute, the ratio

$$z = \frac{\substack{\text{difference of sample proportions} - \\ \text{difference of population proportions}}}{\text{standard error of difference of sample proportions}}$$

is distributed approximately according to the normal distribution so long as the sample sizes are large enough.

If p_1 and p_2 are the actual proportions of members of each of the two populations with the attribute, and if the corresponding estimates computed from the samples are $\hat{p}_1$ and $\hat{p}_2$, respectively,

$$z = \frac{(\hat{p}_1 - \hat{p}_2) - (p_1 - p_2)}{s_{\hat{p}_1 - \hat{p}_2}}$$

We can use this equation to define the $100(1 - \alpha)$ percent confidence interval for the difference in proportions by substituting z_α for z in this equation and solving just as we did before. z_α is the value that defines the most extreme α proportion of the values in the normal distribution;* $z_\alpha = z_{.05} = 1.960$ is commonly used, since it is used to define the 95 percent confidence interval. Thus,

---

*This value can also be obtained from a t table, e.g., Table 4-1, by taking the value of t corresponding to an infinite number of degrees of freedom.

$$(\hat{p}_1 - \hat{p}_2) - z_\alpha s_{\hat{p}_1 - \hat{p}_2} < p_1 - p_2 < (\hat{p}_1 - \hat{p}_2) + z_\alpha s_{\hat{p}_1 - \hat{p}_2}$$

for $100(1 - \alpha)$ percent of all possible samples.

Difference in Mortality Associated with Anesthesia for Open-Heart Surgery

In Chap. 5 we tested the hypothesis that the mortality rates associated with halothane and morphine anesthesia were no different. What is the 95 percent confidence interval for the difference in mortality rate for these two agents?

The mortality rates observed with these two anesthetic agents were 13.1 percent (8 of 61 people) and 14.9 percent (10 of 67 people). Therefore, the difference in observed mortality rates is $\hat{p}_{hlo} - \hat{p}_{mor}$ = .131 - .15 = -.020 and the standard error of the difference, based on a pooled estimate of the proportion of all patients who died, is

$$\hat{p} = \frac{8 + 10}{61 + 67} = .14$$

$$s_{\hat{p}_{hlo} - \hat{p}_{mor}} = \sqrt{\hat{p}(1 - \hat{p})\left(\frac{1}{n_{hlo}} + \frac{1}{n_{mor}}\right)}$$

$$= \sqrt{.14(1 - .14)\left(\frac{1}{61} + \frac{1}{67}\right)} = .062 = 6.2\%$$

Therefore, the 95 percent confidence interval for the difference in mortality rates is

$$(\hat{p}_{hlo} - \hat{p}_{mor}) - z_{.05} s_{\hat{p}_{hlo} + \hat{p}_{mor}} < p_{hlo} - p_{mor} < (\hat{p}_{hlo} - \hat{p}_{mor})$$
$$+ z_{.05} s_{\hat{p}_{hlo} + \hat{p}_{mor}}$$
$$-.020 - 1.960(.062) < p_{hlo} - p_{mor} < -.020 + 1.960(.062)$$
$$-.142 < p_{hlo} - p_{mor} < .102$$

We can be 95 percent confident that the true difference in mortality rate lies between a 14.2 percent better rate for morphine and a 10.2 percent better rate for halothane. Since the confidence interval contains zero, there is not sufficient evidence to reject the hypothesis that the two anesthetic agents are associated with the same mortality rate. Furthermore, the confidence interval ranges about equally on both sides of zero, so there is not even a suggestion that one agent is superior to the other.

Difference in Thrombosis with Aspirin in People Receiving Hemodialysis

Chapter 5 also discussed the evidence that administering low-dose aspirin to people receiving regular kidney dialysis reduces the proportion of people who develop thromboses. Of the people taking the placebo, 72 percent developed thromboses, and 32 percent of the people taking aspirin did. Given only this information, we would report that aspirin reduced the proportion of patients who developed thrombosis by 50 percent. What is the 95 percent confidence interval for the improvement?

The standard error of the difference in proportion of patients who developed thromboses is .15 (from Chap. 5). So the 95 percent confidence interval for the true difference in proportion of patients who developed thromboses is

$$.40 - 1.96(.15) < p_{pla} - p_{asp} < .40 + 1.96(.15)$$
$$.11 < p_{pla} - p_{asp} < .69$$

We can be 95 percent confident that aspirin reduces the rate of thrombosis somewhere between 21 and 79 percent compared with placebo.

How Negative Is a "Negative" Clinical Trial?

Chapter 6 discussed the study of 71 randomized clinical trials that did not demonstrate a statistically significant improvement in clinical outcome (mortality, complications, or the number of patients who showed no improvement, depending on the study). Most of these trials involved too few patients to have sufficient power to be confident that the failure to detect a treatment effect was not due to an inadequate sample size. To get a feeling for how compatible the data are with the hypothesis of no treatment effect, let us examine the 90 percent confidence intervals for the proportion of "successful" cases (the definition of success varied with the study) for all 71 trials. Figure 7-2 shows these confidence intervals.

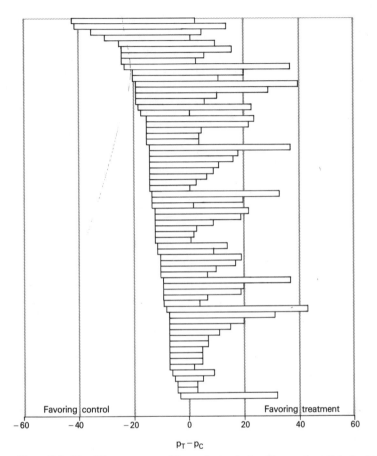

Figure 7-3 The 90 percent confidence intervals for 71 negative clinical trials. Since all the intervals contain zero, there is not sufficient evidence that the success rate is different for the treatment and control groups. Nevertheless, the data are also compatible with the treatment producing a substantial improvement in success rate in many of the trials. (*Data from fig. 2 of J. A. Freiman, T. C. Chalmers, H. Smith, Jr., and R. R. Keubler, "The Importance of Beta, the Type II Error and Sample Size in the Design and Interpretation of the Randomized Control Trial: Survey of 71 'Negative' Trials," N. Engl. J. Med., 299:690-694, 1978.*)

All the confidence intervals include zero, so we cannot rule out the possibility that the treatments had no effect. Note, however, that some of the trials are also compatible with the possibility that the treatments produced sizable improvements in the success rate. Remember that while we can be 90 percent confident that the true change in pro-portion of successes lies in the interval, it could be anywhere. Does this prove that some of these treatments improved clinical outcome? No. The important point is that the confidence with which we can assert that there was no treatment effect is often the same as the confidence with which we can assert that the treatment produced a sizable im-provement. While the size and location of the confidence interval cannot be used as part of a formal statistical argument to prove that the treatment had an effect, it certainly can help you look for trends in the data.

CONFIDENCE INTERVAL FOR RATES AND PROPORTIONS

It is possible to use the normal distribution to compute approximate confidence intervals for proportions from observations, so long as the sample size is large enough to make the approximation reasonably accurate.* When it is not possible to use this approximation, we will compute the exact confidence intervals based on the binomial distribu-tion. While we will not go into the computational details of this pro-cedure, we will present the necessary results in graphical form because papers often present results based on small numbers of subjects. Ex-amining the confidence intervals as opposed to only the observed pro-portion of patients with a given attribute is especially useful in thinking about such studies, because a change of *a single patient* from one group to the other often makes a large difference in the observed proportion of patients with the attribute of interest.

Just as there was an analogous way to use the *t* distribution to re-late the difference of means and the confidence interval for a single sample mean, it is possible to show that if the sample size is large enough

$$z = \frac{\text{observed proportion} - \text{true proportion}}{\text{standard error of proportion}}$$

In other words

---

*As discussed in Chap. 5, $n\hat{p}$ and $n(1 - \hat{p})$ must both exceed about 5, where $\hat{p}$ is the proportion of the observed sample having the attribute of interest.

$$z = \frac{\hat{p} - p}{s_{\hat{p}}}$$

approximately follows the normal distribution. Hence, we can use this equation to define the $100(1 - \alpha)$ percent confidence interval for the true proportion p with

$$\hat{p} - z_{\alpha} s_{\hat{p}} < p < \hat{p} + z_{\alpha} s_{\hat{p}}$$

The Fraction of Articles with Statistical Errors

Figure 1-3 showed that since 1950 the fraction of articles published in medical journals that include errors in the use of statistical procedures has remained around 50 percent. The points in the figure show the proportion of articles examined by each of the reviewers that had errors. Since the articles that were actually analyzed represent only a sample of all articles published that year, let us compute the 95 percent confidence intervals for the proportion of articles containing mistakes to get a better feeling for how large the potential problem is and how much, if at all, things seem to be changing. Chapter 8 will develop formal methods for testing for trends, but simply looking at Fig. 1-3 suggests that the chance that any given article selected at random from a good medical journal has an error in the use of statistical procedures has remained roughly constant at about 40 to 60 percent since 1960.

We will illustrate how to compute the 95 percent confidence interval for the last point in Fig. 1-3. Gore and her colleagues* found that 32 of the 77 original papers published in the *British Medical Journal* between January and March 1976 contained at least one error in their use of statistical procedures. What is the 95 percent confidence interval for the proportion of all articles published in journals of comparable quality at that time?

The proportion of articles with errors is $\hat{p} = {}^{32}/_{77} = .42$, and the standard error of the proportion is $s_{\hat{p}} = \sqrt{.42(1 - .42)/77} = .056$. Therefore, the 95 percent confidence interval is

---

*S. M. Gore, I. G. Jones, and E. C. Rytter, "Misuse of Statistical Methods: Critical Assessment of Articles in BMJ from January to March 1976," *Br. Med. J.,* 1(6053):85–87, 1977.

$$.42 - 1.96(.056) < p < .42 + 1.96(.056)$$
$$.31 < p < .53$$

This interval is plotted around the diamond-shaped point in Fig. 1-3.

How potentially serious are these errors? Gore and her colleagues reported that 5 of the 62 analytical reports that made some use of statistical procedures made some claim in the summary that was not supported by the data presented. Thus $\hat{p} = \frac{5}{62} = .081$ and $s_{\hat{p}} = \sqrt{.081(1 - .081)/62} = .035$, so the 95 percent confidence interval for the proportion of papers with conclusions not supported by the data is

$$.081 - 1.960(.035) < p < .081 + 1.960(.035)$$

or from 1.2 to 15 percent.

Exact Confidence Intervals for Rates and Proportions

When the sample size or observed proportion is too small for the approximate confidence interval based on the normal distribution to be reliable, you have to compute the confidence interval based on the exact theoretical distribution of a proportion, the *binomial distribution.** Since results based on small sample sizes with low observed rates of events turn up frequently in the medical literature, we present the results of computation of confidence intervals using the binomial distribution.

To illustrate how the procedure we followed above can fall apart when $n\hat{p}$ is below about 5, we consider an example. Suppose a surgeon says that he has done 30 operations without a single complication. His observed complication rate $\hat{p}$ is $\frac{0}{30} = 0$ percent for the 30 specific patients he operated on. Impressive as this is, it is unlikely that the surgeon will continue operating forever without a complication, so

---

*The reason we could use the normal distribution here and in Chap. 5 is that for large enough sample sizes there is little difference between the binomial and normal distributions. This result is a consequence of the central-limit theorem, discussed in Chap. 2. For the actual derivation of these results, see W. J. Dixon and F. J. Massey, *Introduction to Statistical Analysis,* McGraw-Hill, New York, 1969, sec. 13-5, "Binomial Distribution: Proportion," or B. W. Brown, Jr., and M. Hollander, *Statistics: A Biomedical Introduction,* Wiley, New York, 1977, chap. 7, "Statistical Inference for Dichotomous Variables."

the fact that $\hat{p} = 0$ probably reflects good luck in the randomly selected patients who happened to be operated on during the period in question. To obtain a better estimate of p, the surgeon's true complication rate, we will compute the 95 percent confidence interval for p.

Let us try to apply our existing procedure. Since $\hat{p} = 0$,

$$s_{\hat{p}} = \sqrt{\frac{\hat{p}(1 - \hat{p})}{n}} = \sqrt{\frac{0(1 - 0)}{30}} = 0$$

and the 95 percent confidence interval is from zero to zero. This result does not make sense. There is no way that a surgeon can *never* have a complication. Obviously, the approximation breaks down.

Figure 7-4 gives a graphical presentation of the 95 percent confidence intervals for proportions. The upper and lower limits are read off the vertical axis using the pair of curves corresponding to the size of the sample n used to estimate $\hat{p}$ at the point on the horizontal axis corresponding to the observed $\hat{p}$. For our surgeon, $\hat{p} = 0$ and $n = 30$, so the 95 percent confidence interval for his true complication rate is from 0 to .10. In other words, we can be 95 percent confident that his true complication rate, based on the 30 cases we happened to observe, is somewhere between 0 and 10 percent.

Now, suppose the surgeon had a single complication. Then $\hat{p} = \frac{1}{30}$ = .033 and

$$s_{\hat{p}} = \sqrt{.033(1 - .033)/30} = .033$$

so the 95 percent confidence interval for the true complication rate, computed using the approximate method, is

$$.033 - 1.96(.033) < p < .033 + 1.96(.033)$$

$$-.032 < p < .098$$

Think about this result for a moment. There is no way a surgeon can have a *negative* complication rate.

Figure 7-4 gives the exact confidence interval, from 0 to .13, or 0 to 13 percent. This confidence interval is not too different from that

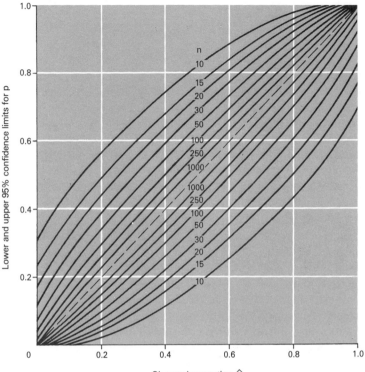

Figure 7-4 Graphical presentation of the exact 95 percent confidence intervals (based on the binomial distribution) for the population proportion. You read this plot by reading the two limits of the lines defined by the sample size at the point on the horizontal axis at the proportion of the sample with the attribute of interest $\hat{p}$. (*Adapted from C. J. Clopper and E. S. Pearson, "The Use of Confidence or Fiducial Limits Illustrated in the Case of the Binomial," Biometrika, 26:404, 1934.*)

computed when there were no complications, as it should be, since there is little real difference between not having any complications and having only one complication in such a small sample.

Notice how important sample size is, especially for small sample sizes. Had the surgeon been bragging that he had a zero complication rate on the basis of only 10 cases, the 95 percent confidence interval for his true complication rate would have extended from zero all the way to 33 percent!

CONFIDENCE INTERVAL FOR THE
ENTIRE POPULATION*

So far we have computed intervals that we can have a high degree of confidence will include a *population parameter*, such as μ or p. It is often desirable to determine a confidence interval for the *population itself*, most commonly when defining the normal range of some variable. The most common approach is to take the range defined by 2 standard deviations about the sample mean on the grounds that this interval contains 95 percent of the members of a population that follows the normal distribution (Fig. 2-5). In fact, in carefully worded language Chap. 2 suggested this rule. When the sample used to compute the mean and standard deviation is large (more than 100 to 200 members), this common rule of thumb is reasonably accurate. Unfortunately, most clinical studies are based on much smaller samples (of the order of 5 to 20 individuals). With such small samples, use of this 2 standard deviations rule of thumb seriously underestimates the range of values likely to be included in the population from which the samples were drawn.

For example, Fig. 2-6 showed the population of the heights of all 200 Martians, together with the results of three random samples of 10 Martians each. Figure 2-6*A* showed that 95 percent of all Martians have heights between 31 and 49 cm. The mean and standard deviation of the heights of population of all 200 Martians are 40 and 5 cm, respectively. The three samples illustrated in Fig. 2-6 yield estimates of the mean of 41.5, 36, and 40 cm, and of the standard deviation of 3.8, 5, and 5 cm, respectively. Suppose we simply compute the range defined by 2 *sample* standard deviations above and below the *sample* mean with the expectation that this range will include 95 percent of the population. Figure 7-5*A* shows the results of this computation for each of the three samples in Fig. 2-5. The light area defines the range of actual heights that covers 95 percent of the Martians' heights. Two of the three samples yield intervals that do not include 95 percent of the population.

---

*Confidence intervals for the population are also called *tolerance limits*. The procedures derived in this section are appropriate for analyzing data obtained from a population that is normally distributed. If the population follows other distributions, there are alternate procedures for computing confidence intervals for the population.

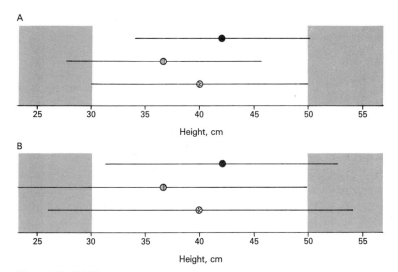

Figure 7-5 (A) The range defined by the sample mean ±2 standard deviations for the three samples of 10 Martians each shown in Fig. 2-6. Two of the three resulting ranges do *not* cover the entire range that includes 95 percent of the population members (indicated by the vertical lines). (B) The 95 percent confidence intervals for the population, computed as the sample mean $\pm K_{.05}$ times the sample standard deviation covers the actual range that includes 95 percent of the actual population; 95 percent of all such intervals will cover 95 percent of the actual population range.

This problem arises because both the sample mean and standard deviation are only *estimates* of the population mean and standard deviation and so cannot be used interchangeably with the population mean and standard deviation when computing the range of population values. To see why, consider the sample in Fig. 2-6B that yielded estimates of the mean and standard deviation of 36 and 5 cm, respectively. By good fortune, the estimate of the standard deviation computed from the sample equaled the population standard deviation. The estimate of the population mean, however, was low. As a result, the interval 2 standard deviations above and below the sample mean did not reach high enough to cover 95 percent of the entire population values. Because of the potential errors in the estimates of the population mean and standard deviation, we must be conservative and use a range greater than 2 standard deviations around the sample mean to be sure of including, say, 95 percent of the entire population. However, as the size of the sample used to estimate the mean and standard deviation increases, the certainty with which we can use these estimates to compute the range spanned by the entire population increases, so we do not have to be as conservative (i.e., take fewer multiples of the sample standard deviation) when computing an interval that contains a specified proportion of the population members.

Specifying the confidence interval for the entire population is more involved than specifying the confidence intervals we have discussed so far because you must specify both the *fraction of the population f* you wish the interval to cover and the *confidence you wish to have that any given interval will cover it.* The size of the interval depends on these two things and the size of the sample used to estimate the mean and standard deviation. The $100(1 - \alpha)$ percent confidence interval for $100f$ percent of the population is

$$\bar{X} - K_\alpha s < X < \bar{X} + K_\alpha s$$

in which $\bar{X}$ and s are the sample mean and standard deviation and K_α is the number of sample standard deviations about the sample mean needed to cover the desired part of the population. Figure 7-6 shows

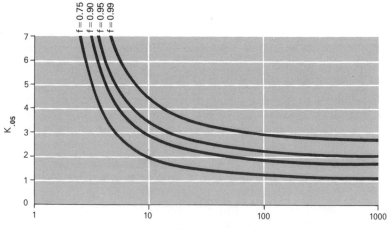

Figure 7-6 $K_{.05}$ depends on the size of the sample n used to estimate the mean and standard deviation and the fraction f of the population you want the interval to include.

$K_{.05}$ as a function of sample size for various values of f. It plays a role similar to t_α or z_α.

K_α is larger than t_α (which is larger than z_α) because it accounts for uncertainty in the estimates of both the mean *and* standard deviation, rather than the mean alone.*

Notice that K_α can be much larger than 2 for samples sizes in the range of 5 to 25, which are common in biomedical research. Thus, simply taking 2 standard deviations about the mean may substantially underestimate the range of the population from which the samples were drawn. Figure 7-5B shows the 95 percent confidence interval for 95 percent of the population of Martians' heights based on the three samples of 10 Martians each shown in Fig. 2-6. All three of the intervals include 95 percent of the population.

As Chap. 2 discussed, many people confuse the standard error of the mean with the standard deviation and consider the range defined by "sample mean ± 2 standard errors of the mean" to encompass about 95 percent of the population. This error leads them to seriously underestimate the possible range of values in the population from which the sample was drawn. We have seen that, for the relatively small sample sizes common in biomedical research, applying the 2 standard deviations rule may underestimate the range of values in the underlying population as well.

PROBLEMS

7-1 Find the 90 and 95 percent confidence intervals for the mean number of authors of articles published in the medical literature in 1946, 1956, 1966, and 1976 using the data from Prob. 2-6.

7-2 Problem 3-1 described an experiment in which women were treated with a gel containing prostaglandin E_2 and a placebo gel to see if the active gel would facilitate softening and dilation of the cervix during an induced labor. One reason for trying to facilitate cervical softening and dilation is to avoid having to do a cesarean section. C. O'Herlihy and H. MacDonald ("Influence of Preinduction Prostaglandin E_2 Vaginal Gel on Cervical Ripening and Labor," *Obstet. Gynecol.*, **54**:708–710, 1979) observed that 15 percent

*For a derivation of K_α that clearly shows how it is related to the confidence limits for the mean and standard deviation, see A. E. Lewis, *Biostatistics,* Reinhold, New York, 1966, chap. 12, "Tolerance Limits and Indices of Discrimination."

of the 21 women in the treatment group required cesarean sections and 23.9 percent of the 21 women in the control group required cesarean sections. Find the 95 percent confidence intervals for the percentage of all women having cesarean sections after receiving each treatment and the difference in cesarean section rate for all women in the two different groups. Can you be 95 percent confident that the prostaglandin E_2 gel reduces the chances that a woman whose labor is being induced will need to be delivered by a cesarean section?

7-3 Find the 95 percent confidence interval for the difference in the mean duration of labor in women treated with prostaglandin E_2 gel compared with women treated with placebo gel using the data in Prob. 3-1. Based on this confidence interval, is the difference statistically significant with $P < .05$?

7-4 Find the 95 percent confidence intervals for the proportion of both groups in Prob. 5-1 for which high-frequency neural modulation was an effective dental analgesic. Compare this result with the hypothesis tests computed in Prob. 5-1.

7-5 Find the 95 percent confidence intervals for the mean forced mid-expiratory flows for the different test groups in Prob. 3-2. Use this information to identify people with different or similar lung function (as we did with Bonferroni t tests in Chap. 4).

7-6 Find the 95 percent confidence intervals for the percentage of articles that reported the results of research based on data collected before deciding on the question to be investigated. Use the data in Prob. 5-6.

7-7 Use the data in Prob. 2-2 to find the 95 percent confidence interval for 90 and 95 percent of the population of exercise times of people who have heart disease. Plot these intervals together with the observations.

How to Test for Trends

The first statistical problem we posed in this book, in connection with Fig. 1-2*A,* dealt with a drug that was thought to be a diuretic, but that experiment cannot be analyzed using our existing procedures. In it, we selected different people and gave them different doses of the diuretic; then we measured their urine output. The people who received larger doses produced more urine. The statistical question is whether the resulting pattern of points relating urine production to drug dose provided sufficient evidence to conclude that the drug increased urine production in proportion to drug dose. This chapter develops the tools for analyzing such experiments. We will estimate how much one variable increases (or decreases) on the average as another variable changes with a *regression line* and quantify the *strength* of the association with *a correlation coefficient.*

MORE ABOUT THE MARTIANS

As in all other statistical procedures, we want to use a sample drawn at random from a population to make statements about the population. Chapters 3 and 4 discussed populations whose members are normally distributed with mean μ and standard deviation σ and used estimates of these parameters to design test statistics (like F and t) that permitted us to examine whether or not some *discrete* treatment was likely to have affected the mean value of a variable of interest. Now, we add another parametric procedure, *linear regression,* to analyze experiments in which the samples were drawn from populations characterized by a mean response varying *continuously* with the size of the treatment. To understand the nature of this population and the associated random samples, we return again to Mars, where we can examine the entire population of 200 Martians.

Figure 2-1 showed that the heights of Martians are normally distributed with a mean of 40 cm and a standard deviation of 5 cm. In addition to measuring the heights of each Martian, let us also weigh each one. Figure 8-1 shows a plot in which each point represents the height x and weight y of one Martian. Since we have observed the *entire population,* there is no question that tall Martians tend to be heavier than short Martians.

There are a number of things we can conclude about the heights and weights of Martians as well as the relationship between these two variables. As noted in Chap. 2, the heights are normally distributed with mean μ = 40 cm and standard deviation σ = 5 cm. The weights are also normally distributed with mean μ = 12 g and standard deviation σ = 2.5 g. The most striking feature of Fig. 8-1, however, is that the *mean weight of Martians at each height* increases as height increases.

For example, the Martians who are 32 cm tall weigh 7.1, 7.9, 8.3 and 8.8 g, so the mean weight of Martians who are 32 cm tall is 8 g. The 8 Martians who are 46 cm tall weigh 13.7, 14.5, 14.8, 15.0, 15.1, 15.2, 15.3 and 15.8 g, so the mean weight of Martians who are 46 cm tall is 15 g. Figure 8-2 shows that the mean weight of Martians at each height increases *linearly* as height increases.

This line does not make it possible, however, to predict the weight of *an individual* Martian if you know his height. Why not? There is variability in weights among Martians at each height. Figure 8-1 reveals that standard deviation of weights of Martians with *any given height* is

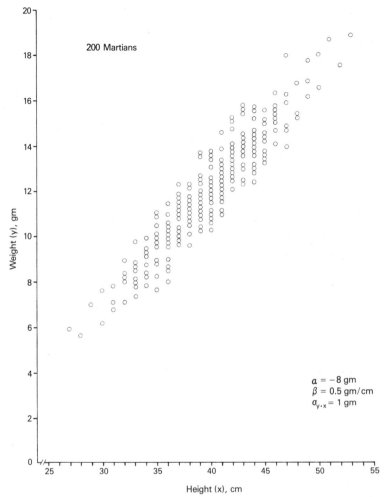

Figure 8-1 The relationship between height and weight in the population of 200 Martians, with each Martian represented by a circle. The heights and weights both follow normal distributions. In addition, the mean weight of Martians at any given height increases linearly with height, and the variability in weight at any given height is the same regardless of height. A population must have these characteristics to be suitable for linear-regression or correlation analysis.

about 1 g. We need to distinguish this standard deviation from the standard deviation of weights of *all* Martians computed without regard for the fact that mean weight varies with height.

The Population Parameters

Now, let us define some new terms and symbols so that we can generalize from Martians to other populations with similar characteristics. Since we are considering how weight varies with height, call height the *independent variable x* and weight the *dependent variable y.* In some instances, including the example at hand, we can only *observe* the independent variable and use it to *predict* the value of the dependent variable (with some uncertainty due to the variability in the dependent variable at each value of the independent variable). In other cases, including controlled experiments, it is possible to *manipulate* the independent variable to control, with some uncertainty, the value of the dependent variable. In the first case, it is only possible to identify an *association* between the two variables, whereas in the second case it is possible to conclude that there is a *causal* link.

For any given value of the independent variable x it is possible to compute the value of the mean of all values of the dependent variable corresponding to that value of x. We denote this mean $\mu_{y \cdot x}$ to indicate that it is the mean of all the values of y in the population at a given value of x. These means fall along a straight line given by

$$\mu_{y \cdot x} = \alpha + \beta x$$

in which α is the intercept and β is the slope* of the *line of means.* For example, Fig. 8-2 shows that, on the average, the average weight of Martians increases by .5 g for every 1-cm increase in height, so the slope β of the $\mu_{y \cdot x}$-versus-x line is .5 g/cm. The intercept α of this line is –8 g. Hence,

$$\mu_{y \cdot x} = -8 \text{ g} + (.5 \text{ g/cm})x$$

There is variability about the line of means. For any given value of the

---

*It is, unfortunately, statistical convention to use α and β in this way even though the same two Greek letters also denote the size of the Type I and Type II errors in hypothesis testing. The meaning of α should be clear from the context. β always refers to the slope of the line of means in this chapter.

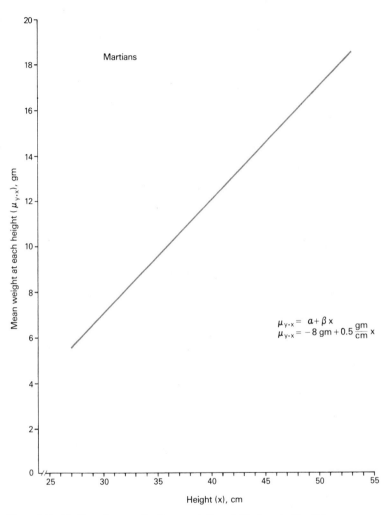

Figure 8-2 The line of means for the population of Martians in Fig. 8-1.

independent variable x, the values of y for the population are normally distributed with mean $\mu_{y \cdot x}$ and standard deviation $\sigma_{y \cdot x}$. This notation indicates that $\sigma_{y \cdot x}$ is the standard deviation of weights (y) computed after allowing for the fact that mean weight varies with height (x). As noted above, the residual variation about the line of means for our Martians is 1 g; $\sigma_{y \cdot x}$ = 1 g. The amount of this variability is an important factor in determining how useful the line of means is for predicting the value of the dependent variable, e.g., weight, when you know the value of the independent variable, e.g., height. The methods we develop below require that this standard deviation be *the same* for all values of x. In other words, the variability of the dependent variable about the line of means is the same regardless of the value of the independent variable.

In sum, we will be analyzing the results of experiments in which the observations were drawn from populations with these characteristics:

• *The mean of the population of the dependent variable at a given value of the independent variable increases (or decreases) linearly as the independent variable increases.*
• *For any given value of the independent variable, the possible values of the dependent variable are distributed normally.*
• *The standard deviation of population of the dependent variable about its mean at any given value of the independent variable is the same for all values of the independent variable.*

The parameters of this population are α and β, which define the line of means, the dependent-variable population mean at each value of the independent variable, and $\sigma_{y \cdot x}$, which defines the variability about the line of means. Now let us turn our attention to the problem of estimating these parameters from samples drawn at random from such populations.

HOW TO ESTIMATE THE TREND FROM A SAMPLE

Since we observed the entire population of Mars, there was no uncertainty how weight varied with height. This situation contrasts with real problems, in which we cannot observe all members of a population and must infer things about it from a limited sample which we hope is representative. To understand the information that such samples contain, let us consider a sample of 10 individuals selected at random from the population of 200 Martians. Figure 8-3A shows the members of the population that happened to be selected; Fig. 8-3B shows what an investigator or reader would see. What do the data in Fig. 8-3B allow you to say about the underlying population? How certain can you be about the resulting statements?

A

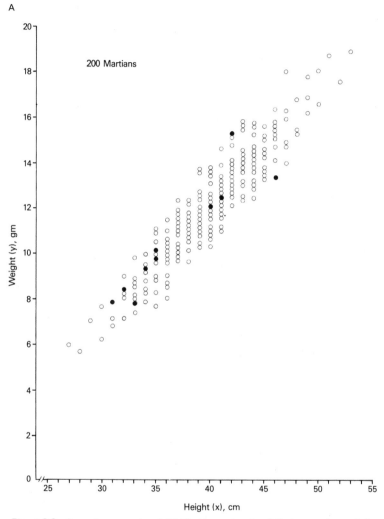

Figure 8-3 A random sample of 10 Martians, showing (A) the members of the population that were selected together with (B) the sample as it appears to the investigator.

Simply looking at Fig. 8-3B reveals that weight increases as height increases among the 10 specific individuals in *this* sample. The real question of interest, however, is: Does weight vary with height in the population the sample came from? After all, there is always a chance

B

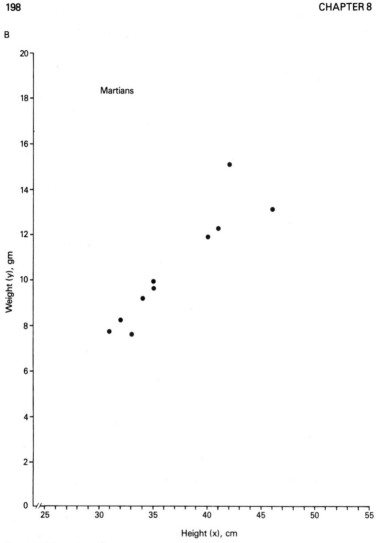

Figure 8-3 (continued)

that we could draw an unrepresentative sample, just as in Fig. 1-2. Before we can test the hypothesis that the apparent trend in the data is due to chance rather than a true trend in the population, we need to estimate the population trend from the sample. This task boils down to estimating the intercept α and slope β of the line of means.

The Best Straight Line through the Data

We will estimate the two population parameters α and β with the intercept and slope, a and b, of a straight line placed through the sample points. Figure 8-4 shows the same sample as Fig. 8-3B with four proposed lines, labeled I, II, III, and IV. Line I is obviously not appropriate; it does not even pass through the data. Line II passes through the data but has a much steeper slope than the data suggest is really the case. Lines III and IV seem more reasonable; they both pass along the cloud defined by the data points. Which one is best?

To select the best line and so get our estimates a and b of α and β, we need to define precisely what "best" means. To arrive at such a definition, first think about why line II seems better than line I and line III seems better than line II. The "better" a straight line is, the closer it comes to all the points taken as a group. In other words, we want to select the line that minimizes the total variability between the data and the line. The farther any one point is from the line, the more the line varies from the data, so let us select the line that leads to the smallest total variability between the observed values and the values predicted from the straight line.

In other words, the problem becomes one of defining a measure of variability, then selecting values of a and b to minimize this quantity. Recall that we quantified variability in a population with the variance (or standard deviation) by computing the sum of the squared deviations from the mean and then divided by the sample size minus 1. Now we will use the same idea and use *sum of the squared differences between the observed values of the dependent variable and the value on the line at the same value of the independent variable* as our measure of how much any given line varies from the data. We square the deviations so that positive and negative deviations contribute equally. Figure 8-5 shows the deviations associated with lines III and IV in Fig. 8-4. The sum of squared deviations is smaller for line IV than line III, so it is the best line. In fact, it is possible to prove mathematically that line IV is the one with the smallest sum of squared deviations between the observations and the line.* For this reason, this procedure is often called the *method of least squares* or *least-squares regression*.

---

*For this proof and a derivation of the formulas for the slope and intercept of this line, see S. A. Glantz *Mathematics for Biomedical Applications,* University of California Press, Berkeley, 1979, pp. 322–325.

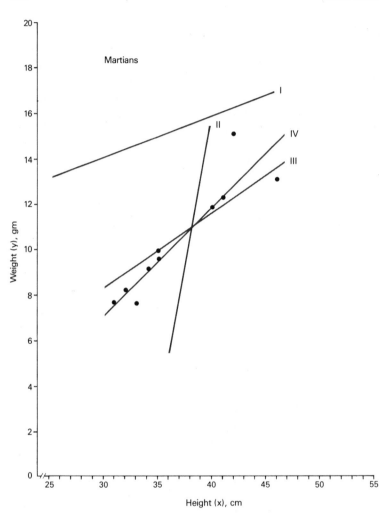

Figure 8-4 Four different possible lines to estimate the line of means from the sample in Fig. 8-3. Lines I and II are unlikely candidates because they fall so far from most of the observations. Lines III and IV are more promising.

The resulting line is called the *regression line* of y on x (in this case the regression line of weight on height). Its equation is

$$\hat{y} = a + bx$$

A

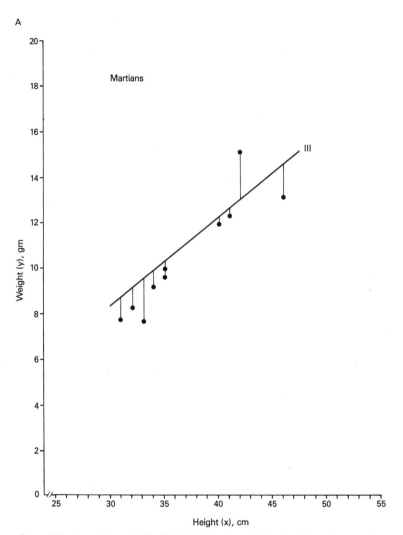

Figure 8-5 Lines III and IV in Fig. 8-4, together with the deviations between the lines and the observations. Line IV is associated with the smallest sum of squared deviations between the regression line and the observed values of the dependent variable. The vertical lines indicate the deviations. The light line is the line of means for the population of Martians in Fig. 8-1. The regression line approximates the line of means but does not precisely coincide with it. Line III in Fig. 8-4 is associated with larger deviations than line IV.

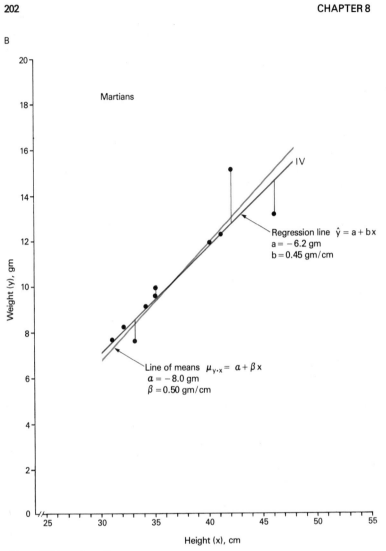

Figure 8-5 (continued)

$\hat{y}$ denotes the value of y on the regression for a given value of x. This notation distinguishes it from the observed value of the dependent variable Y. The intercept a is given by

Table 8-1   Computation of Regression Line in Fig. 8-5B

Observed height X, cm	Observed weight Y, g	X^2, cm^2	XY, g · cm
31	7.8	961	241.8
32	8.3	1,024	265.6
33	7.6	1,089	250.8
34	9.1	1,156	309.4
35	9.6	1,225	336.0
35	9.8	1,225	343.0
40	11.8	1,600	472.0
41	12.1	1,681	496.1
42	14.7	1,764	617.4
46	13.0	2,116	598.0
369	103.8	13,841	3,930.1

$$a = \frac{(\Sigma Y)(\Sigma X^2) - (\Sigma X)(\Sigma XY)}{n(\Sigma X^2) - (\Sigma X)^2}$$

and the slope is given by

$$b = \frac{n(\Sigma XY) - (\Sigma X)(\Sigma Y)}{n(\Sigma X^2) - (\Sigma X)^2}$$

in which X and Y are the coordinates of the n points in the sample.*

Table 8-1 shows these computations for the sample of 10 points in Fig. 8-3B. From this table, $n = 10$, $\Sigma X = 369$ cm, $\Sigma Y = 103.8$ g, $\Sigma X^2 = 13,841$ cm^2, and $\Sigma XY = 3930.1$ g · cm. Substitute these values into the equations for the intercept and slope of the regression line to find

$$a = \frac{(103.8 \text{ g})(13,841 \text{ cm}^2) - (369 \text{ cm})(3930.1 \text{ g} \cdot \text{cm})}{10(13,841 \text{ cm}^2) - (369 \text{ cm})^2} = -6.0 \text{ g}$$

*The calculations can be simplified by computing b first, then finding a from $a = \bar{Y} - b\bar{X}$, in which $\bar{X}$ and $\bar{Y}$ are the means of all observations of the independent and dependent variables, respectively.

and

$$b = \frac{10(3930.1 \text{ gm} \cdot \text{cm}) - (369 \text{ cm})(103.8 \text{ g})}{10(13{,}841 \text{ cm}^2) - (369 \text{ cm})^2} = .44 \text{ g/cm}$$

Line IV in Figs. 8-4 and 8-5B is this regression line,

$$\hat{y} = -6.0 \text{ g} + (.44 \text{ g/cm})x$$

These two values are estimates of the population parameters, $\alpha = -8$ g and $\beta = .5$ g/cm, the intercept and slope of the line of means. The light line in Fig. 8-5B shows the line of means.

Variability about the Regression Line

We have the regression line to estimate the line of means, but we still need to estimate the variability of population members about the line of means, $\sigma_{y \cdot x}$. We estimate this parameter by computing the square root of the "average" squared deviation of the data about the regression line

$$s_{y \cdot x} = \sqrt{\frac{\Sigma [Y - (a + bX)]^2}{n - 2}}$$

where $a + bX$ is the value $\hat{y}$ on the regression line corresponding to the observation at X; Y is the actual observed value of y; $Y - (a + bX)$ is the amount that the observation deviates about the regression line; and Σ denotes the sum, over all the data points, of the squares of these deviations $[Y - (a + bX)]^2$. We divide by $n - 2$ rather than n for reasons analogous to dividing by $n - 1$ when computing the sample standard deviation as an estimate of the population standard deviation. Since the sample will not show as much variability as the population, we need to decrease the denominator when computing the "average" squared deviation from the line to compensate for this tendency to underestimate the population variability.

$s_{y \cdot x}$ is called the *standard error of the estimate.* It can be related to the standard deviations of the dependent and independent variables and the slope of the regression line with

$$s_{y \cdot x} = \sqrt{\frac{n-1}{n-2}(s_Y^2 - b^2 s_X^2)}$$

For the sample shown in Fig. 8-3B (and Table 8-1), $s_X = 5.0$ cm and $s_Y = 2.4$ g, so

$$s_{y \cdot x} = \sqrt{\frac{9}{8}[2.4^2 - .45^2 (5.0^2)]} = .89 \text{ g}$$

This number is an estimate of the actual variability about the line of means, $\sigma_{y \cdot x} = 1$ g.

Standard Errors of the Regression Coefficients

Just as the sample mean is only an estimate of the true population mean, the slope and intercept of the regression line are only estimates of the slope and intercept of the line of means in the population. In addition, just as different samples yield different estimates for the population mean, different samples will yield different regression lines. After all, there is nothing special about the sample in Fig. 8-3. Figure 8-6A shows another sample of 10 individuals drawn at random from the population of all Martians. Figure 8-6B shows what you would see. Like the sample in Fig. 8-3B, the results of this sample also suggest that taller Martians tend to be heavier, but the relationship looks a little different from that associated with our first sample. This sample yields estimates of $a = -4.0$ g and $b = .38$ g/cm as estimates of the intercept and slope of the line of means. There is a population of possible values of a and b corresponding to all possible samples of a given size drawn from the population in Fig. 8-1. These distributions of all possible values of a and b have means α and β, respectively, and standard deviations σ_a and σ_b that we will call the *standard error of the intercept* and *standard error of the slope,* respectively.

These standard errors can be used just as we used the standard error of the mean and standard error of a proportion. Specifically, we will use them to test hypotheses about, and compute confidence intervals for, the regression coefficients and the regression equation itself.

The standard deviation of the population of all possible values of the regression line intercept, the standard error of the intercept, can be estimated from the sample with*

$$s_a = s_{y \cdot x} \sqrt{\frac{1}{n} + \frac{\bar{X}^2}{(n-1)s_X^2}}$$

The *standard error of the slope* of the regression line is the standard deviation of the population of all possible slopes. Its estimate is

$$s_b = \frac{1}{\sqrt{n-1}} \frac{s_{y \cdot x}}{s_X}$$

From the data in Fig. 8-3*B* and Table 8-1 it is possible to compute the standard errors for the slope and intercept as

$$s_a = (.89 \text{ g}) \sqrt{\frac{1}{10} + \frac{(36.9 \text{ cm})^2}{(10-1)(5.0 \text{ cm})^2}} = 2.2 \text{ g}$$

and

$$s_b = \frac{1}{\sqrt{10-1}} \frac{.89 \text{ g}}{5.0 \text{ cm}} = .056 \text{ g/cm}$$

Like the sample mean, both *a* and *b* are computed from sums of the observations. Like the distributions of all possible values of the sample mean, the distributions of all possible values of *a* and *b* tend to be normally distributed. (This result is another consequence of the central-limit theorem.) The specific values of *a* and *b* associated with the regression line are then randomly selected from normally distributed populations. Therefore, these standard errors can be used to compute confidence intervals and test hypotheses using the *t* distribution, just as we did for the sample mean in Chap. 7.

*For a derivation of these formulas, see J. Neter and W. Wasserman, *Applied Statistical Models,* Irwin, Homewood, Ill., 1974, chap. 3, "Inferences in Regression Analysis."

A

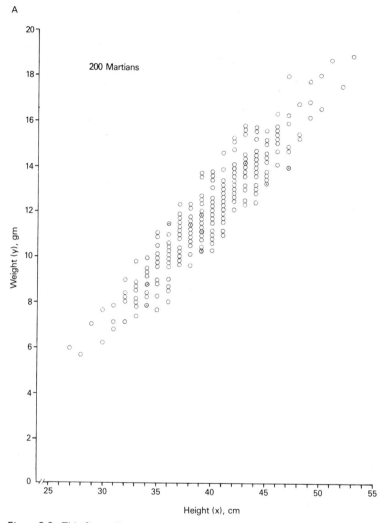

Figure 8-6 This figure illustrates a second random sample of 10 Martians drawn from the population in Fig. 8-1. This sample is associated with a different regression line from that computed from the first sample, shown in Fig. 8-5A.

HOW CONVINCING IS THE TREND?

There are many hypotheses we can test about regression lines, but the most common and important one is that the slope of the line of means

B

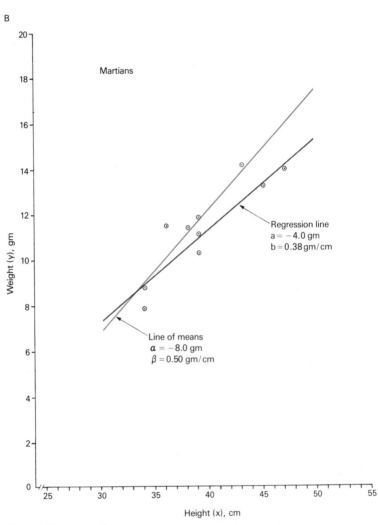

Figure 8-6 (continued)

is zero. This hypothesis is equivalent to estimating the chance that we would observe a trend as strong or stronger than the data show *when there is actually no relationship* between the dependent and independent variables. The resulting *P* value quantifies the certainty with which you can reject the hypothesis that there is no *linear* trend relating the two variables.*

Since the population of possible values of the regression slope is approximately normally distributed, we can use the general definition of the t statistic

$$t = \frac{\text{parameter estimate} - \text{true value of population parameter}}{\text{standard error of parameter estimate}}$$

to test this hypothesis. The equivalent mathematical statement is

$$t = \frac{b - \beta}{s_b}$$

This equation permits testing the hypothesis that there is no trend in the population from which the sample was drawn, that is, $\beta = 0$, using either of the approaches to hypothesis testing developed earlier.

To take a classical hypothesis-testing approach (as in Chap. 4), set β to zero in the equation above and compute

$$t = \frac{b}{s_b}$$

then compare the resulting value of t with the critical value t_α defining the 100α percent most extreme values of t that would occur if the hypothesis of no trend in the population was true. (Use the value corresponding to $\nu = n - 2$ degrees of freedom.)

For example, the data in Fig. 8-3B (and Table 8-1) yielded $b = .45$ g/cm and $s_b = .057$ g/cm from a sample of 10 points. Hence, $t = .45/.057 = 7.894$, which exceeds 5.041, the value of t for $P < .001$ with $\nu = 10 - 2 = 8$ degrees of freedom (from Table 4-1). Hence, it is unlikely that this sample was drawn from a population in which there was no relationship between the independent and dependent variables, i.e., height and weight. We can use these data to assert that as height increases, weight increases ($P < .001$).

---

*This restriction is important. As discussed later in this chapter, it is possible for there to be a strong *nonlinear* relationship in the observations and for the procedures we discuss here to miss it.

Of course, like all statistical tests of hypotheses, this small P value does not guarantee that there is really a trend in the population. For example, the sample in Fig. 1-2A is associated with $P < .001$. Nevertheless, as Fig. 1-2B shows, there is no trend in the underlying population.

If we wish to test the hypothesis that there is no trend in the population using confidence intervals, we use the definition of t above to find the $100(1 - \alpha)$ percent confidence interval for the slope of the line of means,

$$b - t_\alpha s_b < \beta < b + t_\alpha s_b$$

We can compute the 95 percent confidence interval for β by substituting the value of $t_{.05}$ with $\nu = n - 2 = 10 - 2 = 8$ degrees of freedom, 2.306, into this equation together with the observed values of b and s_b

$$.45 - 2.306(.057) < \beta < .45 + 2.306(.057)$$

$$.32 \text{ g/cm} < \beta < .58 \text{ g/cm}$$

Since this interval does not contain zero, we can conclude that there is a trend in the population ($P < .05$).* Note that the interval contains the true value of the slope of the line of means, $\beta = .5$ g/cm.

It is likewise possible to test hypotheses about, or compute confidence intervals for, the intercept using the fact that

$$t = \frac{a - \alpha}{s_a}$$

is distributed according to the t distribution with $\nu = n - 2$ degrees of freedom. For example, the 95 percent confidence interval for the intercept based on the observations in Fig. 8-3B is

$$a - t_{.05} s_a < \alpha < a + t_{.05} s_a$$

$$-6.2 - 2.306(2.2) < \alpha < -6.2 + 2.306(2.2)$$

$$-11.3 \text{ g} < \alpha < -1.1 \text{ g}$$

which includes the true intercept of the line of means, $\alpha = -8$ g.

---

*The 1 percent confidence interval does not contain zero either, so we could obtain the same P value as with the first method using confidence intervals.

A number of other useful confidence intervals associated with regression analysis, such as the confidence interval for the line of means, will be discussed later.

How to Compare Two Regression Lines

It is also possible to use the t test to test hypotheses about two regression lines. For example, to test the hypothesis that two samples were drawn from populations with the same slope of the line of means, we compute

$$t = \frac{\text{difference of regression slopes}}{\text{standard error of difference of regression slopes}}$$

This test is exactly analogous to the definition of the t test to compare two sample means. The standard error of the difference of two regression slopes is *

$$s_{b_1 - b_2} = \sqrt{s_{b_1}^2 + s_{b_2}^2}$$

and so

$$t = \frac{b_1 - b_2}{s_{b_1 - b_2}}$$

The resulting value of t is compared with the critical value of t cor-

---

*This equation provides the best estimate of the standard error of the difference of the slopes if both regression lines are computed from the same number of data points. If there are a different number of points, use the pooled estimate of the difference of slopes (analogous to the pooled estimate of the variance in the t test in Chapter 4):

$$s_{y \cdot x_p}^2 = \frac{(n_1 - 2) s_{y \cdot x_1}^2 + (n_2 - 2) s_{y \cdot x_2}^2}{n_1 + n_2 - 4}$$

in

$$s_{b_1 - b_2} = \sqrt{\frac{s_{y \cdot x_p}^2}{(n_1 - 1) s_{x_1}^2} + \frac{s_{y \cdot x_p}^2}{(n_2 - 1) s_{x_2}^2}}$$

where subscripts 1 and 2 refer to the data for the first and second regression data samples.

responding to $\nu = (n_1 - 2) + (n_2 - 2) = n_1 + n_2 - 4$ degrees of freedom. Similar tests can be constructed to compare intercepts and entire regression lines. There are also procedures analogous to analysis of variance to compare more than two regression lines, but we will not discuss them.*

Dietary Fat and Breast Cancer

Diet influences the development and growth of certain cancers, such as cancer of the breast, in experimental animals. To see whether or not people show the same tendency to develop breast cancer as laboratory mice and rats fed diets high in fat, Carroll[†] plotted the age-adjusted death rate for breast cancer against daily animal-fat intake (Fig. 8-7A) and daily vegetable-fat intake (Fig. 8-7B) for people in 39 different countries.

The regression line associated with the data in Fig. 8-7A is

$$\hat{y} = 2.5 + .16/(g/day)x_A$$

in which $\hat{y}$ represents the age-adjusted death rate (per 100,000 population) on the regression line and x_A represents the animal fat intake, in grams per day. The standard error of the slope s_b is $.013/(g/day)$. To test the hypothesis that there is no relationship between animal-fat intake and death rate from breast cancer compute

$$t = \frac{b}{s_b} = \frac{.16}{.013} = 12$$

This value exceeds 3.574, the value that defines the .1 percent most extreme values of the t distribution with $\nu = 39 - 2 = 37$ degrees of freedom. Thus, with less than 1 chance in 1000 of being wrong ($P < .001$) we can report that the death rate from breast cancer increases as dietary animal-fat consumption increases.

What about the relationship between vegetable fat and death rate

---

*See J. H. Zar, *Biostatistical Analysis,* Prentice-Hall, Englewood Cliffs, N.J., 1974, chap. 17, "Comparing Simple Linear Regression Equations," for a concise discussion of these procedures.

†K. K. Carroll, "Experimental Evidence of Dietary Factors and Hormone-Dependent Cancers," *Cancer Res.* **35**:3375–3383, 1975.

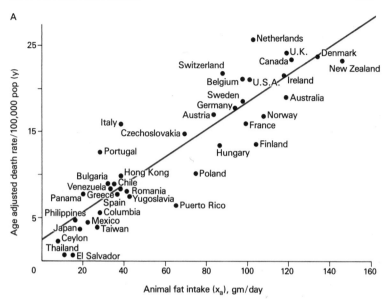

Figure 8-7 Relationship between per capita consumption of animal fat (A) and vegetable fat (B) and age-adjusted death rate from breast cancer in 39 different countries. There appears to be a strong relationship for animal fat but not vegetable fat. (*Adapted from fig. 4 of K. K. Carroll, "Experimental Evidence of Dietary Factors and Hormone-Dependent Cancers," Cancer Res., 35:3374–3383, 1975.*)

from breast cancer? The observations in Fig. 8-7B are associated with the regression equation

$$\hat{y} = 10.4 + .084/(\text{g/day})x_V$$

and the standard error of the slope is .056/(g/day). To test the hypothesis that there is no relationship between death rate and vegetable fat intake, compute

$$t = \frac{b}{s_b} = \frac{.084}{.056} = 1.5$$

which is not sufficient to reject the hypothesis of no linear trend. Notice that the regression line in Fig. 8-7B is essentially flat, indicating no trend between the two variables.

B

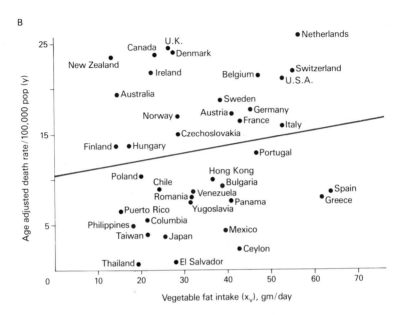

These two studies suggest that animal fat, as opposed to vegetable fat, is an important environmental determinant of the likelihood that a woman will develop breast cancer. Does this prove that eating animal fat *causes* cancer? Not at all. Carroll could not manipulate the diets of the women in the 39 countries he observed, so these data are results of observational rather than experimental studies. There may not be a direct causal link between animal-fat consumption and the development of breast cancer; these two variables may both be related to some third, underlying variable that makes both of them change simultaneously.* The important thing that strengthens the link between fat intake and

*For example, the incidence of breast cancer also increases with a wide variety of other variables, including income, automobiles, and television sets, although these factors are not as closely related to death rate as dietary fat intake. (For more details, see B. S. Drasar and D. Irving, "Environmental Factors and Cancer of the Colon and Breast," *Br. J. Cancer,* 27:167–172, 1973.) Does this mean that television causes cancer? Probably not, although there is always the chance that low-level x-ray or other radiation leaks may be a factor. Rather, all these observations, taken together, suggest that the constellation of factors related to a sedentary and affluent life style are important factors in determining the risk of developing breast cancer.

cancer in people is the fact that fat consumption affects cancer development in animal experiments where the investigator *can* actively manipulate the diet. Note, however, that this link in human beings rests on scientific, as opposed to purely statistical, reasoning.

When interpreting the results of regression analysis, it is important to keep the distinction between observational and experimental studies in mind. When investigators can actively manipulate the independent variable and observe changes in the dependent variable, they can draw strong conclusions about how changes in the independent variable *cause* changes in the dependent variable. On the other hand, when investigators only observe the two variables changing together, they can only observe an *association* between them in which one changes as the other changes. It is impossible to rule out the possibility that both variables are independently responding to some third factor and that the independent variable does not causally affect the dependent variable.

USING REGRESSION LINES TO MAKE PREDICTIONS

Linear-regression analysis has two general uses. The first use, discussed above, is as a scientific tool to identify potentially causal relationships between two variables, like height and weight or death rate from breast cancer and dietary habits. The second use is in applications when there is no question that the two variables are causally related and you wish to use one to predict the other.

Measuring Heart Size with an Angiogram

The heart's ability to pump blood depends on how large it is as it begins to contract; cardiologists are therefore interested in the volume of the heart's chambers, especially the left ventricle, in their patients. One way to estimate the volume of the left ventricle is to take an *angiogram,* i.e., inject fluid that is opaque to x-rays into the ventricle and film it in two perpendicular x-ray views. Given these two views of the heart, it is possible to estimate the ventricle's volume. Since this method involves some assumptions, cardiologists and radiologists usually calibrate the angiographic volumes by filming casts of left ventricles of known volume obtained from cadavers, computing their volume from the films, then computing the regression line of true (cast) volume on angiographic volume. They then use the result to estimate each patient's

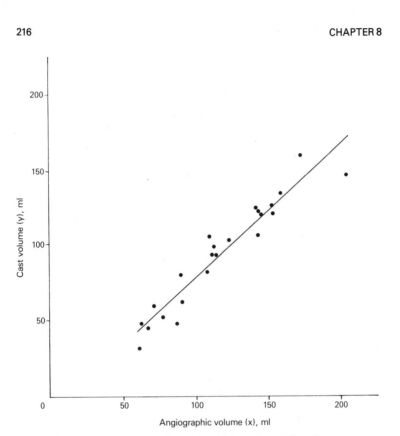

Figure 8-8 Results of an experiment in which angiographic volume was computed from casts of human left ventricles to calibrate the technique for clinical use. (*Data from fig. 5 of M. J. Lipton, T. T. Hayashi, D. Boyd, and E. Carlsson, "Measurement of Left Ventricular Cast Volumes by Computed Tomography," Radiology, 127:419–423, 1978.*)

ventricular volume using the angiographic volume and the regression line.

Figure 8-8 shows one such set of calibration measurements obtained by Lipton and his colleagues.* To use this information to predict the true volume of the left ventricle from the angiographically measured volume, we need to compute the regression of true (cast) volume on

*M. J. Lipton, T. T. Hayashi, D. Boyd, and E. Carlsson, "Measurement of Left Ventricle Cast Volume by Computed Tomography," *Radiology,* **127**:419–423, 1978.

angiographic volume together with some measure of the uncertainty in true volume.

The first part of the problem is easy. Using the methods we have developed above, the regression line is

$$y = -9.94 \text{ mL} + .90x$$

in which y equals the true volume of the cast and x equals the volume computed from the angiogram. This regression line tells how cast volume changes on the average as angiographically determined volume changes.

The points corresponding to the individual casts do not fall precisely on the regression line, however, because of random errors associated with computation of the angiographic volume. (The systematic errors are reflected by the fact that the regression line does not have intercept 0 and slope 1.) The standard error of the estimate $s_{y \cdot x}$ is 10.8 mL for these casts. It may be tempting to use this number to define an interval 2 standard errors of the estimate below and above the regression line as a measure of the range that is likely to include the true cast volume for any given angiographic volume.

The problem with this approach is that it ignores the possible difference between the regression line and the line of means. Therefore, when computing a confidence interval for the value of cast volume at any given angiographic volume, it is necessary to consider two components: uncertainty due to the fact that there is variability in the population about the line of means *and* uncertainty in the actual location of the line of means.

Confidence Interval for the Regression Line

There is uncertainty in the estimates of the slope and intercept of the regression line. The standard errors of the slope and the intercept, s_a and s_b, quantify this uncertainty. These standard errors are $s_a = 7.28$ mL and $s_b = .060$ for the regression of cast volume on angiographic volume. Thus, the line of means could lie slightly above or below the observed regression line or have a slightly different slope. It nevertheless is likely that it lies within a band surrounding the observed regression line. Figure 8-9A shows this region. It is wider at the ends than in the middle because the regression line must be straight and must go through

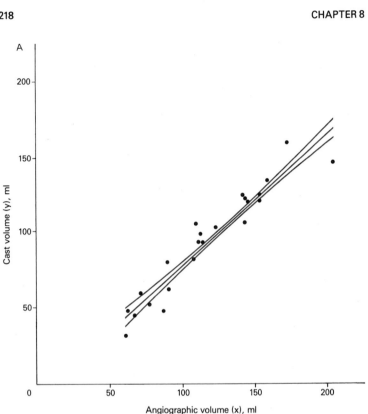

Figure 8-9 (A) The 95 percent confidence interval for the regression line relating angiographic volume to cast volume using the data in Fig. 8-8. (B) The 95 percent confidence interval for an additional observation of cast volume given angiographic volume. This is the confidence interval that should be used to estimate true left ventricular volume from an angiogram to be 95 percent confident that the range includes the true volume.

the point defined by the means of the independent and dependent variables.

There is a distribution of possible values for the regression line at each value of the independent variable x. Since these possible values are normally distributed about the line of means, it makes sense to talk about the standard error of the regression line. (This is another consequence of the central-limit theorem.) Unlike the other standard errors we have discussed so far, this standard error is not constant but depends on the value of the independent variable x:

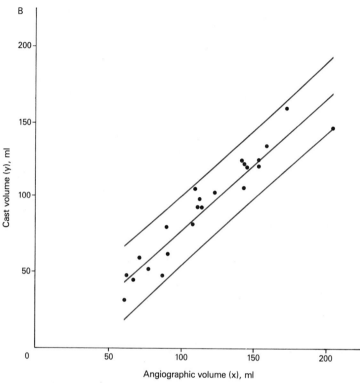

Figure 8-9 (continued)

$$s_{\hat{y}} = s_{y \cdot x} \sqrt{\frac{1}{n} + \frac{(x - \bar{X})^2}{(n - 1)s_X^2}}$$

Since the distribution of possible values of the regression line is normally distributed, we can compute the $100(1 - \alpha)$ percent confidence interval for the regression line with

$$\hat{y} - t_\alpha s_{\hat{y}} < y < \hat{y} + t_\alpha s_{\hat{y}}$$

in which t_α has $\nu = n - 2$ degrees of freedom and $\hat{y}$ is the point on the regression line for each value of x,

$$\hat{y} = a + bx$$

Figure 8-9*A* shows the *95 percent confidence interval for the line of means.* It is wider at the ends than the middle, as it should be. Note also that it is much narrower than the range of the data because it is the confidence interval for the line of means, not the population as a whole.

It is not uncommon for investigators to present the confidence interval for the regression line and discuss it as though it were the confidence interval for the population. This practice is analogous to reporting the standard error of the mean instead of the standard deviation to describe population variability. For example, Fig. 8-9*A* shows that we can be 95 percent confident that the *mean* volume of all casts that resulted in an angiographic volume of 100 mL is between 77 and 81 mL. We cannot be 95 percent confident that the volume of any one cast that has an angiographic volume of 100 mL falls in this narrow range.

Confidence Interval for an Observation

To compute a confidence interval for an individual observation, we must combine the total variability that arises from the variation in the underlying population about the line of means, estimated with $s_{y \cdot x}$, *and* the variability due to uncertainty in the location of the line of means $s_{\hat{y}}$. Since the variance of a sum is the sum of the variances, the standard deviation of the predicted value of the observation will be

$$s_{Y_{new}} = \sqrt{s_{y \cdot x}^2 + s_{\hat{y}}^2}$$

We can eliminate $s_{\hat{y}}$ from this equation by replacing it with the equation for $s_{\hat{y}}$ in the last section

$$s_{Y_{new}} = s_{y \cdot x} \sqrt{1 + \frac{1}{n} + \frac{(x - \bar{X})^2}{(n-1)s_X^2}}$$

This standard error can be used to define the $100(1 - \alpha)$ percent confidence interval for an observation according to

$$\hat{y} - t_\alpha s_{Y_{new}} < y < \hat{y} + t_\alpha s_{Y_{new}}$$

(Remember that both $\hat{y}$ and $s_{Y_{new}}$ depend on the value of the independent variable x.)

The two lines around the regression line in Fig. 8-9*B* show the 95 percent confidence interval for an additional observation. This band includes both the uncertainty due to random variation in the population and variation due to uncertainty in the estimate of the true line of means. Notice that most members of the sample fall in this band. It quantifies the uncertainty in using angiographic volumes to estimate the volumes of casts of human hearts and hence the uncertainty in the true volume of a patient's left ventricle when measured angiographically. For example, it shows that if the angiogram yields a volume of 100 mL, we can be 95 percent confident that the true volume of that patient's left ventricle is between 60 and 105 mL. This confidence interval describes the precision with which it is possible to estimate the true volume of the left ventricle from an angiogram. This information is much more useful than the fact that there is a statistically significant* relationship between the angiographically determined volume and cast volume ($P < .001$).

CORRELATION AND CORRELATION COEFFICIENTS

Linear-regression analysis of a sample provides an estimate of how, on the average, a dependent variable changes when an independent variable changes and an estimate of the variability in the dependent variable about the line of means. These estimates, together with their standard errors, permit computing confidence intervals to show the certainty with which you can predict the value of the dependent variable for a given value of the independent variable. In some experiments, however, two variables are measured that change together, but neither can be considered to be the dependent variable. In such experiments, we abandon all premise of making a statement about causality and simply seek to describe the strength of the relationship between the two variables. The *correlation coefficient*, a number between -1 and +1, is often used to quantify the strength of this association. Figure 8-10 shows that the tighter the relationship between the two variables, the closer the magnitude of *r* to 1; the weaker the relationship between the two variables, the closer *r* is to 0. We will examine two different correlation coefficients.

The first, called the *Pearson product-moment correlation coefficient*, quantifies the strength of association between two variables that

---

*$t = b/s_b = .90/.060 = 15$ for the data in Fig. 8-8. $t_{.001}$ for $\nu = 23 - 2 = 21$ degrees of freedom is 3.819.

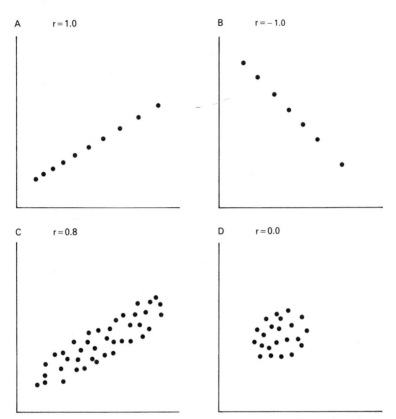

Figure 8-10 The closer the magnitude of the correlation coefficient is to 1, the less scatter there is in the relationship between the two variables. The closer the correlation coefficient is to 0, the weaker the relationship between the two variables.

are normally distributed like those in Fig. 8-1. It therefore provides an alternative perspective on the same data we analyzed using linear regression. When people refer to *the* correlation coefficient, they almost always mean the Pearson product-moment correlation coefficient.

The second, called the *Spearman rank correlation coefficient,* is used to quantify the strength of a trend between two variables that are measured on an *ordinal scale.* In an ordinal scale responses can be graded, but there is no arithmetic relationship between the different possible responses. For example, Pap smears, the common test for cervical cancer, are graded according to this scale: (1) normal, (2) cervicitis (inflammation, usually due to infection), (3) mild to moderate dysplasia (abnormal but noncancerous cells), (4) moderate to severe dysplasia, and (5) cancerous cells present. In this case, a rating of 4 denotes a more serious condition than a rating of 2, but it *is not* necessarily *twice* as serious. This situation contrasts with observations quantified on an *interval scale* where there are arithmetic relationships between the responses. For example, a Martian who weighs 16 g *is* twice as heavy as one who weighs 8 g. Ordinal scales often appear in clinical practice when conditions are ranked according to seriousness.

The Pearson Product-Moment Correlation Coefficient

The problem of describing the strength of association between two variables is closely related to the linear-regression problem, so why not simply arbitrarily make one variable dependent on the other? Figure 8-11 shows that reversing the roles of the two variables when computing the regression line results in *different* regression lines. This situation arises because in the process of computing the slope and intercept of the regression line we minimize the sum of squared deviations between the regression line and the observed values of the *dependent* variable. If we reverse the roles of the two variables, there is a different dependent variable, so different values of the regression-line intercept and slope minimize the sum of squared deviations. We need a measure of association that does not require arbitrarily deciding that one of the variables is the independent variable.

The Pearson product-moment correlation coefficient r, defined by

$$r = \frac{\Sigma(X - \bar{X})(Y - \bar{Y})}{\sqrt{\Sigma(X - \bar{X})^2 \ \Sigma(Y - \bar{Y})^2}}$$

in which the sums are over all the observed (X, Y) points, has this property. Its value does not depend on which variable we call x and y. The magnitude of r describes the *strength of the association* between the two variables, and sign of r tells the direction of this association: $r = +1$ when the two variables increase together (Fig. 8-10A), and $r = -1$ when one decreases as the other increases (Fig. 8-10B). Figure 8-10C also shows the more common case of two variables that are correlated,

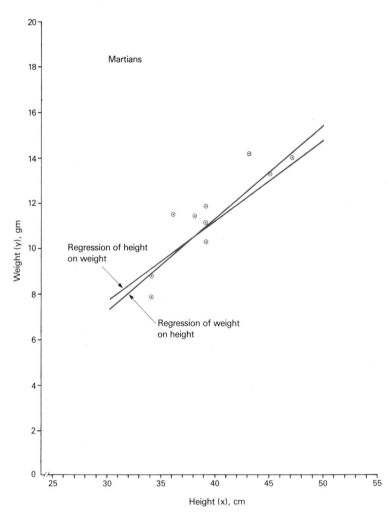

Figure 8-11 The regression of *y* on *x* yields a different regression line than the regression of *x* on *y* for the same data. The correlation coefficient is the same in either case.

though not perfectly. Figure 8-10*D* shows two variables that do not appear to relate to each other at all; $r = 0$.

Table 8-2 illustrates how to compute the correlation coefficient using the sample of 10 points in Fig. 8-3*B*. (These are the same data used

Table 8-2 Computation of Correlation Coefficient for Sample in Fig. 8-3*B*.

Observed weight X, cm	Observed weight Y, g	$(X - \bar{X})$, cm	$(Y - \bar{Y})$, g	$(X - \bar{X})(Y - \bar{Y})$, cm · g	$(X - \bar{X})^2$, cm^2	$(Y - \bar{Y})^2$, g^2
31	7.8	−5.9	−2.6	15.2	34.8	6.7
32	8.3	−4.9	−2.1	10.2	24.0	4.3
33	7.6	−3.9	−2.8	10.8	15.2	7.7
34	9.1	−2.9	−1.3	3.7	8.4	1.6
35	9.6	−1.9	−0.8	1.5	3.6	0.3
35	9.8	−1.9	−0.6	1.1	3.6	2.0
40	11.8	3.1	1.4	4.4	9.6	2.0
41	12.1	4.1	1.7	7.1	16.8	3.0
42	14.7	5.1	4.3	22.0	26.0	18.7
46	13.0	9.1	2.6	23.8	82.8	6.9
369	103.8	0.0	0.0	99.9	224.9	51.8

to illustrate the computation of the regression line in Table 8-1 and Fig. 8-5*B*.) From Table 8-2, $n = 10$, $\bar{X} = \Sigma X/n = 369/10$ cm $= 36.9$ cm, and $\bar{Y} = \Sigma Y/n = 103.8/10$ g $= 10.38$ g, so $\Sigma(X - \bar{X})(Y - \bar{Y}) = 99.9$ g $\cdot$ cm, $\Sigma(X - \bar{X})^2 = 224.9$ cm^2, and $\Sigma(Y - \bar{Y})^2 = 51.8$ g^2. Substitute these numbers into the definition of the correlation coefficient to obtain

$$r = \frac{99.9 \text{ g} \cdot \text{cm}}{\sqrt{224.9 \text{ cm}^2 \cdot 51.8 \text{ g}^2}} = .925$$

To gain more feeling for the meaning to the magnitude of a correlation coefficient, Table 8-3 lists the values of the correlation coefficients for the observations in Figs. 8-2*A*, 8-7, and 8-8.

The Relationship between Regression and Correlation

Obviously, it is possible to compute a correlation coefficient for any data suitable for linear-regression analysis. Indeed, the correlation coefficients in Table 8-3 all were computed from the same examples we used to illustrate regression analysis. In the context of regression analysis it is possible to add to the meaning of the correlation coefficient. Recall that we selected the regression equation that minimized the sum of squared deviations between the points on the regression line and the value of the dependent variable at each observed value of the independent variable. It can be shown that the correlation coefficient also equals

$$r = \sqrt{1 - \frac{\text{sum of squared deviations from regression line}}{\text{sum of squared deviations from mean}}}$$

where the deviations are all measured for the dependent variable.

Let SS$_{res}$ equal the sum of squared deviations (residuals) from the regression line and SS$_{tot}$ equal the total sum of squared deviation from the mean of the dependent variable. Then

$$r = \sqrt{1 - \frac{\text{SS}_{res}}{\text{SS}_{tot}}}$$

Table 8-3 Correlations between Variables in Examples

Fig.	Variables	Correlation coefficient r	Sample size n
8-2A	Height and weight of Martians	.92	10
8-7A	Daily animal-fat consumption and breast cancer death rate	.90	39
8-7B	Daily vegetable-fat consumption and breast cancer death rate	.15	39
8-8	Volume determined from angiogram and true volume of left ventricle cast	.94	23

When there is no variation in the observations about the regression line $SS_{res} = 0$, the correlation coefficient equals 1 (or –1), indicating the dependent variable can be predicted with no uncertainty from the independent variable. On the other hand, when the residual variation about the regression line is the same as the variation about the mean value of the dependent variable, $SS_{res} = SS_{tot}$, there is no trend in the data and $r = 0$. The dependent variable cannot be predicted at all from the independent variable.

The square of the correlation coefficient, r^2, is known as the *coefficient of determination*. Since, from the preceding equation,

$$r^2 = 1 - \frac{SS_{res}}{SS_{tot}}$$

and SS_{tot} is a measure of the total variation in the dependent variable, people say that the coefficient of determination is the fraction of the total variance in the dependent variable "explained" by the regression equation. This is rather unfortunate terminology, because the regression line does not "explain" anything in the sense of providing a mechanistic understanding of the relationship between the dependent and independent variables. Nevertheless, the coefficient of determination is a good description of how clearly a straight line describes the relationship between the two variables.

Likewise, the sum of squared deviations from the regression line, SS_{res}, is just $(n - 2)s_{y \cdot x}^2$ and the sum of squared deviations about the mean, SS_{tot}, is just $(n - 1)s_y^2$. (Recall the definition of sample variance or standard deviation.) Hence, the correlation coefficient is related to the results of regression analysis according to

$$r = \sqrt{1 - \frac{n-2}{n-1} \frac{s_{y \cdot x}^2}{s_y^2}}$$

Thus, as the standard deviation of the residuals about the regression line $s_{y \cdot x}$ decreases with respect to the total variation in the dependent variable, quantified with s_y, the ratio $s_{y \cdot x}/s_y$ decreases and the correlation coefficient increases. Thus, the greater the value of the correlation coefficient, the more precisely the dependent variable can be predicted from the independent variable.

This approach must be used with caution, however, because the absolute uncertainty as described with the confidence interval is usually more informative in that it allows you to gauge the size of the uncertainty in the prediction relative to the size of effect that is of clinical or scientific importance. As Fig. 8-9B showed, it is possible to have correlations well above .9 (generally considered quite respectable in biomedical research) and still have substantial uncertainty in the value of an additional observation for a given value of the independent value.

The correlation coefficient is also related to the slope of the regression equation according to

$$r = b \frac{s_X}{s_Y}$$

We can use the following intuitive argument to justify this relationship. When there is no relationship between the two variables under study, both the slope of the regression line and the correlation coefficient are zero.

How to Test Hypotheses about Correlation Coefficients

Earlier in this chapter we tested for a trend by testing the hypothesis that the slope of the line of means was zero using the t test

$$t = \frac{b}{s_b}$$

with $\nu = n - 2$ degrees of freedom. Since we have just noted that the correlation coefficient is zero when the slope of the regression line is zero, we will test the hypothesis that there is no trend relating two variables by testing the hypothesis that the correlation coefficient is zero with the t test

$$t = \frac{r}{\sqrt{(1 - r^2)/(n - 2)}}$$

with $\nu = n - 2$ degrees of freedom. While this statistic looks quite foreign, it is just another way of writing the t statistic used to test the hypothesis that $b = 0$.*

Dietary Fat and Breast Cancer

To illustrate how to use the correlation coefficient to test for trends, let us return to the observations in Fig. 8-7. From Table 8-2, the correlation between daily animal-fat intake and the age-adjusted death rate from breast cancer, based on data from 39 countries, is .90. To test the

---

*To see this, recall that

$$r = \sqrt{1 - \frac{n - 2}{n - 1} \frac{s_{y \cdot x}^2}{s_Y^2}}$$

so

$$s_{y \cdot x}^2 = \frac{n - 1}{n - 2}(1 - r^2)s_Y^2$$

Use this result to eliminate $s_{y \cdot x}$ from

$$s_b = \frac{1}{\sqrt{n - 1}} \frac{s_{y \cdot x}}{s_X}$$

to obtain

$$s_b = \frac{s_Y}{s_X} \sqrt{\frac{1 - r^2}{n - 2}}$$

Substitute this result, together with $b = r(s_Y/s_X)$ into $t = b/s_b$ to obtain the t test for the correlation coefficient

$$t = \frac{r(s_Y/s_X)}{(s_Y/s_X)\sqrt{(1 - r^2)/(n - 2)}} = \frac{r}{\sqrt{(1 - r^2)/(n - 2)}}$$

hypothesis that there is no linear relationship between breast cancer death rate and animal dietary fat, compute

$$t = \frac{.90}{\sqrt{(1 - .90^2)/(39 - 2)}} = 12$$

Note that this value is exactly the same as the value of t obtained testing for a trend using the slope of the linear regression earlier in the chapter. It must be, since, as just noted, this definition of t is mathematically identical to the one we used to test the slope. The computed value of t exceeds, $t_{.001}$ for $\nu = 39 - 2 = 37$ degrees of freedom, so we can conclude that there is a correlation between dietary fat and breast cancer death rate ($P < .001$).

The correlation coefficient between breast cancer mortality rate and vegetable-fat intake is .15 (from Table 8-2), so

$$t = \frac{.15}{\sqrt{(1 - .15^2)/(39 - 2)}} = .92$$

This value is not large enough to reject the hypothesis that there is no trend relating these two variables.

THE SPEARMAN RANK CORRELATION COEFFICIENT

It is often desirable to test the hypothesis that there is a trend in a clinical state, measured on an ordinal scale, as another variable changes. The Pearson product-moment correlation coefficient is designed to use on data distributed normally along interval scales, so it cannot be used. In addition, it is a parametric statistic that requires that the sample be drawn from a population in which both variables are normally distributed. It also requires that the trend relating the two variables be linear. When the sample suggests that the population in which both variables was drawn from does not meet these criteria, it is often possible to compute a measure of association based on the *ranks* rather than the values of the observations. This new correlation coefficient, called the *Spearman rank correlation coefficient r_S*, is based on ranks and can be used for data quantified with an ordinal scale.* The Spearman rank

---

*Another rank correlation coefficient, known as the Kendall rank correlation coefficient τ, can be generalized to the case in which there are multiple independent variables. For problems involving only two variables it yields conclusions

correlation coefficient is a *nonparametric* statistic because it does not require that the observations be drawn from a normally distributed population.

The idea behind the Spearman rank correlation coefficient is simple. The values of the two variables are ranked in ascending (or descending) order. Next, the Pearson product-moment correlation between the *ranks* (as opposed to the observations) is computed using the same formula as before. A mathematically equivalent formula for the Spearman rank correlation coefficient that is easier to compute is

$$r_S = 1 - \frac{6\Sigma d^2}{n^3 - n}$$

in which d is the difference of the two ranks associated with each point. The resulting correlation coefficient can then be compared with the population of all possible values it would take on if there were in fact no association between the two variables. If the value of r_S associated with the data is larger than this critical value, we conclude that the observations are not compatible with the hypothesis of no association between the two variables.

Table 8-4 illustrates how to compute r_S for the observations in Fig. 8-3. Both the variables (height and weight) are ranked from 1 to 10 (since there are 10 data points), 1 being assigned to the smallest value and 10 to the largest value. When there is a tie, as there is when the height equals 35 cm, both values are assigned the mean of the ranks that would be used if there were no tie. Since the weight tends to increase as height increases, the ranks of both variables increase together. The correlation of these two lists of ranks is the Spearman rank correlation coefficient.

The Spearman rank correlation coefficient for the data in Table 8-3 is

$$r_S = 1$$

$$- \frac{6[(-1)^2 + (-1)^2 + 2^2 + 0^2 + .5^2 + (-.5)^2 + 0^2 + 0^2 + 0^2 + 0^2]}{10^3 - 10} = .96$$

---

identical to the Spearman rank correlation coefficient, although the value of τ associated with a given set of observations differs from the value of r_S associated with the same observations. For a discussion of both procedures, see S. Siegel, *Nonparametric Statistics for the Behavioral Sciences,* McGraw-Hill, New York, 1956, chap. 9, "Measures of Correlation and Their Tests of Significance."

Table 8-4   Computation of Spearman Rank Correlation Coefficient for
Observations in Fig. 8-3

Height		Weight		Difference of
Value, cm	Rank*	Value, g	Rank*	ranks d
31	1	7.7	2	−1
32	2	8.3	3	−1
33	3	7.6	1	2
34	4	9.1	4	0
35	5.5	9.6	5	.5
35	5.5	9.9	6	− .5
40	7	11.8	7	0
41	8	12.2	8	0
42	9	14.8	9	0
46	10	15.0	10	0

*1 = smallest value; 10 = largest value.

Table 8-5 gives various risks of making a Type I error. The observed
value of r_S exceeds .903, the critical value for the most extreme .1 percent of values when there are $n = 10$ data points, so we can report that
there is an association between height and height ($P < .001$).

In this example, of course, we could just as well have used the Pearson product-moment correlation. Had we been dealing with data measured on an ordinal scale, we would have had to use the Spearman rank
correlation coefficient.

Variation among Interns in Use of Laboratory Tests: Relation to Quality of Care

Is extensive use of laboratory tests a mark of a careful and thorough
physician or one who carelessly wastes the patients' money? To study
this question, Schroeder and his colleagues* studied the use of laboratory tests among 21 medical interns. Each intern's clinical ability was
ranked with respect to the rest of the interns by a panel of faculty
members. These ranks form an ordinal scale. The intern who was judged

*S. A. Schroeder, A. Schliftman, and T. E. Piemine, "Variation among Physi-
cians in Use of Laboratory Tests; Relation to Quality of Care," *Medical Care*,
12:709–713, 1974.

Table 8-5   Critical Values for Spearman Rank Correlation Coefficient[*]

	Probability of greater value P								
n	.50	.20	.10	.05	.02	.01	.005	.002	.001
4	.600	1.000	1.000						
5	.500	.800	.900	1.000	1.000				
6	.371	.657	.829	.886	.943	1.000	1.000		
7	.321	.571	.714	.786	.893	.929	.964	1.000	1.000
8	.310	.524	.643	.738	.833	.881	.905	.952	.976
9	.267	.483	.600	.700	.783	.833	.867	.917	.933
10	.248	.455	.564	.648	.745	.794	.830	.879	.903
11	.236	.427	.536	.618	.709	.755	.800	.845	.873
12	.217	.406	.503	.587	.678	.727	.769	.818	.846
13	.209	.385	.484	.560	.648	.703	.747	.791	.824
14	.200	.367	.464	.538	.626	.679	.723	.771	.802
15	.189	.354	.446	.521	.604	.654	.700	.750	.779
16	.182	.341	.429	.503	.582	.635	.679	.729	.762
17	.176	.328	.414	.485	.566	.615	.662	.713	.748
18	.170	.317	.401	.472	.550	.600	.643	.695	.728
19	.165	.309	.391	.460	.535	.584	.628	.677	.712
20	.161	.299	.380	.447	.520	.570	.612	.662	.696
21	.156	.292	.370	.435	.508	.556	.599	.648	.681
22	.152	.284	.361	.425	.496	.544	.586	.634	.667
23	.148	.278	.353	.415	.486	.532	.573	.622	.654
24	.144	.271	.344	.406	.476	.521	.562	.610	.642
25	.142	.265	.337	.398	.466	.511	.551	.598	.630
26	.138	.259	.331	.390	.457	.501	.541	.587	.619
27	.136	.255	.324	.382	.448	.491	.531	.577	.608
28	.133	.250	.317	.375	.440	.483	.522	.567	.598
29	.130	.245	.312	.368	.433	.475	.513	.558	.589
30	.128	.240	.306	.362	.425	.467	.504	.549	.580
31	.126	.236	.301	.356	.418	.459	.496	.541	.571
32	.124	.232	.296	.350	.412	.452	.489	.533	.563
33	.121	.229	.291	.345	.405	.446	.482	.525	.554
34	.120	.225	.287	.340	.399	.439	.475	.517	.547
35	.118	.222	.283	.335	.394	.433	.468	.510	.539
36	.116	.219	.279	.330	.388	.427	.462	.504	.533
37	.114	.216	.275	.325	.383	.421	.456	.497	.526
38	.113	.212	.271	.321	.378	.415	.450	.491	.519
39	.111	.210	.267	.317	.373	.410	.444	.485	.513

Note: See page 234 for footnote.   (Continued)

Table 8-4 Critical Values for Spearman Rank Correlation Coefficient*
(Continued)

	Probability of greater value P								
n	.50	.20	.10	.05	.02	.01	.005	.002	.001
40	.110	.207	.264	.313	.368	.405	.439	.479	.507
41	.108	.204	.261	.309	.364	.400	.433	.473	.501
42	.107	.202	.257	.305	.359	.395	.428	.468	.495
43	.105	.199	.254	.301	.355	.391	.423	.463	.490
44	.104	.197	.251	.298	.351	.386	.419	.458	.484
45	.103	.194	.248	.294	.347	.382	.414	.453	.479
46	.102	.192	.246	.291	.343	.378	.410	.448	.474
47	.101	.190	.243	.288	.340	.374	.405	.443	.469
48	.100	.188	.240	.285	.336	.370	.401	.439	.465
49	.098	.186	.238	.282	.333	.366	.397	.434	.460
50	.097	.184	.235	.279	.329	.363	.393	.430	.456

*For sample sizes greater than 50, use

$$t = \frac{r_S}{\sqrt{(1 - r_S^2)/(n - 2)}}$$

with $\nu = n - 2$ degrees of freedom to obtain the approximate P value.

Source: Adapted from J. H. Zar, *Biostatistical Analysis* Prentice-Hall, Englewood Cliffs, N.J., 1974, p. 498. Used by permission.

to have the most clinical ability was ranked 1, and the one judged to have the least clinical ability was ranked 21. The investigators measured intensity of laboratory use by computing the total cost of laboratory services ordered by each intern during the patients' first 3 days of hospitalization, when the intern would be most actively formulating a diagnosis. Mean costs of laboratory use were computed for each intern's group of patients and ranked in order of increasing cost. Figure 8-12

Figure 8-12 (*A*) Relationship between the relative clinical skill of 21 interns and the relative amount of money each spent on laboratory tests during the first 3 days of a patient's hospitalization. The Spearman rank correlation coefficient for these data is only −.13, which could be interpreted as showing that there is no relationship between clinical skill and expenditures for laboratory tests. (*B*) Closer examination of the data, however, suggests that the best and the worst interns spend less money than those closer to the midrange of skill. Since correlation techniques generally fail to detect such U-shaped relationships, it is important

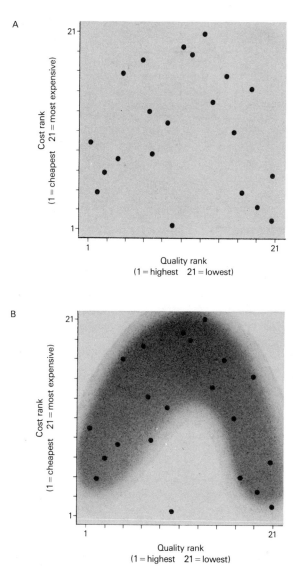

always to examine the raw data as well as the numerical results of a regression or correlation analysis. (*Adapted from fig. 1 of S. A. Schroeder, A. Schliftman, and T. E. Piemine, "Variation in Use of Laboratory Tests: Relation to Quality of Care," Medical Care, 12:709–713, 1974.*)

shows the results of this procedure. Schroeder and his colleagues report that the Spearman rank-order correlation for these two sets of ranks was -.13. This value does not exceed .435, the critical value for r_S to be considered "big" with $P < .05$.

Does this mean that there is no apparent relationship between the quality of an intern and the amount of money spent on laboratory tests? No. Figure 8-12B shows that there is probably a relationship between quality of care and amount of money spent on laboratory tests. The less skilled interns tend to fall at the ends of the cost spectrum; they order many fewer or many more tests than the better interns.

What caused this apparent error? Correlation analysis, whether based on the Pearson or Spearman correlation coefficient, is based on the assumption that if the two variables are related to each other, the relationship takes the form of a consistently upward or downward trend. When the relationship is U-shaped (as in Fig. 8-12) correlation procedures will fail to detect the relationship.

This example illustrates an important rule that should be scrupulously observed when using any form of regression or correlation analysis: Do not just look at the numbers. *Always look at a plot of the raw data* to make sure the data are consistent with the assumptions behind the method of analysis.

PROBLEMS

8-1 Plot the data and compute the linear regression of Y on X and correlation coefficient for each of the following sets of observations:

a X	Y		b X	Y		c X	Y
30	37		30	37		30	37
30	47		30	47		30	47
40	50		40	50		40	50
40	60		40	60		40	60
			20	25		20	25
			20	35		20	35
			50	62		50	62
			50	72		50	72
						10	13
						10	23
						60	74
						60	84

In each case, draw the regression line on the same plot as the data. What stays the same and what changes? Why?

8-2 Plot the data and compute the linear regression of Y on X and correlation coefficient for each of the following sets of observations:

a	X	Y
	15	19
	15	29
	20	25
	20	35
	25	31
	25	41
	30	37
	30	47
	60	40

b	X	Y
	20	21
	20	31
	30	18
	30	28
	40	15
	40	25
	40	75
	40	85
	50	65
	50	75
	60	55
	60	65

In each case, draw the regression line on the same plot as the data. Discuss the results.

8-3 Figure 8-13 shows plots of the following data from four different experiments:

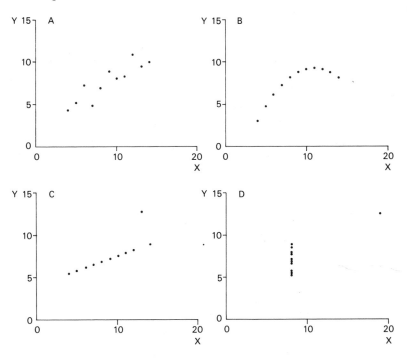

a Experiment 1		b Experiment 2		c Experiment 3		d Experiment 4	
X	Y	X	Y	X	Y	X	Y
10	8.04	10	9.14	10	7.46	8	6.58
8	6.95	8	8.14	8	6.77	8	5.76
13	7.58	13	8.74	13	12.74	8	7.71
9	8.81	9	8.77	9	7.11	8	8.84
11	8.33	11	9.26	11	7.81	8	8.47
14	9.96	14	8.10	14	8.84	8	7.04
6	7.24	6	6.13	6	6.08	8	5.25
4	4.26	4	3.10	4	5.39	19	12.50
12	10.84	12	9.13	12	8.15	8	5.56
7	4.82	7	7.26	7	6.42	8	7.91
5	5.68	5	4.74	5	5.73	8	6.89
ΣX	99		99		99		99
ΣY	82.5		82.5		82.5		82.5
ΣX^2	1001		1001		1001		1001
ΣY^2	660		660		660		660
ΣXY	797.5		797.5		797.5		797.5

Compute the regression and correlation coefficients for each of these four sets of data. Discuss the similarities and differences among these sets of data. Include an examination of the assumptions made in linear regression and correlation analyses.

8-4 As part of the study on retinal permeability of patients with diseased retinas discussed in Prob. 4-2, Gerald Fishman and his coworkers wanted to see if retinal permeability changes were associated with changes in the electrical activity (ERG) of the retinal light-sensing cells as they responded to standardized light stimuli. Do the following data suggest an association?

Penetration ratio, 10^{-6}/min	ERG, μV
19.5	0.0
15.0	38.5
13.5	59.0
23.3	97.4
6.3	119.2
2.5	129.5
13.0	198.7
1.8	248.7
6.5	318.0
1.8	438.5

8-5 There is a continuing search for ways to measure the size of the heart without requiring invasive procedures like angiography that require placing a tube in the heart and injecting contrast medium that will be visible when x-rayed. One promising technique involves infusing a radioactive tracer (such as ^{99m}Tc-HSA) into the circulation. When this material reaches the heart, the radioactive emissions can be recorded with an appropriate sensor and these number of emissions used to estimate the volume of the heart's chambers. Robert Slutsky and his colleagues ("Left Ventricular Volumes by Gated Equilibrium Radionuclide Angiography: A New Method," *Circulation,* **60**:556–564, 1979, by permission of the American Heart Association, Inc.) proposed a method for solving the various technical problems (such as the fact that since the heart is beating the volume is changing during the time it takes to count the radioactive emissions) and compared the resulting volumes computed at end of diastole (when the heart has finished filling and is just about to contract) and the end of systole (when the heart has finished ejecting blood and is about to begin filling again) with those measured in the same people during a conventional angiogram. Here are their results:

Patient	End-diastolic volume, ml		End-systolic volume, ml	
	Radionuclide	Angiographic	Radionuclide	Angiographic
1	75	101	35	47
2	48	75	30	35
3	126	126	52	49
4	93	106	23	23
5	201	195	103	88
6	260	265	182	173
7	40	60	14	12
8	293	288	166	163
9	95	94	27	29
10	58	67	24	25
11	91	81	50	25
12	182	168	139	131
13	91	89	50	49
14	88	102	40	44
15	161	150	57	60
16	118	94	41	18
17	120	129	48	40

240 CHAPTER 8

What is the relationship between the volumes measured using these two techniques at end of diastole? At end of systole? In each case, how good is the correlation? Plot the regression lines and 95 percent confidence intervals for predicting angiographic volume from radionuclide volume in each case. Plot the results. If the radionuclide study indicates an end-diastolic volume of 150 mL, what is the 95 percent confidence interval for the angiographic volume? Compare the slopes and intercepts of the regression lines for the end-diastolic and end-systolic volumes. Are these lines significantly different? If so, propose an explanation; if not, compute a single regression line and confidence intervals for all the data.

8-6 Because daily protein allowances suggested by the World Health Organization and the Japanese Committee on Nutrition are largely based on studies of men, Kayoko Kaneko and Goro Koike studied the utilization of protein in Japanese women ("Utilization and Requirement of Egg Protein in Japanese Women," *J. Nutr. Sci. Vitaminol. (Tokyo)* **31**:43–52, 1985). As part of their study they examined how nitrogen balance depended on nitrogen intake in two groups of women, one on a total daily energy intake of 37 kcal/kg and one on a total daily energy intake of 33 kcal/kg. Here are the data:

Energy intake

37 kcal/kg		33 kcal/kg	
Nitrogen intake	Nitrogen balance	Nitrogen intake	Nitrogen balance
49	−30	32	−32
47	−22	32	−20
50	−29	32	−17
76	−22	51	−10
77	−15	53	−20
99	−10	51	−18
98	−11	52	−21
103	−10	74	4
118	−1	72	−16
105	−4	74	−14
100	−13	98	6
98	−14	97	−7

Compute the linear regressions for each of these groups. Plot the data and draw the regression lines on the same plot. Is there a difference in the relation between nitrogen balance and intake depending on total energy intake?

8-7 It has been suggested that people who are depressed can be identified (or characterized) by their rapid eye movement (REM) patterns during sleep. To further elaborate these patterns, Wojciech
Jernajczyk ("Latency of Eye Movement and Other REM Sleep
Parameters in Bipolar Depression," *Biol. Psychiatry* 21:465–472,
1986) studied 10 patients identified as depressed by history and
clinical psychiatric examination. Part of the examination consisted
of evaluation by two rating systems. Here are the scores of evaluation by two rating systems:

Depression score

Patient	Beck depression inventory	Hamilton rating scale for depression
1	20	22
2	11	14
3	13	10
4	22	17
5	37	31
6	27	22
7	14	12
8	20	19
9	37	29
10	20	15

Do these rating systems give similar assessments of depression?

8-8 Mouthwashes that contain chlorhexidine have been shown to be
effective in preventing formation of dental plaque, but they taste
terrible and may stain the teeth. Ammonium chloride mouthrinses
taste better and do not generally stain the teeth, so they are used in
several commercially available mouthwashes even though they are not
thought to effectively inhibit plaque formation. In light of the continuing use of ammonium chloride–based mouthwashes, F. P. Ashley
and his colleagues ("Effect of a 0.1% Cetylpyridinium Chloride
Mouthrinse on the Accumulation and Biochemical Composition of
Dental Plaque in Young Adults," *Caries Res.* 18:465–471, 1984)
studied the use of such a rinse. Two treatments were studied: a
control inactive rinse over a 48-hour period and an active rinse over
a 48-hour period. Each subject received both treatments in random
order. The amount of plaque was assessed by a clinical score after
24 and 48 hours and by measuring the weight of the plaque accumulation after 48 hours. To see if the clinical scores could be effectively used to assess plaque buildup at 24 hours (when the ac-

tual weight of plaque was not measured), these workers correlated the clinical scores and amount of plaque obtained at 48 hours. Do these data suggest that there is a strong association between the clinical score and the amount of plaque?

Clinical score	Dry weight of plaque, mg
25	2.7
32	1.2
45	2.7
60	2.1
60	3.5
65	2.8
68	3.7
78	8.9
80	5.8
83	4.0
100	5.1
110	5.1
120	4.8
125	5.8
140	11.7
143	8.5
143	11.1
145	7.1
148	14.2
153	12.2

8-9 Normal red blood cells are biconcave. A form of hemoglobin present in some black people makes the red blood cells sickle-shaped. In some individuals, this trait is benign and produces no symptoms. Others develop anemic "crises," in which low concentrations of oxygen in some peripheral circulatory bed produces a change in the red blood cells. This makes them adopt a sickle shape, causing difficulty in passing through the capillaries and impeding the flow of blood through this area. This reduced flow can damage the affected organs by starving them of oxygen; often large quantities of the person's red blood cells are destroyed, resulting in severe anemia that requires several weeks to recover from and sometimes causes death. There is, however, great variability in the clinical severity of problems associated in sickle-cell anemia among people with very similar blood and genetic makeup. Robert Hebbel and his colleagues ("Erythrocyte Adherence to Endothelium in

Sickle-Cell Anemia: A Possible Determinant of Disease Severity,"
N. Engl. J. Med., **302**:992–995, 1980, used by permission) questioned the view that changes in the shape of the red blood cells is the only determinant of sickling crises. In particular, they noticed considerable variability in the tendency of red blood cells to adhere to the inside of the capillaries (the endothelium); they hypothesized that there is a relationship between the clinical severity of disease and the tendency of sickle cells to adhere to the endothelium.

To test this hypothesis, they needed to construct measures of the clinical severity of the disease and the tendency for red blood cells to stick to the endothelium. They constructed a "clinical severity score" that reflects the frequency and severity of each patient's symptoms by assigning points to the following symptoms:

	Points
Crises per year requiring hospitalization or narcotics:	
1–5	1
6–10	2
11–15	3
Skin ulcerations	2
Retinal lesions	1
Central nervous system abnormalities (stroke or unexplained convulsions)	2
Bone lesions (infarcts or aseptic necrosis), per lesion	2

They then summed the points assigned to each patient to obtain an ordinal measure of disease severity, with totally asymptomatic individuals having a score of 0 and progressively sicker individuals having progressively higher scores.

To measure the adherence of sickle cells to endothelium, a blood sample was incubated with endothelium that had been grown in cell culture; then the endothelium was washed with a cell-free solution. They measured the mass of cells that adhered to the endothelium, then divided it by the mass of normal red blood cells that adhered to the same endothelium. Thus, the resulting number, called the *adherence ratio* equaled 1 for normal cells and exceeded 1 when the cells tended to stick to the endothelium.

Hebbel and his colleagues then measured the clinical severity of disease and the adherence ratio in 20 patients. Here is what they found:

Clinical severity score	Adherence ratio
0	1.0
0	1.4
1	1.0
1	1.0
1	1.9
1	2.0
1	2.5
1	3.0
2	2.0
2	3.2
3	3.0
3	3.2
3	6.3
4	2.7
5	3.0
5	5.0
5	17.0
6	5.2
9	19.8
11	25.0

Do these data support the hypothesis that there is a relationship between adherence ratio and clinical severity of sickle-cell anemia?

Experiments When Each Subject Receives More Than One Treatment

The procedures for testing hypotheses discussed in Chaps. 3 to 5 apply to experiments in which the control and treatment groups contain *different* subjects (individuals). It is often possible to design experiments in which *each* experimental subject can be observed *before* and *after* one or more treatments. Such experiments are more sensitive because they make it possible to measure how the treatment *affects each individual.* When the control and treatment groups consist of different individuals, the changes due to the treatment may be masked by variability between experimental subjects. This chapter shows how to analyze experiments in which each subject is repeatedly observed under different experimental conditions.

We will begin with the *paired t test* for experiments in which the subjects are observed before and after receiving a single treatment. Then, we will generalize this test to obtain *repeated-measures analysis of variance,* which permits testing hypotheses about any number of treatments whose effects are measured repeatedly in the same subjects. We will explicitly separate the total variability in the observations into three components: variability between the experimental subjects, variability in each individual subject's response, and variability due to the treatments. Like all analyses of variance (including t tests), these procedures require that the observations come from normally distributed populations. (Chapter 10 presents methods based on ranks that do not require this assumption.) Finally, we will develop *McNemar's test* to analyze data measured on a nominal scale and presented in contingency tables.

EXPERIMENTS WHEN SUBJECTS ARE OBSERVED BEFORE AND AFTER A SINGLE TREATMENT: THE PAIRED t TEST

In experiments in which it is possible to observe each experimental subject *before* and *after* administering a single treatment, we will test a hypothesis about the average *change* the treatment produces instead of the difference in average responses with and without the treatment. This approach reduces the variability in the observations due to differences between individuals and yields a more sensitive test.

Figure 9-1 illustrates this point. Panel A shows daily urine production in *two* samples of 10 different people each; one sample group took a placebo and the other took a drug. Since there is little difference in the mean response relative to the standard deviations, it would be hard to assert that the treatment produced an effect on the basis of these observations. In fact, t computed using the methods of Chap. 4 is only 1.33, which comes nowhere near $t_{.05} = 2.101$, the critical value for $\nu = 2(n - 1) = 2(10 - 1) = 18$ degrees of freedom.

Now consider Fig. 9-1B. It shows urine productions identical to those in Fig. 9-1A but for an experiment in which urine production was measured in *one* sample of 10 individuals *before* and *after* administering the drug. A straight line connects the observations for each individual. Figure 9-1B shows that the drug increased urine production in 8 of the 10 people in the sample. This result suggests that the drug *is* an effective diuretic.

By concentrating on the *change* in each individual that accompanied taking the drug (in Fig. 9-1B) we could detect an effect that was masked by the variability between individuals when different people received the placebo and the drug (in Fig. 9-1A).

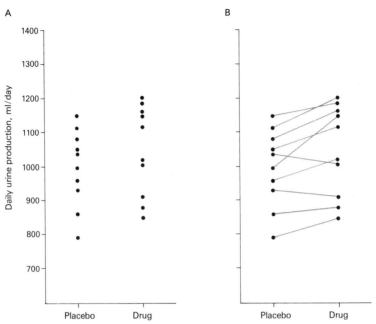

Figure 9-1 (A) Daily urine production in two groups of 10 different people. One group of 10 people received the placebo and the other group of 10 people received the drug. The diuretic does not appear to be effective. (B) Daily urine production in a single group of 10 people before and after taking a drug. The drug appears to be an effective diuretic. The observations are identical to those in panel A; by focusing on changes in each individual's response rather than the response of all the people taken together, it is possible to detect a difference that was masked by the between-subjects variability in panel A.

Now, let us develop a statistical procedure to quantify our subjective impression in such experiments. The *paired t test* can be used to test the hypothesis that there is, on the average, no change in each individual after receiving the treatment under study. Recall that the general definition of the t statistic is

$$t = \frac{\text{parameter estimate} - \text{true value of population parameter}}{\text{standard error of parameter estimate}}$$

The parameter we wish to estimate is the average difference in response δ *in each individual* due to the treatment. If we let d equal the observed change in each individual that accompanies the treatment, we can use $\bar{d}$, the mean change, to estimate δ. The standard deviation of the observed differences is

$$s_d = \sqrt{\frac{\Sigma(d - \bar{d})^2}{n - 1}}$$

So the standard error of the differences is

$$s_{\bar{d}} = \frac{s_d}{\sqrt{n}}$$

Therefore,

$$t = \frac{\bar{d} - \delta}{s_{\bar{d}}}$$

To test the hypothesis that there is, on the average, no response to the treatment, set $\delta = 0$ in this equation to obtain

$$t = \frac{\bar{d}}{s_{\bar{d}}}$$

The resulting value of t is compared with the critical value of $\nu = n - 1$ degrees of freedom.

To recapitulate, when analyzing data from an experiment in which it is possible to observe each individual before and after applying a single treatment:

   ● *Compute the change in response that accompanies the treatment in each individual d.*
   ● *Compute the mean change $\bar{d}$ and the standard error of the mean changes $s_{\bar{d}}$.*
   ● *Use these numbers to compute $t = \bar{d}/s_{\bar{d}}$.*
   ● *Compare this t with the critical value for $\nu = n - 1$ degrees of freedom, where n is the number of experimental subjects.*

Of course, this t test, like all t tests, is predicated on a normally distributed population. In the t test for unpaired observations Chap. 4 developed the responses needed to be normally distributed. In the paired t test the changes associated with the treatment need to be normally distributed.

Cigarette Smoking and Platelet Function

Smokers are more likely to develop diseases caused by abnormal blood clots (thromboses), including heart attacks and occlusion of peripheral arteries, than nonsmokers. Platelets are small bodies that circulate in the blood and stick together to form blood clots. Since smokers experience more disorders related to undesirable blood clots than nonsmokers, Levine* drew blood samples in 11 people before and after they smoked a single cigarette and measured the extent to which platelets aggregated when exposed to a standard stimulus. This stimulus, adenosine diphosphate, makes platelets release their granular contents, which, in turn, makes them stick together and form a blood clot.

Figure 9-2 shows the results of this experiment, with platelet stickiness quantified as the maximum percentage of all the platelets that aggregated after being exposed to adenosine diphosphate. The *pair* of observations made in each individual before and after smoking the cigarette is connected by straight lines. The mean percentage aggregations were 43.1 before smoking and 53.5 after smoking, with standard deviations of 15.9 and 18.7 percent, respectively. Simply looking at these numbers does not suggest that smoking had an effect on platelet aggregation. This approach, however, omits an important fact about the experiment: the platelet aggregations were not measured in two different groups of people, smokers and nonsmokers, but in a single group of people who were observed both before and after smoking the cigarette.

In all but one individual, the maximum platelet aggregation increased after smoking the cigarette, suggesting that smoking facilitates thrombus formation. The means and standard deviations of platelet aggregation before and after smoking for all people taken together did not suggest this pattern because the variability between individuals

*P. H. Levine, "An Acute Effect of Cigarette Smoking on Platelet Function: A Possible Link between Smoking and Arterial Thrombosis," *Circulation,* 48:619–623, 1973.

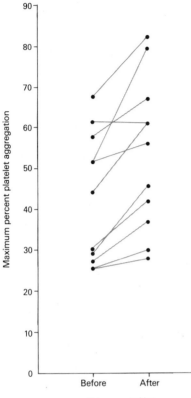

Figure 9-2 Maximum percentage platelet aggregation before and after smoking a tobacco cigarette in 11 people. (*Adapted from fig. 1 of P. H. Levine, "An Acute Effect of Cigarette Smoking on Platelet Function: A Possible Link between Smoking and Arterial Thrombosis," Circulation, 48:619–623, 1973. By permission of the American Heart Association, Inc.*)

masked the variability in platelet aggregation that was due to smoking the cigarette. When we took into account the fact that the observations actually consisted of pairs of observations done before and after smoking in each individual, we could focus on the *change* in response and so remove the variability that was due to the fact that different people have different platelet-aggregation tendencies regardless of whether they smoked a cigarette or not.

The changes in maximum percent platelet aggregation that accompany smoking are (from Fig. 9-2) 2, 4, 10, 12, 16, 15, 4, 27, 9, -1, and 15 percent. Therefore, the mean change in percent platelet aggregation with smoking in these 11 people is $\bar{d}$ = 10.3 percent. The standard deviation of the change is 8.0 percent, so the standard error of the change is $s_{\bar{d}}$ = $8.0/\sqrt{11}$ = 2.41 percent. Finally, our test statistic is

$$t = \frac{\bar{d}}{s_{\bar{d}}} = \frac{10.3}{2.41} = 4.27$$

This value exceeds 3.169, the value that defines the most extreme 1 percent of the t distribution with $\nu = n - 1 = 11 - 1 = 10$ degrees of freedom (from Table 4-1). Therefore, we report that smoking increases platelet aggregation ($P < .01$).

How convincing is this experiment that a constituent of the *tobacco* smoke, as opposed to other chemicals common to smoke in general (e.g., carbon monoxide), or even the stress of the experiment produced the observed change? To investigate this question, Levine also had his subjects "smoke" an unlit cigarette and a lettuce leaf cigarette that contained no nicotine. Figure 9-3 shows the results of these experiments, together with the results of smoking a standard cigarette (from Fig. 9-2).

When the experimental subjects merely pretended to smoke or smoked a nonnicotine cigarette made of dried lettuce, there was no discernible change in platelet aggregation. This situation contrasts with the increase in platelet aggregation that followed smoking a single tobacco cigarette. This experimental design illustrates an important point:

In a well-designed experiment the only difference between the treatment group and the control group, chosen to represent a population of interest, is the treatment.

In this experiment the treatment of interest was tobacco constituents in the smoke, so it was important to compare the results with observations obtained after exposing the subjects to nontobacco smoke. This step helped ensure that the observed changes were due to the tobacco rather than smoking in general. The more carefully the investigator can isolate the treatment effect, the more convincing the conclusions will be.

There are also subtle biases that can cloud the conclusions from an

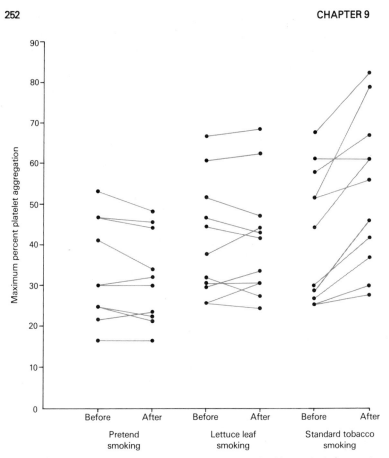

Figure 9-3 Maximum percentage platelet aggregation in 11 people before and after pretending to smoke ("sham smoking"), before and after smoking a lettuce-leaf cigarette that contained no nicotine, and before and after smoking a tobacco cigarette. These observations, taken together, suggest that it was something in the tobacco smoke, rather than the act of smoking or other general constituents of smoke, that produced the change in platelet aggregation. (*Redrawn from fig. 1 of P. H. Levine, "An Acute Effect of Cigarette Smoking on Platelet Function: A Possible Link between Smoking and Arterial Thrombosis," Circulation, 48:619–623, 1973. By permission of the American Heart Association, Inc.*)

experiment. Most investigators, and their colleagues and technicians, want the experiments to support their hypothesis. In addition, the experimental subjects, when they are people, generally want to be helpful and wish the investigator to be correct, especially if the study is evaluating a new treatment that the experimental subject hopes will provide a cure. These factors can lead the people doing the study to tend to slant judgment calls (often required when collecting the data) toward making the study come out the way everyone wants. For example, the laboratory technicians who measure platelet aggregation might read the control samples on the low side and the smoking samples on the high side without even realizing it. Perhaps some psychological factor among the experimental subjects (analogous to a placebo effect) led their platelet aggregation to increase when they smoked the tobacco cigarette. Levine avoided these difficulties by doing the experiments in a *double-blind* manner in which the investigator, the experimental subject, and the laboratory technicians who analyzed the blood samples did not know the content of the cigarettes being smoked until after all experiments were complete and specimens analyzed. Double-blind studies are the most effective way to eliminate bias due to both the observer and experimental subject.

Double-blind indicates that neither the investigator nor the experimental subject knows which treatment (or placebo) the subject is taking at any given time. In *single-blind* studies one party, usually the investigator, knows which treatment is being administered. This approach controls biases due to the placebo effect but not observer biases. Some studies are also partially blind, in which the participants know something about the treatment but do not have full information. For example, the blood platelet study might be considered partially blind because both the subject and the investigator obviously knew when the subject was only pretending to smoke. It was possible, however, to withhold this information from the laboratory technicians who actually analyzed the blood samples to avoid biases in their measurements of percent platelet aggregation.

The paired t test can be used to test hypotheses when observations are taken before and after administering a single treatment to a group of individuals. To generalize this procedure to experiments in which the same individuals are subjected to a number of treatments, we now develop repeated-measures analysis of variance. To do so, we must first introduce some new nomenclature for analysis of variance. To ease the transition, we begin with the analysis of variance presented in Chap. 3, in which each treatment was applied to *different* individuals. After reformulating this type of analysis of variance, we will go on to the case of repeated measurements on the same individual.

ANOTHER APPROACH TO ANALYSIS OF VARIANCE*

When we developed the analysis of variance in Chap. 3, we assumed that all the samples were drawn from a single population (i.e., that the treatments had no effect), estimated the variability in that population from the variability within the sample groups and between the sample groups, then compared these two estimates to see how compatible they were with the original assumption that all the samples were drawn from a single population. When the two estimates of variability were unlikely to arise if the samples had been drawn from a single population, we concluded that at least one of the samples represented a different population (i.e., that at least one treatment had an effect). We used estimates of the population *variance* to quantify variability. In Chap. 8, we used a slightly different method to quantify the variability of observed data points about a regression line. We used the *sum of squared deviations* about the regression line to quantify variability. The variance and sum of squared deviations, of course, are intimately related. One obtains the variance by dividing the sum of squared deviations by the appropriate number of degrees of freedom. We now will recast analysis of variance using sums of squared deviations to quantify variability. This new nomenclature forms the basis of all forms of analysis of variance, including repeated-measures analysis of variance.

In Chap. 3, we considered the following experiment. To determine whether diet affected cardiac output in people living in a small town, we randomly selected four groups of seven people each. People in the control group continued eating normally; people in the second group ate only spaghetti; people in the third group ate only steak; and people in the fourth group ate only fruit and nuts. After 1 month, each person was cathéterized and his cardiac output measured. Figure 3-1 showed that diet did not, in fact, affect cardiac output. Figure 3-2 showed the results of the experiment as they would appear to you as an investigator or reader. Table 9-1 presents the same data in tabular form. The

*This and the following section, which develops repeated-measures analysis of variance (the multitreatment generalization of the paired *t* test), are more mathematical than the rest of the text. Some readers may wish to skip this section until they encounter an experiment that should be analyzed with repeated-measures analysis of variance. Despite the fact that such experiments are common in the biomedical literature, this test is rarely used. This omission leads to the same kinds of multiple-*t*-test errors discussed in Chaps. 3 and 4 for the unpaired *t* test.

Table 9-1 Cardiac Output (L/min) in Different Groups of Seven People Fed Different Diets

	Treatment			
	Control	Spaghetti	Steak	Fruit and nuts
	4.6	4.6	4.3	4.3
	4.7	5.0	4.4	4.4
	4.7	5.2	4.9	4.5
	4.9	5.2	4.9	4.9
	5.1	5.5	5.1	4.9
	5.3	5.5	5.3	5.0
	5.4	5.6	5.6	5.6
Treatment (column) means	4.96	5.23	4.93	4.80
Treatment (column) sums of squares	.597	.734	1.294	1.200

Grand mean = 4.98   Total sum of squares = 4.501

four different groups did show some variability in cardiac output. The question is: How consistent is this observed variability with the hypothesis that diet did not have any effect on cardiac output?

Some New Notation

Tables 9-1 and 9-2 illustrate the notation we will now use to answer this question; it is required for more general forms of analysis of variance. The four different diets are called the *treatments* and are represented by the columns in the table. We denote the four different treatments with the numbers 1 to 4 (1 = control, 2 = spaghetti, 3 = steak, 4 = fruit and nuts). Seven *different* people receive each treatment. Each particular experimental subject (or, more precisely, the observation or data point associated with each subject) is represented by X_{ts}, where t represents the treatment and s represents a specific subject in that treatment group. For example, $X_{11} = 4.6$ L/min represents the observed cardiac output for the first subject ($s = 1$) who received the control diet ($t = 1$). $X_{35} = 5.1$ L/min represents the fifth subject ($s = 5$) who had the steak diet ($t = 3$).

Tables 9-1 and 9-2 also show the mean cardiac outputs for all

Table 9-2   Notation for One-Way Analysis of Variance in Table 9-1

	Treatment			
	1	2	3	4
	X_{11}	X_{21}	X_{31}	X_{41}
	X_{12}	X_{22}	X_{32}	X_{42}
	X_{13}	X_{23}	X_{33}	X_{43}
	X_{14}	X_{24}	X_{34}	X_{44}
	X_{15}	X_{25}	X_{35}	X_{45}
	X_{16}	X_{26}	X_{36}	X_{46}
	X_{17}	X_{27}	X_{37}	X_{47}
Treatment (column) means	$\bar{X}_1$	$\bar{X}_2$	$\bar{X}_3$	$\bar{X}_4$
Treatment (column) sums of squares	$\sum_s (X_{1s}-\bar{X}_1)^2$	$\sum_s (X_{2s}-\bar{X}_2)^2$	$\sum_s (X_{3s}-\bar{X}_3)^2$	$\sum_s (X_{4s}-\bar{X}_4)^2$

Grand mean = $\bar{X}$ Total sum of squares = $\sum_t \sum_s (X_{ts} - \bar{X})^2$

subjects (in this case, people) receiving each of the four treatments, labeled $\bar{X}_1$, $\bar{X}_2$, $\bar{X}_3$, and $\bar{X}_4$. For example, $\bar{X}_2 = 5.23$ L/min is the mean cardiac output observed among people who were treated with spaghetti. The tables also show the variability within each of the treatment groups, quantified by the *sum of squared deviations about the treatment mean,*

Sum of squares for treatment t = sum, over all subjects who received treatment t, of (value of observation for subject – mean response of all individuals who receive treatment t)^2

The equivalent mathematical statement is

$$SS_t = \sum_s (X_{ts} - \bar{X}_t)^2$$

The summation symbol, Σ, has been modified to indicate that we sum over all s subjects who received treatment t. We need this more explicit notation because we will be summing up the observations in different ways. For example, the sum of squared deviations from the mean cardiac output for the seven people who ate the control diet ($t = 1$) is

$$SS_1 = \sum_s (X_{1s} - \bar{X}_1)^2$$
$$= (4.6 - 4.96)^2 + (4.7 - 4.96)^2 + (4.7 - 4.96)^2 + (4.9 - 4.96)^2$$
$$+ (5.1 - 4.96)^2 + (5.3 - 4.96)^2 + (5.4 - 4.96)^2$$
$$= .597 \ (L/min)^2$$

Recall that the definition of sample variance is

$$s^2 = \frac{\sum(X - \bar{X})^2}{n - 1}$$

where n is the size of the sample. The expression in the numerator is just the sum of squared deviations from the sample mean, so we can write

$$s^2 = \frac{SS}{n - 1}$$

Hence, the variance in treatment group t equals the sum of squares for that treatment divided by the number of individuals who received the treatment (i.e., the sample size) minus 1:

$$s_t^2 = \frac{SS_t}{n - 1}$$

In Chap. 3, we estimated the population variance from within the groups for our diet experiment with the average of the variances computed from within each of the four treatment groups

$$s_{wit}^2 = \frac{1}{4}(s_{con}^2 + s_{spa}^2 + s_{st}^2 + s_{fn}^2)$$

In the notation of Table 9-1, we can rewrite this equation as

$$s_{\text{wit}}^2 = \frac{1}{4}(s_1^2 + s_2^2 + s_3^2 + s_4^2)$$

Now, replace each of the variances in terms of sums of squares

$$s_{\text{wit}}^2 = \frac{1}{4}\left[\frac{\sum_s(X_{1s} - \bar{X}_1)^2}{n-1} + \frac{\sum_s(X_{2s} - \bar{X}_2)^2}{n-1} + \frac{\sum_s(X_{3s} - \bar{X}_3)^2}{n-1}\right.$$
$$\left. + \frac{\sum_s(X_{4s} - \bar{X}_4)^2}{n-1}\right]$$

or

$$s_{\text{wit}}^2 = \frac{1}{4}\left(\frac{SS_1}{n-1} + \frac{SS_2}{n-1} + \frac{SS_3}{n-1} + \frac{SS_4}{n-1}\right)$$

in which $n = 7$ represents the size of each sample group. Factor $n - 1$ out of the four expressions for variance computed from within each of the four separate treatment groups, and let $m = 4$ represent the number of treatments (diets), to obtain

$$s_{\text{wit}}^2 = \frac{1}{m}\frac{SS_1 + SS_2 + SS_3 + SS_4}{n-1}$$

The numerator of this fraction is just the total of the sums of squared deviations of the observations about the means of their respective treatment groups. Call it the *within-treatments (or within-groups) sum* of squares SS_{wit}. Note that the within-treatments sum of squares is a measure of variability in the observations that is independent of whether or not the mean responses to the different treatments are the same.

For the data from our diet experiment in Table 9-1

$$SS_{wit} = .597 + .734 + 1.294 + 1.200 = 3.825 \ (L/min)^2$$

Given our definition of SS_{wit} and the equation for s_{wit}^2 above, we can write

$$s_{wit}^2 = \frac{SS_{wit}}{m(n-1)}$$

s_{wit}^2 appears in the denominator of the F ratio associated with $\nu_d = m(n-1)$ degrees of freedom. In general, analysis-of-variance degrees of freedom are generally denoted by DF rather than ν, so let us replace $m(n-1)$ with DF_{wit} in the equation for s_{wit}^2 to obtain

$$s_{wit}^2 = \frac{SS_{wit}}{DF_{wit}}$$

For the diet experiment, $DF_{wit} = m(n-1) = 4(7-1) = 24$ degrees of freedom.

Finally, recall that in Chap. 2 we defined the variance as the "average" squared deviation from the mean. In this spirit, statisticians call the ratio SS_{wit}/DF_{wit} the within-groups *mean square* and denote it MS_{wit}. This notation is clumsy, since SS_{wit}/DF_{wit} is not really a mean in the standard statistical meaning of the word, and it obscures the fact that MS_{wit} is the estimate of the variance computed from within the groups (that we have been denoting s^2_{wit}). Nevertheless, it is so ubiquitous that we will adopt it. Therefore, we will estimate the variance from within the sample groups with

$$MS_{\text{wit}} = \frac{SS_{\text{wit}}}{DF_{\text{wit}}}$$

We will replace s^2_{wit} in the definition of F with this expression.

For the data in Table 9-1

$$MS_{\text{wit}} = \frac{3.825}{24} = .159 \; (\text{L/min})^2$$

Next, we need to do the same thing for the variance estimated from between the treatment groups. Recall that we estimated this variance by computing the standard deviation of the sample means as an estimate of the standard error of the mean, then estimated the population variance with

$$s^2_{\text{bet}} = ns^2_{\bar{X}}$$

The square of the standard deviation of treatment means is

$$s^2_{\bar{X}} = \frac{(\bar{X}_1 - \bar{X})^2 + (\bar{X}_2 - \bar{X})^2 + (\bar{X}_3 - \bar{X})^2 + (\bar{X}_4 - \bar{X})^2}{m - 1}$$

in which m again denotes the number of treatment groups (4) and $\bar{X}$ denotes the mean of *all* the observations (which also equals the mean of the sample means when the samples are all the same size). We can write this equation more compactly as

$$s^2_{\bar{X}} = \frac{\sum_t (\bar{X}_t - \bar{X})^2}{m - 1}$$

so that

$$s^2_{\text{bet}} = \frac{n\sum_t (\bar{X}_t - \bar{X})^2}{m - 1}$$

(Notice that we are now summing over treatments rather than experimental subjects.) The between-groups variance can be written as the sum of squared deviations of the treatment means about the mean of all observations times the sample size divided by $m - 1$. Denote this sum of squares the *between-groups* or *treatment* sum of squares

$$\text{SS}_{\text{bet}} = \text{SS}_{\text{treat}} = n\sum_t (\bar{X}_t - \bar{X})^2$$

The treatment sum of squares is a measure of the variability between the groups, just as the within-groups sum of squares is a measure of the variability within the groups.

For the data for the diet experiment in Table 9-1

$$
\begin{aligned}
\text{SS}_{\text{treat}} &= n\sum_t (\bar{X}_t - \bar{X})^2 \\
&= 7\,[(4.96 - 4.98)^2 + (5.23 - 4.98)^2 + (4.93 - 4.98)^2 \\
&\qquad\qquad\qquad\qquad\qquad\qquad\qquad + (4.80 - 4.98)^2\,] \\
&= .685\ (\text{L/min})^2
\end{aligned}
$$

The treatment (between-groups) variance appears in the numerator of the F ratio and is associated with $\nu = m - 1$ degrees of freedom; we therefore denote $m - 1$ with

$$\text{DF}_{\text{bet}} = \text{DF}_{\text{treat}} = m - 1$$

in which case

$$s^2_{\text{bet}} = \frac{\text{SS}_{\text{bet}}}{\text{DF}_{\text{bet}}} = \frac{\text{SS}_{\text{treat}}}{\text{DF}_{\text{treat}}}$$

Just as statisticians call the ratio SS_{wit} the within-groups mean square, they call the estimate of the variance from between the groups (or treatments) the treatment (or between-groups) mean square MS_{treat} (or MS_{bet}). Therefore,

$$MS_{bet} = \frac{SS_{bet}}{DF_{bet}} = \frac{SS_{treat}}{DF_{treat}} = MS_{treat}$$

For the data in Table 9-1, $DF_{treat} = m - 1 = 4 - 1 = 3$, so

$$MS_{treat} = \frac{.685}{3} = .228 \ (L/min)^2$$

We can write the F-test statistic as

$$F = \frac{MS_{bet}}{MS_{wit}} = \frac{MS_{treat}}{MS_{wit}}$$

and compare it with the critical value of F for numerator degrees of freedom, DF_{treat} (or DF_{bet}), and denominator degrees of freedom, DF_{wit}.

Finally, for the data in Table 9-1

$$F = \frac{MS_{treat}}{MS_{wit}} = \frac{.228}{.159} = 1.4$$

the same value of F we obtained from these data in Chap. 3.

We have gone far afield into a computational procedure that is more complex and, on the surface, less intuitive than the one developed in Chap. 3. This approach is necessary, however, to analyze the results obtained in more complex experimental designs. Surprisingly, there are intuitive meanings which can be attached to these sums of squares and which are very important.

Accounting for All the Variability in the Observations

The sums of squares within and between the treatment groups, SS_{wit} and SS_{treat}, quantify the variability observed within and between the treatment groups. In addition, it is possible to describe the total variability observed in the data by computing the *sum of squared devi-*

ations of all observations about the grand mean $\bar{X}$ of all the observations, called *the total sum of squares*

$$SS_{tot} = \sum_t \sum_s (X_{ts} - \bar{X})^2$$

The two summation symbols indicate the sums over all subjects in all treatment groups.

The total number of degrees of freedom associated with this sum of squares is $DF_{tot} = mn - 1$, or 1 less than the total sample size (m treatment groups times n subjects in each treatment group). For the observations in Table 9-1,

$$SS_{tot} = 4.501 \ (L/min)^2 \quad \text{and} \quad DF_{tot} = 4(7) - 1 = 27$$

Notice that the variance estimated from all the observations, without regard for the fact that there are different experimental groups, is just

$$\frac{\sum_t \sum_s (X_{ts} - \bar{X})^2}{mn - 1} = \frac{SS_{tot}}{mn - 1}$$

The three sums of squares discussed so far are related in a very simple way:

The total sum of squares is the sum of the treatment (between-groups) sum of squares and the within-groups sum of squares

$$SS_{tot} = SS_{bet} + SS_{wit}$$

In other words, the total variability, quantified with appropriate sums of squared deviations, can be *partitioned* into two components, one due to variability between the experimental groups and another component due to variability within the groups.* It is common to sum-

---

*To see why this is true, first decompose the amount that any given observation deviates from the grand mean, $X_{ts} - \bar{X}$, into two components, the deviation of the treatment group mean from the grand mean and the deviation of the observation from the mean of its treatment group.

$$(X_{ts} - \bar{X}) = (\bar{X}_t - \bar{X}) + (X_{ts} - \bar{X}_t)$$

(Continued)

marize all these computations in an *analysis-of-variance table* such as Table 9-3. Notice that the treatment and within-groups sums of squares do indeed add up to the total sum of squares.

F is the ratio of MS_{treat} over MS_{wit} and should be compared with the critical value of F with DF_{treat} and DF_{wit} degrees of freedom for the numerator and denominator, respectively, to test the hypothesis that all the samples were drawn from a single population.

Note also that the treatment and within-groups degrees of freedom also add up to the total number of degrees of freedom. This is not a

---

* (Continued)

Square both sides

$$(X_{ts} - \bar{X})^2 = (\bar{X}_t - \bar{X})^2 + (X_{ts} - \bar{X}_t)^2 + 2(\bar{X}_t - \bar{X})(X_{ts} - \bar{X}_t)$$

and sum over all observations to obtain the total sum of squares

$$SS_{tot} = \sum_t \sum_s (X_{ts} - \bar{X})^2$$
$$= \sum_t \sum_s (\bar{X}_t - \bar{X})^2 + \sum_t \sum_s (X_{ts} - \bar{X}_t)^2 + \sum_t \sum_s 2(\bar{X}_t - \bar{X})(X_{ts} - \bar{X}_t)$$

Since $\bar{X}_t - \bar{X}$ does not depend on which of the n individuals in each sample are being summed over,

$$\sum_s (\bar{X}_t - \bar{X})^2 = n(\bar{X}_t - \bar{X})^2$$

The first term on the right of the equals sign can be written

$$\sum_t \sum_s (\bar{X}_t - \bar{X})^2 = n \sum_t (\bar{X}_t - \bar{X})^2$$

which is just SS_{treat}. Furthermore, the second term on the right of the equals sign is just SS_{wit}.

It only remains to show that the third term on the right of the equals sign equals zero. To do this, note again that $\bar{X}_t - \bar{X}$ does not depend on which member of each sample is being summed, so we can factor it out of the sum over the member of each sample, in which case

$$\sum_t \sum_s 2(\bar{X}_t - \bar{X})(X_{ts} - \bar{X}_t) = 2 \sum_t (\bar{X}_t - \bar{X}) \sum_s (X_{ts} - \bar{X}_t)$$

But $\bar{X}_t$ is the mean of the n members of treatment group t, so

$$\sum_s (X_{ts} - \bar{X}_t) = \sum_s X_{ts} - \sum_s \bar{X}_t = \sum_s X_{ts} - n\bar{X}_t = n(\sum_s X_{ts}/n - \bar{X}_t) = n(\bar{X}_t - \bar{X}_t) = 0$$

Therefore,

$$SS_{tot} = SS_{treat} + SS_{wit} + 0 = SS_{treat} + SS_{wit}$$

chance occurrence; it will always be the case. Specifically, if there are m experimental groups with n members each,

$$DF_{treat} = m - 1 \qquad DF_{wit} = m(n - 1) \qquad \text{and} \qquad DF_{tot} = mn - 1$$

so that

$$DF_{treat} + DF_{wit} = (m - 1) + m(n - 1) = m - 1 + mn - m$$
$$= mn - 1 = DF_{tot}$$

In other words, just as it was possible to partition the total sum of squares into components due to treatment (between-group) and within-group variability, it is possible to partition the degrees of freedom. Figure 9-4 illustrates how the sums of squares and degrees of freedom are partitioned in this analysis of variance.

Now we are ready to attack the original problem, that of developing an analysis of variance suitable for experiments in which each experimental subject receives more than one treatment.

EXPERIMENTS WHEN SUBJECTS ARE OBSERVED AFTER MANY TREATMENTS: REPEATED-MEASURES ANALYSIS OF VARIANCE

When each experimental subject receives more than one treatment, it is possible to partition the total variability in the observations into three mutually exclusive components: variability between all the experi-

Table 9-3 Analysis-of-Variance Table for Diet Experiment

Source of variation	SS	DF	MS
Between groups	.685	3	.228
Within groups	3.816	24	.159
Total	4.501	27	

$$F = \frac{MS_{bet}}{MS_{wit}} = \frac{.228}{.159} = 1.4$$

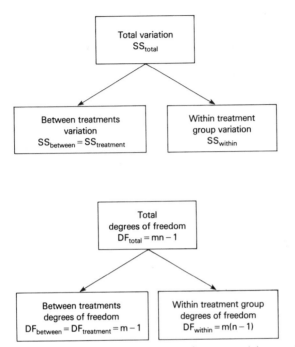

Figure 9-4 Partitioning of the sums of squares and degrees of freedom for a one-way analysis of variance.

mental subjects, variability due to the treatments, and variability within the subjects' response to the treatments. The last component of variability represents the fact there is some random variation in how a given individual responds to a given treatment, together with measurement errors. Figure 9-5 shows this breakdown. The resulting procedure is called a *repeated-measures* analysis of variance because the measurements are repeated under all the different experimental conditions (treatments) in each of the experimental subjects.

Now, let us write expressions for these three kinds of variability. As Fig. 9-5 suggests, the first step is to divide the total variability into variability within subjects and between subjects.

Table 9-4 illustrates the notation we will use for repeated-measures analysis of variance. (In this case it is for an experiment in which four experimental subjects each receive three different treatments.) At first glance, this table appears quite similar to Table 9-2, used to analyze

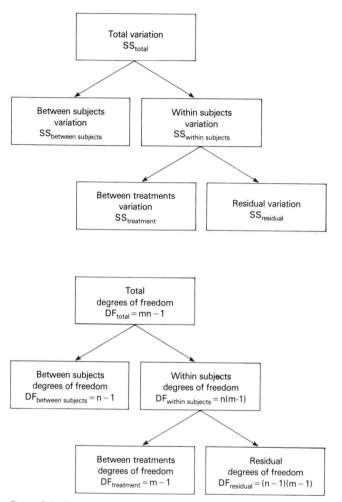

Figure 9-5 Partitioning of the sums of squares and degrees of freedom for a repeated-measures analysis of variance. Notice that this procedure allows us to concentrate on the variation within experimental subjects.

experiments in which *different* subjects received each of the treatments. There is one important difference: in Table 9-4 *the same* subjects receive all the treatments. For example, X_{11} represents how the first experimental subject responded to the first treatment; X_{21} represents

Table 9-4 Notation for Repeated-Measures Analysis of Variance

Experimental subject, $n = 4$	Treatment, $m = 3$			Subject	
	1	2	3	Mean	SS
1	X_{11}	X_{21}	X_{31}	$\bar{S}_1$	$\sum_t (X_{t1} - \bar{S}_1)^2$
2	X_{12}	X_{22}	X_{32}	$\bar{S}_2$	$\sum_t (X_{t2} - \bar{S}_2)^2$
3	X_{13}	X_{23}	X_{33}	$\bar{S}_3$	$\sum_t (X_{t3} - \bar{S}_3)^2$
4	X_{14}	X_{24}	X_{34}	$\bar{S}_4$	$\sum_t (X_{t4} - \bar{S}_4)^2$
Mean	$\bar{T}_1$	$\bar{T}_2$	$\bar{T}_3$		

$$\text{Grand mean } \bar{X} = \frac{\sum_t \sum_s X_{ts}}{mn} \qquad SS_{tot} = \sum_t \sum_s (X_{ts} - \bar{X})^2$$

how the (same) first experimental subject responded to the second treatment. In general, X_{ts} is the response of the sth experimental subject to the tth treatment.

$\bar{S}_1, \bar{S}_2, \bar{S}_3$, and $\bar{S}_4$ are the mean responses of each of the four subjects to all (three) treatments

$$\bar{S}_s = \frac{\sum_t X_{ts}}{m}$$

in which there are $m = 3$ treatments. Likewise, $\bar{T}_1, \bar{T}_2$, and $\bar{T}_3$ are the mean responses to each of the three treatments of all (four) experimental subjects.

$$\bar{T}_t = \frac{\sum_s X_{ts}}{n}$$

in which there are $n = 4$ experimental subjects.

As in all analyses of variance, we quantify the total variation with the total sum of squared deviations of all observations about the grand mean. The grand mean of all the observations is

$$\bar{X} = \frac{\sum\limits_{t}\sum\limits_{s} X_{ts}}{mn}$$

and the total sum of squared deviations from the grand mean is

$$SS_{tot} = \sum_{t}\sum_{s}(X_{ts} - \bar{X})^2$$

This sum of squares is associated with $DF_{tot} = mn - 1$ degrees of freedom.

Next, we partition this total sum of squares into variation within subjects and variation between subjects. The variation of observations within subject 1 about the mean observed for subject 1, $\bar{S}_1$, is

$$SS_{wit\ subj\ 1} = \sum_{t}(X_{t1} - \bar{S}_1)^2$$

Likewise, the variation in observations within subject 2 about the mean observed in subject 2 is

$$SS_{wit\ subj\ 2} = \sum_{t}(X_{t2} - \bar{S}_2)^2$$

We can write similar sums for the other two experimental subjects. The total variability observed within all subjects is just the sum of the variability observed within each subject

$$SS_{wit\ subjs} = SS_{wit\ subj\ 1} + SS_{wit\ subj\ 2} + SS_{wit\ subj\ 3} + SS_{wit\ subj\ 4}$$

$$= \sum_{s}\sum_{t}(X_{ts} - \bar{S}_s)^2$$

Since the sum of squares within each subject is associated with $m - 1$ degrees of freedom (where m is the number of treatments) and there are n subjects, $SS_{wit\ subjs}$ is associated with $DF_{wit\ subjs} = n(m-1)$ degrees of freedom.

The variation between subjects is quantified by computing the sum of squared deviations of the mean response of each subject about the grand mean

$$SS_{bet\ subjs} = m\sum_{s}(\bar{S}_s - \bar{X})^2$$

The sum is multiplied by m because each subject's mean is the mean response to the m treatments. (This situation is analogous to the computation of the between-groups sum of squares as the sum of squared deviations of the sample means about the grand mean in the analysis of variance developed in the last section.) This sum of squares has $DF_{bet\,subjs} = n - 1$ degrees of freedom.

It is possible to show that

$$SS_{tot} = SS_{wit\,subjs} + SS_{bet\,subjs}$$

i.e., that the total sum of squares can be partitioned into the within- and between-subjects sums of squares.*

Next, we need to partition the within-subjects sum of squares into two components, variability in the observations due to the treatments and the *residual* variation due to random variation in how each individual responds to each treatment. The sum of squares due to the treatments is the sum of squared differences between the treatment means and the grand mean,

$$SS_{treat} = n \sum_t (\bar{T}_t - \bar{X})^2$$

We multiply by n, the number of subjects used to compute each treatment mean, just as we did above when computing the between-subjects sum of squares. Since there are m different treatments, there are $DF_{treat} = m - 1$ degrees of freedom associated with SS_{treat}.

Since we are partitioning the within-subjects sum of squares into the treatment sum of squares and the residual sum of squares,

$$SS_{wit\,subjs} = SS_{treat} + SS_{res}$$

and so

$$SS_{res} = SS_{wit\,subjs} - SS_{treat}$$

The same partitioning for the degrees of freedom yields

*For a derivation of this equation, see B. J. Winer, *Statistical Principles in Experimental Design,* 2d ed., McGraw-Hill, New York, 1971, chap. 4, "Single-Factor Experiments Having Repeated Measures on the Same Elements."

$$DF_{res} = DF_{wit\ subjs} - DF_{treat} = n(m-1) - (m-1) = (n-1)(m-1)$$

Finally, our estimate of the population variance from the treatment sum of squares is

$$MS_{treat} = \frac{SS_{treat}}{DF_{treat}}$$

and the estimate of the population variance from the residual sum of squares is

$$MS_{res} = \frac{SS_{res}}{DF_{res}}$$

Since MS_{treat} and MS_{res} are both estimates of the same (unknown) population variance, compute

$$F = \frac{MS_{treat}}{MS_{res}}$$

to test the hypothesis that the treatments do not change the experimental subjects. If the hypothesis of no treatment effect is true, this F ratio will follow the F distribution with DF_{treat} numerator degrees of freedom and DF_{res} denominator degrees of freedom.

This development has been, by necessity, more mathematical than most of the explanations in this book. Let us apply it to a simple example to make the concepts more concrete.

Oral Hydralazine Therapy for Pulmonary Hypertension

High pressure in the blood vessels in the lungs, called pulmonary hypertension, is a debilitating and potentially fatal condition. The high pressure in the circulation can force fluid into the lungs, which inhibits gas transport and makes breathing difficult. In addition, the elevated blood pressure in the lungs requires the right side of the heart to work harder, and this increased workload can, over time, damage the heart. Hydralazine is a drug that causes blood vessels to relax and dilate, reducing blood pressure. Since it is used to treat high blood pressure of the gen-

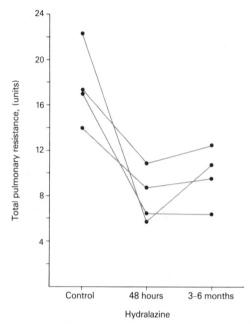

Figure 9-6 Total pulmonary resistance in four people with pulmonary hypertension before, 48 h after, and 3 to 6 months after beginning treatment with hydralazine. Each individual's responses are connected by straight lines. (*Adapted from fig. 1 of L. J. Rubin and R. H. Peter, "Oral Hydralazine Therapy for Primary Pulmonary Hypertension," N. Engl. J. Med., 302:69–73, 1980. Used by permission.*)

eral circulation, Rubin and Peter* thought that this drug might also reduce blood pressure in the lungs of people with pulmonary hypertension. To investigate this question, they measured a variety of variables 3 times (before administering hydralazine to four people with pulmonary hypertension, again 48 h after administering the drug, and again 3 to 6 months later).

Figure 9-6 shows one of their measurements, total pulmonary resistance. Total pulmonary resistance is a measure of how much pressure it requires to produce a given flow of blood through the lungs. The more serious the pulmonary hypertension, the greater the total pulmonary

*L. J. Rubin and R. H. Peter, "Oral Hydralazine Therapy for Primary Pulmonary Hypertension," *N. Engl. J. Med.,* **302**:69–73, 1980.

Table 9-5   Total Pulmonary Resistance before and during Treatment with Hydralazine

Person (subject)	No drug (control)	Hydralazine 48 h	Hydralazine 3–6 mo	Subject Mean	Subject SS
1	22.2	5.4	10.6	12.73	147.95
2	17.0	6.3	6.2	9.83	77.05
3	14.1	8.5	9.3	10.63	18.35
4	17.0	10.7	12.3	13.33	21.45
Treatment mean	17.58	7.73	9.60		

Grand mean = 11.63   Total SS = 289.82

Source: L. J. Rubin and R. H. Peter "Oral Hydralazine Therapy for Primary Pulmonary Hypertension," *N. Engl. J. Med.,* **302**:69–73, 1980, table 1. Reprinted by permission.

resistance. Simply looking at Fig. 9-6 suggests that hydralazine lowers total pulmonary resistance, but there are only four people in the study. How confident can we be when asserting that the drug actually lowers resistance? To answer this question, we perform a repeated-measures analysis of variance.

Table 9-5 shows the same data as Fig. 9-6, together with the mean pulmonary artery resistance observed for each of the $n = 4$ experimental subjects (people) and each of the $m = 3$ treatments (control, 48 h, 3 to 6 months). For example, subject 2's mean response to all three treatments is

$$\bar{S}_2 = \frac{17.0 + 6.3 + 6.2}{3} = 9.83 \text{ units}$$

and the mean response of all four subjects to treatment 1 (control) is

$$\bar{T}_1 = \frac{22.2 + 17.0 + 14.1 + 17.0}{4} = 17.58 \text{ units}$$

The grand mean of all observations $\bar{S}$ is 11.63 units, and the total sum of squares is $SS_{tot} = 289.82$ units^2.

Table 9-5 also includes the sums of squares within each subject; e.g., for subject 2

$$SS_{\text{wit subj 2}} = (17.0 - 9.83)^2 + (6.3 - 9.83)^2 + (6.2 - 9.83)^2$$
$$= 77.05 \text{ units}^2$$

Adding the within-subjects sums of squares for the four subjects in the study yields

$$SS_{\text{wit subjs}} = 147.95 + 77.05 + 18.35 + 21.45 = 264.80 \text{ units}^2$$

We obtain the sum of squares between subjects by adding up the squares of the deviations between the subjects' means and the grand mean and multiplying by the number of treatments ($m = 3$, the number of numbers used to compute each subject's mean response)

$$SS_{\text{bet subjs}} = 3[(12.73 - 11.63)^2 + (9.83 - 11.63)^2$$
$$+ (10.63 - 11.63)^2 + (13.33 - 11.63)^2]$$
$$= 25.02 \text{ units}^2$$

(Note that $SS_{\text{wit subjs}} + SS_{\text{bet subjs}} = 264.80 + 25.02 = 289.82$, the total sum of squares, as it should.)

We obtain the sum of squares for the treatments by multiplying the squares of the differences between the treatment means and the grand mean times the number of subjects ($n = 4$, the number of numbers used to compute each mean),

$$SS_{\text{treat}} = 4[(17.58 - 11.63)^2 + (7.73 - 11.63)^2 + (9.60 - 11.63)^2]$$
$$= 218.93 \text{ units}^2$$

There are $DF_{\text{treat}} = m - 1 = 3 - 1 = 2$ degrees of freedom associated with the treatments. Therefore, the residual sum of squares is

$$SS_{\text{res}} = SS_{\text{wit subjs}} - SS_{\text{treat}} = 264.80 - 218.93 = 45.87 \text{ units}^2$$

and $DF_{\text{res}} = (n - 1)(m - 1) = (4 - 1)(3 - 1) = 6$ degrees of freedom.

Table 9-6, the analysis-of-variance table for this experiment, sum-

Table 9-6   Analysis-of-Variance Table for One-Way Repeated-Measures Analysis of Hydralazine in Pulmonary Hypertension

Source of variation	SS	DF	MS
Between subjects	25.02	3	
Within subjects	264.80	8	
Treatments	218.93	2	109.47
Residual	45.87	6	7.65
Total	289.82	11	

$$F = \frac{MS_{treat}}{MS_{res}} = \frac{109.47}{7.65} = 14.31$$

marizes the results of all these calculations. Notice that we have partitioned the sums of squares into more components than we did in Table 9-3. We were able to do this because we made repeated measurements on the same experimental subjects.

From Table 9-6 our two estimates of the population variance are

$$MS_{treat} = \frac{SS_{treat}}{DF_{treat}} = \frac{218.93}{2} = 109.47 \text{ units}^2$$

and

$$MS_{res} = \frac{SS_{res}}{DF_{res}} = \frac{45.87}{6} = 7.65 \text{ units}^2$$

so our test statistic is

$$F = \frac{MS_{treat}}{MS_{res}} = \frac{109.47}{7.65} = 14.31$$

This value exceeds $F_{.01} = 10.92$, the critical value that defines the largest 1 percent of possible values of F with 2 and 6 degrees of freedom for the numerator and denominator, respectively. Therefore, these data permit concluding that hydralazine alters total pulmonary resistance ($P < .01$).

So far we can conclude that at least one of the treatments produced a change. To isolate which one, we need to use a multiple-comparisons procedure analogous to the Bonferroni t test developed in Chap. 4.

How to Isolate Differences in Repeated-Measures Analysis of Variance

In Chap. 4 we made multiple pairwise comparisons between groups with the Bonferroni t test

$$t = \frac{\bar{X}_1 - \bar{X}_2}{\sqrt{2s^2_{\text{wit}}/n}}$$

To keep the total chance of making a Type I error below α_T, for k pairwise comparisons, we required t to exceed the value required for $P < \alpha_T/k$. To use the Bonferroni t test to isolate differences following a repeated-measures analysis of variance we simply replace s^2_{wit} with our estimate of the variance computed from the residual sum of squares MS_{res}

$$t = \frac{\bar{T}_i - \bar{T}_j}{\sqrt{2MS_{\text{res}}/n}}$$

in which $\bar{T}_i$ and $\bar{T}_j$ represent the mean treatment responses of the pair of treatments (treatments i and j) you are comparing. The resulting value of t is compared with the critical value for DF_{res} degrees of freedom.

For example, there are three comparisons, that is, $k = 3$, we can make in the hydralazine experiment. To compare total pulmonary resistance before taking the drug to total pulmonary resistance 48 h later

$$t = \frac{17.58 - 7.73}{\sqrt{2(7.65)/4}} = 5.036$$

To compare control resistance to resistance at 3 to 6 months

$$t = \frac{17.58 - 9.60}{\sqrt{2(7.65)/4}} = 4.080$$

and to compare 48-h resistance to 3- to 6-month resistance

$$t = \frac{7.73 - 9.60}{\sqrt{2(7.65)/4}} = -.9561$$

To keep the total chances of erroneously reporting a difference below 5 percent, we compare the values of t with the critical value for $\frac{5}{3} = 1.6$ percent and $DF_{res} = 6$ degrees of freedom, approximately 3.37 (by interpolating in Table 4-1). The first two values of t above exceed 3.37, whereas the third one does not. These results allow us to conclude that the hydralazine lowers total pulmonary resistance within 48 h and continued use of the drug for 3 to 6 months will maintain this lowered resistance $(P < .05)$.

EXPERIMENTS WHEN OUTCOMES ARE MEASURED ON A NOMINAL SCALE: McNEMAR'S TEST

The paired t test and repeated-measures analysis of variance can be used to analyze experiments in which the variable being studied can be measured on an interval scale (and satisfies the other assumptions required of parametric methods). What about experiments, analogous to the ones in Chap. 5, in which outcomes are measured on a *nominal* scale? This problem often arises when asking whether or not an individual responded to a treatment or when comparing the results of two different diagnostic tests that are classified as positive or negative in the same individuals. We will develop a procedure to analyze such experiments, *McNemar's test for changes,* in the context of one such study.

Skin Reactivity in People with Cancer

It is generally believed that a person's immune system plays an important role in combating cancer. In particular, patients with a compromised immune system seem to be less responsive to therapy than those with a strong immune system. Dinitrochlorobenzene (DNCB) is a chemical irritant that provokes a reaction when left in contact with the skin. Since this reaction requires a functioning immune system, it has been proposed as a diagnostic test to assess the status of a person's immune system. Other investigators questioned this conclusion and asserted that the reaction seen was actually due to local tissue damage, independent of the immune system.

To investigate this question Roth and his colleagues* applied DNCB and croton oil, an irritating extract made from seeds of a tropical shrub, to the skin of 173 people suffering from cancer. Croton oil produces an immediate effect due to local damage of the skin and blood vessels which does not depend on the immune system. If DNCB and croton oil produced similar effects, it would be evidence against the view that the ability of a patient to react to DNCB indicates an active immune system rather than local damage to the skin and blood vessels.

Table 9-7 shows the results of this study, with the plus sign indicating a positive reaction to the irritant and a minus sign indicating no reaction.

This table looks very much like the 2×2 contingency tables analyzed in Chap. 5. In fact, most people simply compute a χ^2 statistic from these data and look the P value up in Table 5-5. The numbers in this table are associated with a value of $\chi^2 = 1.107$ (computed including the Yates correction for continuity). This value is well below 3.841, the value of χ^2 that defines the largest 5 percent of possible values of χ^2 with 1 degree of freedom. As a result, one might report "no significant difference" between responses to DNCB and croton oil and conclude that the reaction to DNCB is as likely to be due to local tissue damage as a functioning immune system, so that the test is worthless.

There is, however, a serious problem with this approach. The χ^2 test statistic developed for contingency tables in Chap. 5 was used to test the hypothesis that the *rows and columns of the tables are independent*. In Table 9-7 the rows and columns are *not* independent because they represent the responses of the *same* individuals to two different treatments. (This situation is analogous to the difference between the unpaired t test presented in Chap. 4 and the paired t test presented in this chapter.) In particular, the 81 people who responded to *both* DNCB and croton oil and the 21 people who responded to *neither* DNCB nor croton oil do not tell you anything about whether or not people with cancer respond differently to these two irritants. We need a

*J. A. Roth, F. R. Eilber, J. A. Nizze, and D. L. Morton, "Lack of Correlation between Skin Reactivity to Dinitrochlorobenzene and Croton Oil in Patients with Cancer," *N. Engl. J. Med.,* **293**:388–389, 1975.

Table 9-7 Skin-Test Reaction to DNCB and Croton Oil in People with Cancer

Croton oil	DNCB	
	+	-
+	81	48
-	23	21

Source: J. A. Roth, F. R. Eilber, J. A. Nizze, and D. L. Morton, "Lack of Correlation between Skin Reactivity to Dinitrochlorobenzene and Croton Oil in Patients with Cancer," *N. Engl. J. Med.,* **293**:388–389, 1975, table 1. Reprinted by permission.

statistical procedure that focuses on the 71 people who responded to *one* of the irritants but not the other.

If there is no difference in the effects of DNCB and croton oil in these people, we would expect half of the 71 people who reacted to only one of the irritants to respond to DNCB and not croton oil and the other half to respond to croton oil but not DNCB. Table 9-7 shows that the observed number of people who fell into each of these two categories was 23 and 48, respectively. To compare these observed and expected frequencies, we can use the χ^2 test statistic to compare these observed frequencies with the expected frequency of $^{71}/_2 = 35.5$

$$\chi^2 = \Sigma \frac{(|O - E| - \frac{1}{2})^2}{E}$$

$$= \frac{(|23 - 35.5| - \frac{1}{2})^2}{35.5} + \frac{(|48 - 35.5| - \frac{1}{2})^2}{35.5} = 8.113$$

(Notice that this computation of χ^2 includes the Yates correction for continuity because it has only 1 degree of freedom.)

This value exceeds 6.635, the value of χ^2 that defines the biggest 1 percent of the possibe values of χ^2 with 1 degree of freedom (from Table 5-7) if the differences in observed and expected are simply the effects of random sampling. This analysis leads to the conclusion that there *is* a difference in response to DNCB and croton oil ($P < .01$). In fact, Roth and his colleagues went on to show that DNCB activity correlates with clinical course, whereas no such relationship could be demonstrated for croton oil reactivity.

This example illustrates that it is entirely possible to compute values of test statistics and look up P values in tables that are meaningless when the experimental design and underlying populations are not compatible with the assumptions used to derive the statistical procedure.

In sum, McNemar's test for changes consists of the following procedure:

- *Ignore individuals who responded the same way to both treatments.*
- *Compute the total number of individuals who responded differently to the two treatments.*
- *Compute the expected number of individuals who would have responded positively to each of the two treatments (but not the other) as half the total number of individuals who responded differently to the two treatments.*
- *Compare the observed and expected number of individuals that responded to one of the treatments by computing a χ^2 test statistic (including Yates correction for continuity).*
- *Compare this value of χ^2 with the critical values of the χ^2 distribution with 1 degree of freedom.*

This procedure yields a P value that quantifies the probability that the differences in treatment response is due to chance rather than actual differences in how the two treatments affect the same individuals.

PROBLEMS

9-1 In Prob. 8-8 you analyzed data from the study F. P. Ashley and his colleagues completed on the effectiveness of an ammonium chloride-based mouthrinse. A group of people was randomly given either an inactive control rinse for 48 hours or the active rinse for 48 hours. When that period was over, those given the active rinse were given the inactive rinse, and vice versa. Ashley and his coworkers measured a clinical score for the amount of plaque at 48 hours for each rinse and found:

Plaque score

Active rinse	Control rinse
32	14
60	39
25	24
45	13
65	9
60	3
68	10
83	14
120	1
110	36

Do these two rinses have different abilities to suppress plaque?

9-2 Young infants often develop streptococcal infections. There is some evidence that if the mother's blood contains antibodies to these infectious agents, the antibodies cross the placenta and also provide the infant with protection against these infections. There is also evidence that immunization against pneumococcus may produce antibodies that also protect against streptococcal infections because of structural similarities between pneumococcus and streptococcus. If these three statements are true, it would be possible to protect the newborn children against common streptococcal infections by immunizing their mothers with pneumococcal vaccine (while they are still pregnant). Carol Baker and her colleagues ("Influence of Preimmunization Antibody Levels on the Specificity of the Immune Response to Related Polysaccharide Antigens," *N. Engl. J. Med.* **303**:173–178, 1980, used by permission) tested the final statement in this chain of logic by administering pneumococcal vaccine to healthy (nonpregnant) volunteers who had low native concentrations of antipneumococcal antibodies and measured how their concentrations of streptococcal antibodies changed. They found:

Antibody Concentration before and after Immunization

Pneumococcus, mg/mL		Streptococcus, µg/mL	
Before	4 weeks after	Before	4 weeks after
79	163	.4	.4
100	127	.4	.5
133	288	.4	.5
141	1154	.4	.9
43	666	.5	.5
63	156	.5	.5
127	644	.5	.5
140	273	.5	.5
145	231	.5	.5
217	1097	.6	12.2
551	227	.6	.6
170	310	.7	1.1
1049	1189	.7	1.2
986	1695	.8	.8
436	1180	.9	1.2
1132	1194	.9	1.9
129	1186	1.0	2.0
228	444	1.0	.9
135	2690	1.6	8.1
110	95	2.0	3.7

Did the antibody concentration to pneumococcus change following immunization? Did the antibody concentration to streptococcus change following immunization?

9-3 What are the chances of detecting a doubling of the antibody concentrations to pneumococcus and streptococcus in Prob. 9-2 (also 95 percent confidence)? Note that the power chart in Fig. 6-9 applies to the paired t test by setting n equal to *twice* the sample size. Why do you set n equal to twice the sample size?

9-4 Rework Prob. 9-2 as a repeated-measures analysis of variance. What is the arithmetic relationship between F and t?

9-5 In addition to measuring total pulmonary resistance, Rubin and Peter measured the rate at which the heart pumped blood (cardiac output) in the four people they gave hydralazine. Their results are:

Patient no.	Control	Cardiac output after hydralazine, L/min	
		48 h later	3–6 mo later
1	3.5	8.6	5.1
2	3.3	5.4	8.6
3	4.9	8.8	6.7
4	3.6	5.6	5.0

Did hydralazine affect cardiac output? If so, are the effects the same immediately (48 h) and 3 to 6 months after giving the drug? (Data from Rubin and Peter, loc. cit., table 1.)

9-6 People with coronary artery disease develop chest pain (angina pectoris) soon after smoking a cigarette for at least two reasons: nicotine increases the heart's demand for oxygen, and carbon monoxide binds to the blood and reduces its ability to deliver oxygen to the heart. There is, however, some question whether other constituents of the smoke also play an important role in precipitating angina in people who smoke. To investigate this question, Wilbert Aronow ("Effect of Non-nicotine Cigarettes and Carbon Monoxide on Angina," *Circulation,* **61**:262–265, 1979, by permission of the American Heart Association, Inc.) measured how long 12 people with heart disease could exercise before and after smoking five nonnicotine cigarettes and before and after inhaling an equivalent amount of carbon monoxide. Here are his data:

Length of Time (Seconds) Subject Could Exercise before Developing Chest Pain

Patient	Smoking		Carbon monoxide	
	Before	After	Before	After
1	289	155	281	177
2	203	117	186	125
3	359	187	372	238
4	243	¯134	254	165

(Continued)

Length of Time (Seconds) Subject Could Exercise before Developing Chest Pain *(Continued)*

Patient	Smoking		Carbon monoxide	
	Before	After	Before	After
5	232	135	219	153
6	210	119	225	148
7	251	145	264	180
8	246	121	237	144
9	224	136	212	152
10	239	124	250	147
11	220	118	209	138
12	211	107	226	141

What conclusions can be drawn from these observations?

9-7 Animal studies have demonstrated that compression and distension of the stomach trigger nerves that signal the brain to turn off the desire to eat. This fact has led some to propose surgery to reduce stomach size in clinically obese people as a way of reducing food intake and, ultimately, body weight. This surgery, however, has significant risks—including death—associated with it. Alan Geliebter and his colleagues ("Extra-abdominal Pressure Alters Food Intake, Intragastric Pressure, and Gastric Emptying Rate," *Am. J. Physiol.* **250**:R549–R552, 1986) sought to limit expansion of the stomach (and so increase pressure within the stomach) by placing a large inflatable cuff around the abdomen of experimental subjects, inflating the cuff to a specified pressure to limit abdominal (and, presumably, stomach) expansion, and then measuring the volume of food consumed at a meal following a control period during which diet was controlled. Subjects were told that the main purpose of the study was to detect expansion of the abdomen during eating by monitoring the air pressure in the cuff around their abdomen, with several pressure levels used to determine the one most sensitive to abdominal expansion. They were asked to drink a liquid lunch from a reservoir until they felt full. The subjects did not know that food intake was being measured. Here are the data:

Subject	Food intake (milliliters) at abdominal pressure of:		
	0 mmHg	10 mmHg	20 mmHg
1	448	470	292
2	472	424	390
3	631	538	508
4	634	498	560
5	643	547	602
6	734	578	508
7	820	711	724

What do you conclude from these data? Why did Geliebter and his colleagues lie to the subjects about the purpose and design of the experiment?

9-8 In the fetus, there is a connection between the aorta and the artery going to the lungs called the ductus arteriosus that permits the heart to bypass the nonfunctioning lungs and circulate blood to the placenta to obtain oxygen and nourishment and dispose of wastes. After the infant is born and begins breathing, these functions are served by the lungs and the ductus arteriosus closes. Occasionally, especially in premature infants, the ductus arteriosus remains open and shunts blood around the lungs. This shunting prevents the infant from getting rid of carbon dioxide and taking on oxygen. As a result the infant does not receive adequate oxygen. The drug indomethacin has been used to make the ductus arteriosus close. It is very likely that the outcome (with or without drugs) depends on gestational age, age after birth, fluid intake, other illnesses, and other drugs the infant is receiving. For these reasons, an investigator might decide to pair infants who are as alike as possible in each of these identified variables, and randomly treat one member of each pair with indomethacin or placebo, then judge the results as improved or not improved. Suppose the findings are:

		Indomethacin	
		Improved	Not improved
Placebo	Improved	65	13
	Not improved	27	40

Do these data support the hypothesis that indomethacin is no better than a placebo?

9-9 The data in Prob. 9-8 could also be presented in the following form:

	Improved	Not improved
Indomethacin	92	53
Placebo	78	67

How would these data be analyzed? If this result differs from the analysis in Prob. 9-8, explain why and decide which approach is correct.

9-10 Review all original articles published in the *New England Journal of Medicine* during the last 12 months. How many of these articles present the results of experiments that should be analyzed with a repeated-measures analysis of variance? What percentage of these articles actually did such an analysis? Of those which did not, how did the authors analyze their data? Comment on potential difficulties with the conclusions that are advanced in these papers.

Alternatives to Analysis of Variance and the *t* Test Based on Ranks

Analysis of variance, including the *t* tests, is widely used to test the hypothesis that one or more treatments had no effect on the mean of some observed variable. All forms of analysis of variance, including the *t* tests, are based on the assumptions that the observations are drawn from normally distributed populations in which the variances are the same even if the treatments change the mean responses. These assumptions are often satisfied well enough to make analysis of variance an extremely useful statistical procedure. On the other hand, experiments often yield data that are not compatible with these assumptions. In addition, there are often problems in which the observations are measured on an ordinal rather than an interval scale and may not be amenable to an analysis of variance. This chapter develops analogs to the *t* tests and analysis of variance based on *ranks* of the observations rather than the observations themselves. This approach uses information about the relative sizes of the observations without assuming anything about the specific nature of the population they were drawn from. We will begin with the nonparametric analog to the unpaired and paired t tests, the *Mann-Whitney rank-sum test,* and *Wilcoxon's signed-rank test.* Then we will present the analogs of one-way analysis of variance, the *Kruskal-Wallis statistic,* and repeated-measures analysis-of-variance *Friedman statistic.*

HOW TO CHOOSE BETWEEN PARAMETRIC AND NONPARAMETRIC METHODS

As already noted, analysis of variance is called a *parametric* statistical method because it is based on estimates of the two population parameters, the mean and standard deviation (or variance), that completely define a normal distribution. Given the assumption that the samples are drawn from normally distributed populations, one can compute the distributions of the F- or t-test statistics that will occur in all possible experiments of a given size when the treatments have no effect. The critical values that define a value of F or t can then be obtained from that distribution. When the assumptions of parametric statistical methods are satisfied, they are the most powerful tests available.

If the populations the observations were drawn from are not normally distributed (or are not reasonably compatible with other assumptions of a parametric method, such as equal variances in all the treatment groups), parametric methods become quite unreliable because the mean and standard deviation, the key elements of parametric statistics, no longer completely describe the population. In fact, when the population substantially deviates from normality, interpreting the mean and standard deviation in terms of a normal distribution produces a very misleading picture.

For example, recall our discussion of the distribution of heights of the entire population of Jupiter. The mean height of all Jovians is 37.6 cm in Fig. 2-3*A,* and the standard deviation is 4.5 cm. Rather than being equally distributed about the mean, the population is *skewed* toward taller heights. Specifically, the heights of Jovians range from 31 to 52 cm, with most heights around 35 cm. Figure 2-3*B* shows what the population of heights would have been if, instead of being skewed toward taller heights, they had been normally distributed with the same mean and standard deviation as the actual population (in Fig. 2-3*A*). The heights would have ranged from 26 to

49 cm, with most heights around 37 to 38 cm. Simply looking at Fig. 2-3 should convince you that envisioning a population on the basis of the mean and standard deviation can be quite misleading if the population does not, at least approximately, follow the normal distribution.

The same thing is true of statistical tests that are based on the normal distribution. When the population the samples were drawn from does not at least approximately follow the normal distribution, these tests can be quite misleading. In such cases, it is possible to use the *ranks* of the observations rather than the observations themselves to compute statistics that can be used to test hypotheses. By using ranks rather than the actual measurements, it is possible to retain much of the information about the relative size of responses without making any assumptions about how the population the samples were drawn from is distributed. Since these tests are not based on the parameters of the underlying population, they are called *nonparametric* or *distribution-free* methods.* All the methods we will discuss require only that the distributions under the different treatments have similar shapes, but there is no restriction on what those shapes are.† When the observations are drawn from normally distributed populations, the nonparametric methods in this chapter are 95 to 96 percent as powerful as the analogous parametric methods. When the observations are drawn from populations that are not normally distributed, nonparametric methods are not only more reliable but also more powerful than parametric methods.

Unfortunately, you can never observe the entire population. So how can you tell whether the assumptions such as normality are met, to permit using the parametric tests like analysis of variance? The simplest approach is to plot the observations and look at them. Do they seem compatible with the assumptions that they were drawn from normally distributed populations with roughly the same variances, i.e., within a

---

*The methods in this chapter are obviously not the first nonparametric methods we have encountered. The χ^2 for analysis of nominal data in contingency tables in Chap. 5, the Spearman rank correlation to analyze ordinal data in Chap. 8, and McNemar's test in Chap. 9 are three widely used nonparametric methods.

†They also require that the distributions be continuous (so that ties are impossible) to derive the mathematical forms of the sampling distributions used to define the critical values of the various test statistics. In practice, however, this restriction is not important, and the methods can be applied to observations with tied measurements.

factor of 2 to 3 of each other? If so, you are probably safe in using parametric methods. If, on the other hand, the observations are heavily skewed (suggesting a population like the Jovians in Fig. 2-3A) or appear to have more than one peak, you probably will want to use a nonparametric method. When the standard deviation is about the same size or larger than the mean and the variable can take on only positive values, this is an indication that the distribution is skewed. (A normally distributed variable would have to take on negative values.) In practice, these simple rules of thumb are often all you will need.

There are two ways to make this procedure more objective. The first is to plot the observations on *normal-probability graph paper*. Normal-probability graph paper has a distorted scale that makes normally distributed observations plot as a straight line (just as exponential functions plot as a straight line on semilogarithmic graph paper). Examining how straight the line is will show how compatible the observations are with a normal distribution. One can also construct a χ^2 statistic to test how closely the observed data agree with those expected if the population is normally distributed with the same mean and standard deviation. Since in practice simply looking at the data is generally adequate, we will not discuss these approaches in detail.*

Unfortunately, none of these methods is especially convincing one way or the other for the small sample sizes common in biomedical research, and your choice of approach (i.e., parametric versus nonparametric) often has to be based more on judgment and preference than hard evidence.

Things basically come down to the following difference of opinion. Some people think that in the *absence* of evidence that the data were *not* drawn from a normally distributed population, one should use parametric tests because they are more powerful and more widely used. These people say that you should use a nonparametric test only when there is positive evidence that the populations under study are not normally distributed. Others point out that the nonparametric methods discussed in this chapter are 95 percent as powerful as parametric methods when the data are from normally distributed popula-

*For discussions and examples of these procedures, see J. H. Zar, *Biostatistical Analysis,* Prentice-Hall, Englewood Cliffs, N.J., 1974, chap. 7, "The Normal Distribution," or W. J. Dixon and F. J. Massey, Jr., *Introduction to Statistical Analysis,* McGraw-Hill, New York, 1969, chap. 5, "The Normal Distribution."

tions and more reliable when the data are not from normally distributed populations. They also believe that investigators should assume as little as possible when analyzing their data; they therefore recommend that nonparametric methods be used except when there is positive evidence that parametric methods are suitable. At the moment there is no definitive answer stating which attitude is preferable. And there probably never will be such an answer.

TWO DIFFERENT SAMPLES: THE MANN-WHITNEY RANK-SUM TEST

When we developed the analysis of variance, t test, and Pearson product-moment correlation, we began with a specific (normally distributed) population and examined the values of the test statistic associated with all possible samples of a given size that could be selected from that population. The situation is different for methods based on ranks rather than the actual observations. We will replace the actual observations with their ranks, then focus on the population of possible combinations of ranks. Since all samples have a finite number of members, we can simply list all the different possible ways to rank the members to obtain the distribution of possible values for the test statistic when the treatment has no effect.

To illustrate this process but keep this list relatively short, let us analyze a small experiment in which three people take a placebo and four people take a drug that is thought to be a diuretic. Table 10-1

Table 10-1 Observations in Diuretic Experiment

Placebo (control)		Drug (treatment)	
Daily urine production, mL/day	Rank*	Daily urine production, mL/day	Rank*
1000	1	1400	6
1380	5	1600	7
1200	3	1180	2
		1220	4
	$T = 9$		

*1 = smallest, 7 = largest

shows the daily urine production observed in this experiment. Table 10-1 also shows the ranks of all the observations without regard to which experimental group they fall in; the smallest observed urine production is ranked 1, and the largest one is ranked 7. If the drug affected daily urine production, we would expect the rankings in the control group to be lower (or higher, if the drug decreased urine production) than the ranks for the treatment group. We will use the sum of ranks in the smaller group (in this case, the control group) as our test statistic T. The control-group ranks add up to 9.

Is the value of $T = 9$ sufficiently extreme to justify rejecting the hypothesis that the drug had no effect?

To answer this question, we examine the *population of all possible rankings* to see how likely we are to get a rank sum as extreme as that associated in Table 10-1. Notice that we are no longer discussing the actual observations but their ranks, so our results will apply to *any* experiment in which there are two samples, one containing three individuals and the other containing four individuals, regardless of the nature of the underlying populations.

We begin with the hypothesis that the drug did not affect urine production, so that the ranking pattern in Table 10-1 is just due to chance. To estimate the chances of getting this pattern when the two samples were drawn from a single population, we need not engage in any fancy mathematics, we just *list* all the possible rankings that could have occurred. Table 10-2 shows all 35 different ways the ranks could have been arranged with 3 people in one group and 4 in the other. The crosses indicate a person in the placebo group, and the blanks indicate a person in the treatment group. The right-hand column shows the sum of ranks for the people in the smaller (placebo) group for each possible combination of ranks. Figure 10-1 shows the distribution of possible values of our test statistic, the sum of ranks of the smaller group T that can occur when the treatment has no effect. This distribution looks a little like the t distribution in Fig. 4-5. Except that the distributions are not identical, there is another very important difference. Whereas the t distribution is continuous and, in theory, is based on an infinitely large collection of possible values of the t-test statistic, Fig. 10-1 shows *every possible* value of the sum-of-ranks test statistic T.

Since there are 35 possible ways to combine the ranks, there is 1 chance in 35 of getting rank sums of 6, 7, 17, or 18; 2 chances in 35 of getting 8 or 16; 3 chances in 35 of getting 9 or 15; 4 chances in

Table 10-2 Possible Ranks and Rank Sums for 3 Individuals Out of 7

			Rank				
1	2	3	4	5	6	7	Rank sum T
X	X	X					6
X	X		X				7
X	X			X			8
X	X				X		9
X	X					X	10
X		X	X				8
X		X		X			9
X		X			X		10
X		X				X	11
X			X	X			10
X			X		X		11
X			X			X	12
X				X	X		12
X				X		X	13
X					X	X	14
	X	X	X				9
	X	X		X			10
	X	X			X		11
	X	X				X	12
	X		X	X			11
	X		X		X		12
	X		X			X	13
	X			X	X		13
	X			X		X	14
	X				X	X	15
		X	X	X			12
		X	X		X		13
		X	X			X	14
		X		X	X		14
		X		X		X	15
		X			X	X	16
			X	X	X		15
			X	X		X	16
			X		X	X	17
				X	X	X	18

35 of getting 10, 11, 13 or 14; and 5 chances in 35 of getting 12. What are the chances of getting an extreme value of T? There is a $\frac{2}{35} = .057 = 5.7$ percent chance of obtaining $T = 6$ or $T = 18$ when the treat-

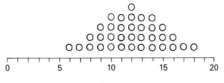

Sum of ranks in smaller group, T

Figure 10-1 Sums of ranks in the smaller group for all possible rankings of seven individuals with three individuals in one sample and four in the other. Each circle represents one possible sum of ranks.

ment has no effect. We use these numbers as the critical values to define extreme values of T and reject the hypothesis of no treatment effect. Hence, the value of $T = 9$ associated with the observations in Table 10-1 is not extreme enough to justify rejecting the hypothesis that the drug had no effect on urine production.

Notice that in this case $T = 6$ and $T = 18$ correspond to $P = .057$. Since T can take on only integer values, P can take on only discrete values. As a result, tables of critical values of T present pairs of values that define the proportion of possible values nearest traditional critical P values, for example, 5 and 1 percent, but the exact P values defined by these critical values generally do not equal 5 and 1 percent exactly. Table 10-3 presents these critical values. n_S and n_B are the number of members in the smaller and larger samples. The table gives the critical values of T that come nearest defining the most extreme 5 and 1 percent of all possible values of T that will occur if the treatment has no effect, as well as the exact proportion of possible T values defined by the critical values. For example, Table 10-3 shows that 7 and 23 define the 4.80 percent most extreme possible values of the rank sum of the smaller of two sample groups T when $n_S = 3$ and $n_B = 6$.

The procedure we just described is the *Mann-Whitney* rank-sum test.* The procedure for testing the hypothesis that a treatment had no effect with this statistic is:

*There is an alternative formulation of this test that yields a statistic commonly denoted by U. U is related to T by the formula $U = T - n_S(n_S + 1)/2$, where n_S is the size of the smaller sample (or either sample if both contain the same number of individuals). For a presentation of the U statistic, see S. Siegel, *Nonparametric Statistics for the Behavioral Sciences,* McGraw-Hill, New York, 1956, pp. 116–127, "The Mann-Whitney U Test." For a detailed derivation and discussion of the Mann-Whitney test as developed here, as well as its relationship to

Table 10-3 Critical Values (Two-Tailed) of the Mann-Whitney Rank-Sum Statistic T

n_S	n_B	.05 Critical values	P	.01 Critical values	P
3	4	6, 18	.057		
	5	6, 21	.036		
	5	7, 20	.071		
	6	7, 23	.048	6, 24	.024
	7	7, 26	.033	6, 27	.017
	7	8, 25	.067		
	8	8, 28	.042	6, 30	.012
4	4	11, 25	.057	10, 26	.026
	5	11, 29	.032	10, 30	.016
	5	12, 28	.063		
	6	12, 32	.038	10, 34	.010
	7	13, 35	.042	10, 38	.012
	8	14, 38	.048	11, 41	.008
	8	. . . . .	. . . .	12, 40	.016
5	5	17, 38	.032	15, 40	.008
	5	18, 37	.056	16, 39	.016
	6	19, 41	.052	16, 44	.010
	7	20, 45	.048	17, 48	.010
	8	21, 49	.045	18, 52	.011
6	6	26, 52	.041	23, 55	.009
	6	. . . . .	. . . .	24, 54	.015
	7	28, 56	.051	24, 60	.008
	7	. . . . .	. . . .	25, 59	.014
	8	29, 61	.043	25, 65	.008
	8	30, 60	.059	26, 64	.013
7	7	37, 68	.053	33, 72	.011
	8	39, 73	.054	34, 78	.009
8	8	49, 87	.050	44, 92	.010

Source: Computed from F. Mosteller and R. Rourke, *Sturdy Statistics: Nonparametrics and Order Statistics,* Addison-Wesley, Reading, Mass., 1973, Table A-9. Used by permission.

U, see F. Mosteller and R. Rourke, *Sturdy Statistics: Nonparametrics and Order Statistics,* Addison-Wesley, Reading, Mass., 1973, chap. 3, "Ranking Methods for Two Independent Samples."

• *Rank all observations according to their magnitude, a rank of 1 being assigned to the smallest observation. Tied observations should be assigned the same rank, equal to the average of the ranks they would have been assigned had there been no tie (i.e., using the same procedure as in computing the Spearman rank correlation coefficient in Chap. 8).*

• *Compute T, the sum of the ranks in the smaller sample. (If both samples are the same size, you can compute T from either one.)*

• *Compare the resulting value of T with the distribution of all possible rank sums for experiments with samples of the same size to see whether the pattern of rankings is compatible with the hypothesis that the treatment had no effect.*

There are two ways to compare the observed value of T with the critical value defining the most extreme values that would occur if the treatment had no effect. The first approach is to compute the exact distribution of T by listing all the possibilities, as we just did, then tabulate the results in a table like Table 10-3. For experiments in which the samples are small enough to be included in Table 10-3, this approach gives the exact P value associated with a given set of experimental observations. For larger experiments, this exact approach becomes quite tedious because the number of possible rankings gets very large. For example, there are 184,756 different ways to rank two samples of 10 individuals each.

Second, when the larger sample contains more than eight members, the distribution of T is very similar to the normal distribution with mean

$$\mu_T = \frac{n_S(n_S + n_B + 1)}{2}$$

and standard deviation

$$\sigma_T = \sqrt{\frac{n_S n_B(n_S + n_B + 1)}{12}}$$

in which n_S is the size of the smaller sample.* Hence, we can transform T into the test statistic

$$z_T = \frac{T - \mu_T}{\sigma_T}$$

and compare this statistic with the critical values of the normal distribution that define the, say 5 percent, most extreme possible values. z_T can also be compared with the t distribution with an infinite number of degrees of freedom (Table 4-1) because it equals the normal distribution. This comparison can be made more accurate by including a *continuity correction* (analogous to the Yates correction for continuity in Chap. 5) to account for the fact that the normal distribution is continuous whereas the rank sum T must be an integer

$$z_T = \frac{|T - \mu_T| - \frac{1}{2}}{\sigma_T}$$

The Leboyer Approach to Childbirth

Generally accepted methods of assisting low-risk women during childbirth have changed dramatically in recent years, with a general trend away from heavy sedation and increased emphasis on a role for the father during labor and delivery. The exact procedures to be used, however, are controversial. The French physician Leboyer heated up this debate with his book *Birth without Violence* in 1975. Leboyer suggested specific maneuvers to minimize the shock of the newborn child's first separation experience. He described the ideal birth as occurring in a dark, quiet room to minimize sensory overstimulation.

---

*When there are tied measurements, the standard deviation needs to be reduced according to the following formula, which depends on the number of ties:

$$\sigma_T = \sqrt{\frac{n_S n_B (N + 1)}{12} - \frac{n_S n_B}{12N(N-1)} \Sigma(\tau_i - 1)\tau_i(\tau_i + 1)}$$

in which $N = n_S + n_B$, τ_i = number of tied ranks in ith set of ties, the sum indicated by Σ is computed over all sets of tied ranks.

He suggested placing the infant on his mother's abdomen and delaying cutting the umbilical cord until it stopped pulsating; calming the infant by gentle massaging; and placing the infant in a warm bath "to insure that this separation is not a shock but a joy." He claimed that children delivered this way were healthier and happier. Many medical practitioners objected to these procedures, saying that they interfered with accepted medical practice and increased risks to both the mother and child. Nevertheless, the Leboyer approach has gained popularity.

Like so many medical procedures, there is surprisingly little evidence to support or refute the claims Leboyer or his critics make. Until Nelson and her colleagues* completed a randomized clinical trial of the methods, the only published evidence consisted of "clinical experience" and a single uncontrolled trial that supported Leboyer's position.

Nelson and her colleagues recruited low-risk pregnant women who were interested in the Leboyer method from an obstetrical practice at McMaster University, Ontario, Canada. The women had to have carried the infant for at least 36 weeks and be available for assessments of the child's development 3 days and 8 months after birth. After acceptance into the study, women were randomly allocated to be delivered by Leboyer techniques or by conventional (control) methods in a normally lit delivery room in which no particular attention was paid to sound levels, the umbilical cord was cut immediately after delivery, and the baby was wrapped in a blanket and given to the mother. In both groups the use of pain killers was minimized, and both parents participated actively in the labor and delivery. Thus, the study was designed to focus on the effects of the specific and controversial aspects of Leboyer's methods rather than the general principles of a gentle delivery.

Obviously the parents, physicians, and nurses who participated in the delivery knew which experimental group they were in. The researchers who were charged with evaluating the mothers and children before and after delivery and over the ensuing months, however, did not know how the children had been delivered. Thus, this is a *single-*

---

*N. Nelson, M. Enkin, S. Saigal, K. Bennett, R. Milner, and D. Sackett, "A Randomized Clinical Trial of the Leboyer Approach to Childbirth," *N. Engl. J. Med.*, **302**:655–660, 1980.

blind protocol that minimizes the effects of observer biases but cannot control for the placebo effect.

Since the prime benefit of the Leboyer method is believed to be better development of the child, the investigators measured infant development on a specially constructed scale. They estimated that 30 percent of conventionally delivered infants would have "superior" scores on this scale. They reasoned that if the Leboyer method is really better, they would want to be able to detect a change that led to 90 percent of infants delivered by the Leboyer technique to rate "superior" in development. Computations using power revealed that the study had to include at least 20 infants in each treatment group to have a 90 percent chance of detecting such a difference with $P < .05$ (i.e., the power of the experiment is .90). Notice that they were, in effect, saying that they were not interested in detecting any smaller effect of the Leboyer treatment.

During the 1 year in which they recruited experimental subjects, they talked to 187 families and explained the trial to them; 34 did not meet the initial eligibility requirements, and 56 of the remaining 153 agreed to be randomized. Among the 97 who refused randomization, 70 insisted on a Leboyer delivery and 23 refused to participate in the study. One woman was delivered prematurely before randomization, and the remaining 55 were randomized. One of the women in the control group dropped out of the study, leaving 26 women in the control group and 28 in the Leboyer (treatment) group. Six women in the control group and eight in the Leboyer group had complications that precluded delivery as planned, leaving the required 20 women in each group. This bit of bookkeeping illustrates how difficult it is to accumulate a sufficient number of cases in clinical studies, even ones as relatively simple and benign as this one.*

Although Nelson and her colleagues examined a wide variety of variables before, during, immediately after, and several months after delivery, we will examine only one of the things they measured, the number of minutes the newborn child was alert during the first hour of

---

*The decision of whom to include and not include in a randomized trial, combined with the effects of people who drop out or are lost to follow up, can have a profound effect on the outcome of the study. For a discussion of this problem, see D. Sackett and M. Gent, "Controversy in Counting and Attributing Events in Clinical Trials," *N. Engl. J. Med.*, **301**:1410–1412, 1979.

life. If the Leboyer method leads to less traumatized newborns, we would expect them to be more alert immediately after delivery. Table 10-4 and Fig. 10-2 show the number of minutes of alertness during the first hour for the 20 infants in each of the two treatment groups.

The first thing that is evident from Fig. 10-2 is that the observations probably do not come from normally distributed populations. The length of time these infants were alert is skewed towards higher times, rather than being equally likely to be above the mean as below it. Since these data are *not* suitable for analysis with a parametric method such as the unpaired t test, we will use the Mann-Whitney rank-sum test.

In addition to the observed number of minutes of alert behavior in the first hour, Table 10-4 shows the ranks of these observations, assigned without regard to which treatment group contains the in-

Table 10-4 Minutes of Alert Activity during First Hour after Birth

Control delivery	Rank	Leboyer delivery	Rank
5.0	2	2.0	1
10.1	3	19.0	5
17.7	4	29.7	10
20.3	6	32.1	12
22.0	7	35.4	15
24.9	8	36.7	17
26.5	9	38.5	19
30.8	11	40.2	20
34.2	13	42.1	22
35.0	14	43.0	23
36.6	16	44.4	24
37.9	18	45.6	26
40.4	21	46.7	27
45.5	25	47.1	28
49.3	31	48.0	29
51.1	33	49.0	30
53.1	36	50.9	32
55.0	38	51.2	34
56.7	39	52.5	35
58.0	40	53.3	37
	$T = 374$		

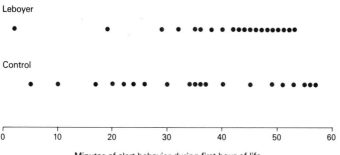

Figure 10-2   Number of minutes of alert behavior during first hour of life among infants delivered by conventional gentle techniques and the Leboyer method. Notice that the times are skewed toward higher values.

dividual infant being ranked. Since both samples are the same size, we can compute the rank sum T from either group. The rank sum for the control group is $T = 374$. Since there are 20 people in each group, we will compute the P value by computing z_T and comparing the resulting value with the normal distribution. The mean of all possible values of T for experiments of this size is

$$\mu_T = \frac{n_S(n_S + n_B + 1)}{2} = \frac{20(20 + 20 + 1)}{2} = 410$$

and the standard deviation is

$$\sigma_T = \sqrt{\frac{n_S n_B (n_S + n_B + 1)}{12}} = \sqrt{\frac{20(20)\,(20 + 20 + 1)}{12}} = 36.97$$

So

$$z_T = \frac{|T - \mu_T| - \frac{1}{2}}{\sigma_T} = \frac{|374 - 410| - \frac{1}{2}}{36.9} = .962$$

This value is smaller than 1.960, the value of z that defines the biggest 5 percent of the normal distribution (from Table 4-1 with an infinite number of degrees of freedom). Hence, this study does not provide sufficient evidence to conclude that the Leboyer method is associated with more alert newborns.*

In fact, except for the feeling by mothers that the Leboyer method had influenced their child's behavior and the tendency of women using the Leboyer method to have shorter active labors, Nelson and her colleagues could find no evidence that the Leboyer method led to outcomes different from those of a conventional gentle birth. These differences may actually be reflections of the placebo effect, since the mothers obviously knew the methods used for delivery and may have wanted better outcomes. The bottom line, for both the method's enthusiasts and critics, however, seems to be that nothing is gained or lost by choosing to use or not to use Leboyer's specific recommendations.

EACH SUBJECT OBSERVED BEFORE AND AFTER ONE TREATMENT: THE WILCOXON SIGNED-RANK TEST

Chapter 9 presented the paired t test to analyze experiments in which each experimental subject was observed before and after a single treatment. This test required that the changes accompanying treatment be normally distributed. We now develop an analogous test based on ranks that does not require this assumption. We compute the differences caused by the treatment in each experimental subject, rank these differences according to their magnitude (without regard for sign), then attach the sign of the difference to each rank, and finally sum the signed ranks to obtain the test statistic W.

This procedure uses information about the sizes of the differences the treatment produces in each experimental subject as well as its direction. Since it is based on ranks, it does not require making any assumptions about the nature of the population of the differences the treatment produces. As with the Mann-Whitney rank-sum test statistic, we can obtain the distribution of all possible values of the test statistic W by simply listing all the possibilities of the signed-rank sum for experiments of a given size. We finally compare the value of W associated with our observations with the distribution of all possible values

---

*It is possible to compute a confidence interval for the median, but we will not discuss this procedure. For a discussion of confidence intervals for the median, see Mosteller and Rourke, op. cit., chap. 14, "Order Statistics: Distributions of Probabilities; Confidence Limits, Tolerance Limits.

of W that can occur in experiments involving the number of individuals in our study. If the observed value of W is "big," the observations are not compatible with the assumption that treatment had no effect.

Remember that observations are ranked based on the *magnitude* of the changes *without regard for signs,* so that the differences which are equal in magnitude but opposite in sign, say –5.32 and +5.32, both have the same rank.

We begin with another hypothetical experiment in which we wish to test a potential diuretic on six people. In contrast to the experiments the last section described, we will observe daily urine production in each person *before* and *after* administering the drug. Table 10-5 shows the results of this experiment, together with the change in urine production that followed administering the drug in each person.

Daily urine production fell in five of the six people. Are these data sufficient to justify asserting that the drug was an effective diuretic?

To apply the signed-rank test, we first rank the magnitudes of each observed change, beginning with 1 for the smallest change and ending with 6 for largest change. Next, we attach the sign of the change to each rank (last column of Table 10-5) and compute the sum of the signed ranks W. For this experiment, $W = -13$.

If the drug has no effect, the ranks associated with positive changes should be similar to the ranks associated with the negative changes and W should be near zero. On the other hand, when the treatment alters

Table 10-5   Effect of a Potential Diuretic on Six People

	Daily urine production mL/day			Rank* of difference	Signed rank of difference
Person	Before drug	After drug	Difference		
1	1600	1490	–110	5	–5
2	1850	1300	–550	6	–6
3	1300	1400	+100	4	+4
4	1500	1410	–90	3	–3
5	1400	1350	–50	2	–2
6	1010	1000	–10	1	–1
					$W = -13$

*1 = smallest magnitude, 6 = largest magnitude.

the variable being studied, the changes with the larger or smaller ranks will tend to have the same sign and the signed rank sum W will be a big positive or big negative number.

As with all test statistics, we need only draw the line between "small" and "big." We do this by listing *all* 64 possible combinations of different ranking patterns, from all negative changes to all positive changes (Table 10-6). There is 1 chance in 64 of getting any one of

Table 10-6 Possible Combinations of Signed Ranks for a Study of Six Individuals

Rank*						Sum of signed ranks
1	2	3	4	5	6	
−	−	−	−	−	−	−21
+	−	−	−	−	−	−19
−	+	−	−	−	−	−17
−	−	+	−	−	−	−15
−	−	−	+	−	−	−13
−	−	−	−	+	−	−11
−	−	−	−	−	+	−9
+	+	−	−	−	−	−15
+	−	+	−	−	−	−13
+	−	−	+	−	−	−11
+	−	−	−	+	−	−9
+	−	−	−	−	+	−7
−	+	+	−	−	−	−11
−	+	−	+	−	−	−9
−	+	−	−	+	−	−7
−	+	−	−	−	+	−5
−	−	+	+	−	−	−7
−	−	+	−	+	−	−5
−	−	+	−	−	+	−3
−	−	−	+	+	−	−3
−	−	−	+	−	+	−1
−	−	−	−	+	+	1
+	+	+	−	−	−	−9
+	+	−	+	−	−	−7
+	+	−	−	+	−	−5
+	+	−	−	−	+	−3
+	−	+	+	−	−	−5
+	−	+	−	+	−	−3

Table 10-6 Possible Combinations of Signed Ranks for a Study of Six Individuals *(Continued)*

1	2	3	4	5	6	Sum of signed ranks
+	−	+	−	−	+	−1
+	−	−	+	+	−	−1
+	−	−	+	−	+	1
+	−	−	−	+	+	3
−	+	+	+	−	−	−3
−	+	+	−	+	−	−1
−	+	+	−	−	+	1
−	+	−	+	+	−	1
−	+	−	+	−	+	3
−	+	−	−	+	+	5
−	−	+	+	+	−	3
−	−	+	+	−	+	5
−	−	+	−	+	+	7
−	−	−	+	+	+	9
+	+	+	+	−	−	−1
+	+	+	−	+	−	1
+	+	+	−	−	+	3
+	+	−	+	+	−	3
+	+	−	+	−	+	5
+	+	−	−	+	+	7
+	−	+	+	+	−	5
+	−	+	+	−	+	7
+	−	+	−	+	+	9
+	−	−	+	+	+	11
−	+	+	+	+	−	7
−	+	+	+	−	+	9
−	+	+	−	+	+	11
−	+	−	+	+	+	13
−	−	+	+	+	+	15
+	+	+	+	+	−	9
+	+	+	+	−	+	11
+	+	+	−	+	+	13
+	+	−	+	+	+	15
+	−	+	+	+	+	17
−	+	+	+	+	+	19
+	+	+	+	+	+	21

*Signs denote whether rank is positive or negative.

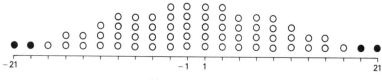

Sum of signed ranks, W

Figure 10-3 All 64 possible sums of signed ranks for observations before and after administering a treatment to six individuals. Table 10-6 lists all the possibilities. The shaded circles show that 4 out of 64 have a magnitude of 19 or more, that is, fall at or below –19 or at or above +19.

these patterns by chance. Figure 10-3 shows all 64 of the signed-rank sums listed in Table 10-6.

To define a "big" value of W, we take the most extreme values of W that can occur when the treatment has no effect. Of the 64 possible rank sums, 4, or $\frac{4}{64}$ = .0625 = 6.25 percent, fall at or beyond 19 (or –19), so we will reject the hypothesis that the treatment has no effect when the magnitude of W exceeds 19 (i.e., W is more negative than –19 or more positive than +19) with P = .0625.

Notice that, as with the Mann-Whitney rank-sum test, the discrete nature of the distribution of possible values of W means that we cannot always obtain P values precisely at traditional levels, like 5 percent. Since the value of W associated with the observations in Table 10-5 is only –13, these data are not sufficiently incompatible with the assumption that the treatment had no effect (that the drug is not an effective diuretic) to justify rejecting that hypothesis.

Table 10-7 presents the values of W that come closest to defining the most extreme 5 and 1 percent of all possible values for experiments with up to 20 subjects. For larger experiments, we use the fact that the distribution of W closely approximates a normal distribution with mean

$$\mu_W = 0$$

and standard deviation

$$\sigma_W = \sqrt{\frac{n(n+1)(2n+1)}{6}}$$

in which n equals the number of experimental subjects.

Table 10-7   Critical Values (Two-Tailed) of Wilcoxon W

n	Critical value	P	n	Critical value	P
5	15	.062	13	65	.022
6	21	.032		57	.048
	19	.062	14	73	.020
7	28	.016		63	.050
	24	.046	15	80	.022
8	32	.024		70	.048
	28	.054	16	88	.022
9	39	.020		76	.050
	33	.054	17	97	.020
10	45	.020		83	.050
	39	.048	18	105	.020
11	52	.018		91	.048
	44	.054	19	114	.020
12	58	.020		98	.050
	50	.052	20	124	.020
				106	.048

Source: Adapted from F. Mosteller and R. Rourke, *Sturdy Statistics: Non-parametrics and Order Statistics,* Addison-Wesley, Reading, Mass., 1973, table A-11. Used by permission.

Therefore, we use

$$z_W = \frac{W - \mu_W}{\sigma_W} = \frac{W}{\sqrt{[n(n+1)(2n+1)]/6}}$$

as our test statistic. This approximation can be improved by including a continuity correction to obtain

$$z_W = \frac{|W| - \frac{1}{2}}{\sqrt{[n(n+1)(2n+1)]/6}}$$

There are two kinds of *ties* that can occur when computing W. First, there can be no change in the observed variable when the treatment is applied, so that the difference is zero. In this case, that individual provides no information about whether the treatment increases or decreases the response variable; so it is simply dropped from the analysis, and the sample size is reduced by 1. Second, the magnitudes of the change the treatment produces can be the same for two or more individuals. As with the Mann-Whitney test, all the individuals with that change are assigned the same rank as the average of the ranks that would be used for the same number of individuals if they were not tied.*

In summary, here is the procedure for comparing the observed effects of a treatment in a single group of experimental subjects before and after administering a treatment:

- *Compute the change in the variable of interest in each experimental subject.*
- *Rank all the differences according to their magnitude without regard for sign. (Zero differences should be dropped from the analysis with a corresponding reduction of sample size. Tied ranks should be assigned the average of the ranks that would be assigned to the tied ranks if they were not tied.)*
- *Apply the sign of each difference to its rank.*
- *Add all the signed ranks to obtain the test statistic W.†*
- *Compare the observed value of W with the distribution of possible values that would occur if the treatment had no effect, and reject this hypothesis if W is "big."*

To further illustrate this process, let us use the *Wilcoxon signed-rank test* to analyze the results of an experiment we discussed in Chap. 9.

---

*When there are tied ranks and you use the normal distribution to compute the P value, σ_W needs to be reduced by a factor that depends on the number of ties according to the formula

$$\sigma_W = \sqrt{\frac{n(n+1)(2n+1)}{6} - \Sigma \frac{(\tau_i - 1)\tau_i(\tau_i + 1)}{12}}$$

in which n is the number of experimental subjects, τ_i is the number of tied ranks in the ith set of ties, and Σ indicates summation over all the sets of tied ranks.

†Note that we have developed W as the sum of *all* the signed ranks of the differences. There are alternative derivations of the Wilcoxon signed-rank test that are based on the sum of only the positively or negatively signed ranks. These alternative forms are mathematically equivalent to the one developed here. You need to be careful when using tables of the critical value W to be sure which way the test statistic was computed when the table was constructed.

Table 10-8 Maximum Percentage Platelet Aggregation before and after Smoking One Cigarette

Person	Before smoking	After smoking	Difference	Rank of difference	Signed rank of difference
1	25	27	2	2	2
2	25	29	4	3.5	3.5
3	27	37	10	6	6
4	44	56	12	7	7
5	30	46	16	10	10
6	67	82	15	8.5	8.5
7	53	57	4	3.5	3.5
8	53	80	27	11	11
9	52	61	9	5	5
10	60	59	-1	1	-1
11	28	43	15	8.5	8.5
					$W = 64$

Cigarette Smoking and Platelet Function

Table 10-8 reproduces the results, shown in Fig. 9-2, of Levine's experiment measuring platelet aggregation of 11 people before and after each one smokes a cigarette. Recall that increased platelet aggregation indicates a greater propensity to form blood clots (capable of causing heart attacks, strokes, and other vascular disorders). The table's fourth column shows the change in platelet aggregation that accompanies smoking a cigarette.

Figure 10-4 shows these differences. While this figure may not present results that preclude using methods based on the normal dis-

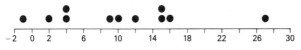
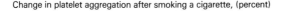

Change in platelet aggregation after smoking a cigarette, (percent)

Figure 10-4 Change in platelet aggregation after smoking a cigarette. These changes do not seem to be normally distributed, especially because of the outlier at 27 percent. This plot suggests that a nonparametric method, such as the Wilcoxon signed-rank test, is preferable to a parametric method, such as the paired *t* test, to analyze the results of this experiment.

tribution (like the paired t test), it does suggest that it would be more prudent to use a nonparametric method like the Wilcoxon signed-rank test because the differences do not appear to be symmetrically distributed about the mean and more likely to be near the mean as far from it. In particular, the severe *outliers* like that at 27 percent can bias methods based on a normal distribution.

To continue with our computation, which does not require the assumption of normally distributed changes, rank the magnitudes of each of these changes, the smallest change (1 percent) being ranked 1 and the largest change (27 percent) being ranked 11. The fifth column in Table 10-8 shows these ranks. The last column shows the same ranks with the sign of the change attached. The sum of the signed ranks W is $2 + 3.5 + 6 + 7 + 10 + 8.5 + 3.5 + 11 + 5 + (-1) + 8.5 = 64$. This value exceeds 44, the value that defines the 5.4 percent most extreme values of W that can occur when the treatment has no effect (from Table 10-7), so we can report that these data support the assertion that smoking increases platelet aggregation ($P = .054$).

EXPERIMENTS WITH THREE OR MORE GROUPS WHEN EACH GROUP CONTAINS DIFFERENT INDIVIDUALS: THE KRUSKAL-WALLIS STATISTIC

Chapter 3 discussed experiments in which three or more different groups of experimental subjects are exposed to different treatments and the observations could be considered to come from normally distributed populations with similar variances. Now we shall develop an analogous procedure to the one-way analysis of variance (Chap. 3) based on ranks that does not require making these assumptions.

The *Kruskal-Wallis statistic* is a direct generalization of the Mann-Whitney rank-sum test. One first ranks all the observations *without regard for which treatment group they are in,* beginning with 1 for the smallest observation. (Ties are treated as before; i.e., they are assigned the average value that would be associated with the tied observations if they were not tied.) Next, compute the rank sum for each group. If the treatments have no effect, the *large and small ranks should be evenly distributed among the different groups,* so the average rank in each group should approximate the average of all the ranks computed without regard of the grouping. The more disparity there is between observed average ranks in each group and what you would expect if the hypothesis of no treatment effect was true, the less likely we will be to accept that hypothesis. Now, let us construct such a test statistic.

For simplicity, let us assume there are only three groups; then generalize the resulting equations to any number of groups when we are finished. The three different treatment groups contain n_1, n_2, and n_3 experimental subjects, and the rank sums for these three groups are R_1, R_2, and R_3. Therefore, the mean ranks observed in the three groups are $\bar{R}_1 = R_1/n_1$, $\bar{R}_2 = R_2/n_2$, and $\bar{R}_3 = R_3/n_3$, respectively. The average rank of all the $n_1 + n_2 + n_3 = N$ observations is the average of the first N integers

$$\bar{R} = \frac{1 + 2 + 3 + \cdots + N}{N} = \frac{N + 1}{2}$$

We will use the sum of squared deviations between each sample group's average rank and the overall average rank, weighted by the sizes of each group, as a measure of variability between the observations and what you would expect if the hypothesis of no treatment effect was true. Call this sum D

$$D = n_1(\bar{R}_1 - \bar{R})^2 + n_2(\bar{R}_2 - \bar{R})^2 + n_3(\bar{R}_3 - \bar{R})^2$$

This sum of squared deviations is exactly analogous to the weighted sum of squared deviations between the sample means and grand mean that define the between-groups sum of squares in the parametric one-way analysis of variance as developed in Chap. 9.

The distribution of possible values of D when the treatments have no effect depends on the size of the sample. It is possible to obtain a test statistic that does not depend on sample size by dividing D by $N(N + 1)/12$,

$$H = \frac{D}{N(N + 1)/12} = \frac{12}{N(N + 1)} \Sigma n_t(\bar{R}_t - \bar{R})^2$$

The summation denoted with Σ is over all the treatment groups, regardless of how many treatment groups there are. It is the *Kruskal-Wallis test statistic*.

The exact distribution of H can be computed by listing all the possibilities, as we did with the Mann-Whitney and Wilcoxon tests, but there are so many different possibilities that the resulting table would be huge. Fortunately, if the sample sizes are not too small, the χ^2 distribution with $\nu = k - 1$ degrees of freedom, where k is the number of treatment groups, closely approximates the distribution of H. Hence, we can test the hypothesis that the treatments had no effect by computing H for the observations and comparing the resulting value with the critical values for χ^2 in Table 5-7. This approximation works well in experiments with three treatment groups when each group contains at least 5 members and for experiments with four treatment groups when there are more than 10 individuals in the entire study. For smaller studies, consult a table of the exact distribution of the H to obtain the P value. (We do not include such a table because of its length and the relatively infrequent need for one; most intermediate statistics texts include one.)

In sum, the procedure for analyzing an experiment in which different groups of experimental subjects receive each treatment is as follows:

• *Rank each observation without regard for treatment group, beginning with a rank of 1 for the smallest observation. (Ties are treated in the same way as the other rank tests.)**

• *Compute the Kruskal-Wallis test statistic H to obtain a normalized measure of how much the average ranks within each treatment group deviate from the average rank of all the observations.*

• *Compare H with the χ^2 distribution with 1 less degree of freedom than the number of treatment groups, unless the sample size is small, in which case you must compare H with the exact distribution. If H exceeds the critical value that defines a "big" H, reject the hypothesis that the treatment has no effect.*

Now let us illustrate this procedure with an example.

---

*When there are ties, the approximation between the distributions of H and x^2 can be improved by dividing H computed above by

$$1 - \frac{\Sigma(\tau_i - 1)\tau_i\,(\tau_i + 1)}{N(N^2 - 1)}$$

where τ_i is the number of ties in the ith set of tied ranks (as before). If there are only a few ties, this correction makes little difference and may be ignored.

Elimination of Caffeine Impaired by Oral Contraceptives

Caffeine, a widely used drug in prescription and nonprescription medications, occurs as well in common foods like coffee, tea, and soft drinks. It acts on the cardiovascular and nervous systems and various metabolic processes. Pregnant women take longer to eliminate caffeine from their bodies than when they are not pregnant, and it is possible that changes in hormone balances during pregnancy change the way caffeine is metabolized to slow its elimination from the body. This observation is important because, in large enough quantities, caffeine may harm an unborn child. To investigate whether there are differences in caffeine metabolism between men and women and between women with elevated estrogen and progesterone concentrations in their blood, such as occur during pregnancy, Patwardhan and his colleagues* administered a pill containing 250 mg of caffeine (equivalent to roughly 3 cups of coffee) to men, women who were not taking oral contraceptives, and women who were taking oral contraceptives. Oral contraceptives artificially change the estrogen and progesterone levels to resemble those during pregnancy. The investigators drew a number of blood samples, measured the caffeine concentrations, and measured how rapidly caffeine disappeared from the blood. They quantified this rate with the half-life, the time it takes the caffeine concentration to fall to one-half its original value. A longer half-life indicates that the caffeine concentration is falling more slowly.

Table 10-9 gives half-lives of caffeine concentration for the 31 people in the study. It also shows the ranks of each observation, together with the sum of ranks and mean ranks for each of the three treatment groups. The mean rank of all 31 observations is

$$\bar{R} = \frac{1 + 2 + 3 + \cdots + 31}{31} = \frac{N+1}{2} = \frac{31+1}{2} = 16$$

Therefore, the weighted sum of squared deviations between the average ranks observed in each treatment group and the average of all ranks is

*R. Patwardhan, P. Desmond, R. Johnson, and S. Schenker, "Impaired Elimination of Caffeine by Oral Contraceptives," *J. Lab. Clin. Med.*, **95**:603–608, 1980.

Table 10-9   Half-Life of Caffeine in the Blood after a Single Dose

| | Males (n_1 = 13) | | Females | | | |
| | | | No oral contraceptives (n_2 = 9) | | Oral contraceptives (n_3 = 9) | |
	Half-life, h	Rank	Half-life, h	Rank	Half-life, h	Rank
	2.04	1	5.30	12	10.36	25
	5.16	10	7.28	19	13.28	29
	6.11	15	8.98	21	11.81	28
	5.82	14	6.59	16	4.54	6
	5.41	13	4.59	8	11.04	26
	3.51	4	5.17	11	10.08	24
	3.18	2	7.25	18	14.47	31
	4.57	7	3.47	3	9.43	23
	4.83	9	7.60	20	13.41	30
	11.34	27				
	3.79	5				
	9.03	22				
	7.21	17				
Sum of ranks R_t		146		128		222
Mean rank $\bar{R}_t = R_t/n_t$		11.23		14.22		24.67

$$D = 13(11.23 - 16)^2 + 9(14.22 - 16)^2 + 9(24.67 - 16)^2$$
$$= 13(-4.77)^2 + 9(-1.78)^2 + 9(8.67)^2 = 1000.82$$

and

$$H = \frac{D}{N(N+1)/12} = \frac{1000.82}{31(31+1)/12} = 12.107$$

This value exceeds 9.201, the value that defines the largest 1 percent of values of the χ^2 distribution with $\nu = k - 1 = 3 - 1 = 2$ degrees of freedom (from Table 5-7). Therefore, we conclude that at least one of these three treatment groups eliminated caffeine at a rate different from that of the others ($P < .01$).

To identify which one, we do the pairwise comparisons with Mann-Whitney rank-sum tests, including a Bonferroni adjustment for the fact that we are making multiple comparisons between the same observations. Since the smallest of the samples contains nine members, the samples are large enough to use the normal approximation to compute the P value for the Mann-Whitney rank-sum test.

To compare the males with the females who did not take oral contraceptives, we note that $n_S = 9$ and $n_B = 13$, so the mean and standard deviation of the normalized test statistic z_T are

$$\mu_T = \frac{n_S(n_S + n_B + 1)}{2} = \frac{9(13 + 9 + 1)}{2} = 103.5$$

and

$$\sigma_T = \sqrt{\frac{n_S n_B (n_S + n_B + 1)}{12}} = \sqrt{\frac{9(13)(9 + 13 + 1)}{12}} = 14.97$$

From Table 10-10, the rank sum of the smaller group is $T = 120$. Therefore, the value of z_T associated with the comparison of the first and second experimental groups is

$$z_T = \frac{|T - \mu_T| - \frac{1}{2}}{\sigma_T} = \frac{|120 - 103.5| - \frac{1}{2}}{14.97} = 1.069$$

To compare the males with the females taking oral contraceptives (the first and third groups), the sizes of the two samples are the same as in the computations just completed, and the rank sum for the smaller group (the females taking contraceptives) is $T = 149$. Therefore,

$$z_T = \frac{|149 - 103.5| - \frac{1}{2}}{14.97} = 3.006$$

Finally, to compare the women taking oral contraceptives with those not taking oral contraceptives (the second and third groups), we need to compute μ_T and σ_T for $n_S = n_B = 9$

$$\mu_T = \frac{9(9 + 9 + 1)}{2} = 85.5 \qquad \sigma_T = \sqrt{\frac{9(9)(9 + 9 + 1)}{12}} = 11.32$$

Table 10-10   Ranks for Pairwise Comparison of Caffeine Half-Life

Males	Females, no OC*	Males	Females, OC	Females, no OC	Females, OC
1	11	1	16	5	13
9	18	8	20	8	16
14	20	11	19	10	15
13	15	10	5	6	2
12	7	9	17	3	14
4	10	3	15	4	12
2	17	2	22	7	18
6	3	6	14	1	11
8	19	7	21	9	17
22		18			
5		4			
21		13			
16		12			
	$T = 120$		$T = 149$	$T = 53$	

*OC = oral contraceptives.

Since both samples contain the same number of members, we can compute T from either sample; if we use the women not taking oral contraceptives, Table 10-10 shows that $T = 53$, so

$$z_T = \frac{|53 - 85.5| - \frac{1}{2}}{11.32} = 2.827$$

Since we made three comparisons, the Bonferroni inequality says that to keep the total chance of erroneously rejecting the hypothesis of no treatment effect below 5 percent, we should compare each of these z_T's with the critical value that defines the $\frac{5}{3} = 1.67$ percent most extreme portions of the normal distribution. Interpolating in Table 4-1 with an infinite number of degrees of freedom, we find that this cutoff value is approximately 2.41. Therefore, we conclude that men and normal women eliminate caffeine from their bodies in similar ways and that women taking oral contraceptives eliminate it more slowly than either women not taking the pill or men ($P < .05$).

Since the rate at which caffeine is removed is slowed in women taking oral contraceptives, presumably because of the increased estrogen levels, even modest amounts of caffeine (2 to 4 cups of coffee per day) will tend to accumulate in such people. To the extent that women taking oral contraceptives metabolize caffeine similarly to pregnant women and to the extent that high caffeine concentrations are potentially harmful to the fetus, this study suggests that physicians and nurses recommend that pregnant women moderate the amount of caffeine they take.

EXPERIMENTS IN WHICH EACH SUBJECT RECEIVES MORE THAN ONE TREATMENT: THE FRIEDMAN TEST

Often it is possible to complete experiments in which each individual is exposed to a number of different treatments. This experimental design reduces the uncertainty due to variability in the responses between individuals and provides a more sensitive test of what the treatments do in a given person. When the assumptions required for parametric methods can be reasonably satisfied, such experiments can be analyzed with the repeated-measures analysis of variance in Chap. 9. Now we will derive an analogous test based on ranks that does not require that the observations be drawn from normally distributed populations. The resulting test statistic is called *Friedman's statistic.*

The logic of this test is quite simple. Each experimental subject receives each treatment, so we rank *each subject's* responses to the treatments without regard for the other subjects. If the hypothesis that the treatment has no effect is true, then, for each subject, the ranks will be randomly distributed, and the sums of the ranks for each *treatment* will be similar. Table 10-11 illustrates such a case, in which 5 different subjects receive 4 treatments. Instead of the measured responses, this table contains the *ranks* of each experimental subject's responses. Hence, the treatments are ranked 1, 2, 3, and 4 separately for each subject. The bottom line in the table gives the sums of the ranks for all people receiving each treatment. These rank sums are all similar and also roughly equal to 12.5, which is the average rank, $(1 + 2 + 3 + 4)/4 = 2.5$, times the number of subjects, 5. This table does not suggest that any of the treatments had any systematic effect on the experimental subjects.

Now consider Table 10-12. The first treatment *always* produces the greatest response in all experimental subjects, the second treatment always produces the smallest response, and the third and fourth treatments always produce intermediate responses, the third treatment

Table 10-11 Ranks of Outcomes for Experiment When 5 Subjects Each Receive 4 Treatments

Experimental subject	Treatment			
	1	2	3	4
1	1	2	3	4
2	4	1	2	3
3	3	4	1	2
4	2	3	4	1
5	1	4	3	2
Rank sum R_t	11	14	13	12

Table 10-12 Ranks of Outcomes for Another Experiment When 5 Subjects Each Receive 4 Treatments

Experimental subject	Treatment			
	1	2	3	4
1	4	1	3	2
2	4	1	3	2
3	4	1	3	2
4	4	1	3	2
5	4	1	3	2
Rank sum R_t	20	5	15	10

producing a greater response than the fourth treatment. The bottom line shows the column rank sums. In this case there is a great deal of variability in the rank sums, some being much larger or smaller than 5 times the average rank, or 12.5. Table 10-12 strongly suggests that the treatments affect the variable being studied.

All we have left to do is to reduce this subjective impression of a difference to a single number. In a way similar to that used in deriving the Kruskal-Wallis statistic, let us compute the sum of squared deviations between the rank sums observed for each treatment and the rank sum that we would expect if each treatment were as likely to have any of the possible rankings. This latter number is the average of the possible ranks.

For the examples in Tables 10-11 and 10-12, there are four possible treatments, so there are four possible ranks. Therefore, the average rank is $(1 + 2 + 3 + 4)/4 = 2.5$. In general, if there are k treatments, the average rank will be

$$\frac{1 + 2 + 3 + \cdots + k}{k} = \frac{k + 1}{2}$$

In our example there are five experimental subjects, so we would expect each of the rank sums to be around 5 times the average rank for each person, or $5(2.5) = 12.5$. In Table 10-11 this is the case whereas in Table 10-12 it is not. If there are n experimental subjects and the ranks are randomly distributed between the treatments, each of the rank sums should be about n times the average rank, or $n(k + 1)/2$. Hence, we can collapse all this information into a single number by computing the sum of squared differences between the observed rank sums and rank sums that would be expected if the treatments had no effect

$$S = \Sigma[R_t - n(k + 1)/2]^2$$

in which Σ denotes the sum over all the treatments and R_t denotes the sum of ranks for treatment t.

For example, for the observations in Table 10-11, $k = 4$ treatments and $n = 5$ experimental subjects, so

$$S = (11 - 12.5)^2 + (14 - 12.5)^2 + (13 - 12.5)^2 + (12 - 12.5)^2$$
$$= (-1.5)^2 + (1.5)^2 + (.5)^2 + (-.5)^2 = 5$$

and for Table 10-12

$$S = (20 - 12.5)^2 + (5 - 12.5)^2 + (15 - 12.5)^2 + (10 - 12.5)^2$$
$$= (7.5)^2 + (-7.5)^2 + (2.5)^2 + (-2.5)^2 = 125$$

In the former case, S is a small number; in the latter S is a big number. The more of a pattern there is relating the ranks within each subject to the treatments, the greater the value of our test statistic S.

We could stop here and formulate a test based on S, but statisticians have shown that we can simplify the problem by dividing this sum of squared differences between the observed and expected rank sums by $nk(k + 1)/12$ to obtain

$$\chi_r^2 = \frac{S}{nk(k + 1)/12} = \frac{12\Sigma[R_t - n(k + 1)/2]^2}{nk(k + 1)}$$

The test statistic χ_r^2 is called *Friedman's statistic* and has the desirable property that, for large enough samples, it follows the χ^2 distribution with $\nu = k - 1$ degrees of freedom, regardless of sample size. When there are three treatments and nine or fewer experimental subjects or four treatments with four or fewer experimental subjects each, the χ^2 approximation is not adequate, so one needs to compare χ_r^2 to the exact distribution of possible values obtained by listing all the possibilities in Table 10-13.

In sum, the procedure for using the Friedman statistic to analyze experiments in which the same individuals receive several treatments is as follows:

• *Rank each observation within each experimental subject, assigning 1 to the smallest respònse. (Treat ties as before.)*
• *Compute the sum of the ranks observed in all subjects for each treatment.*
• *Compute the Friedman test statistic χ_r^2 as a measure of how much the observed rank sums differ from those that would be expected if the treatments had no effect.*
• *Compare the resulting value of the Friedman statistic with the χ^2 distribution if the experiment involves large enough samples or with the exact distribution of χ_r^2 in Table 10-13 if the sample is small.*

Now, let us apply this test to two experiments, one old and one new.

Oral Hydralazine Therapy for Primary Pulmonary Hypertension

Table 10-14 reproduces the observed total pulmonary resistances in Table 9-5 that Rubin, and Peter used to study whether or not hydralazine would also relieve high blood pressure in the lungs. In Chap. 9 we analyzed these data with a repeated-measures one-way analysis of vari-

Table 10-13 Critical Values for Friedman χ_r^2

$k = 3$ treatments			$k = 4$ treatments		
n	χ_r^2	P	n	χ_r^2	P
3	6.00	.028	2	6.00	.042
4	6.50	.042	3	7.00	.054
	8.00	.005		8.20	.017
5	5.20	.093	4	7.50	.054
	6.40	.039		9.30	.011
	8.40	.008	5	7.80	.049
6	5.33	.072		9.96	.009
	6.33	.052			
	9.00	.008	6	7.60	.043
7	6.00	.051		10.20	.010
	8.86	.008	7	7.63	.051
8	6.25	.047		10.37	.009
	9.00	.010	8	7.65	.049
9	6.22	.048		10.35	.010
	8.67	.010			
10	6.20	.046			
	8.60	.012			
11	6.54	.043			
	8.91	.011			
12	6.17	.050			
	8.67	.011			
13	6.00	.050			
	8.67	.012			
14	6.14	.049			
	9.00	.010			
15	6.40	.047			
	8.93	.010			

Source: Adapted from Owen, *Handbook of Statistical Tables,* U.S. Department of Energy, Addison-Wesley, Reading, Mass., 1962. Used by permission.

ance. Now, let us reexamine them using ranks to avoid having to make any assumptions about the population these patients represent.

Table 10-14 shows how the three treatments rank in terms of total pulmonary resistance for each of the four people in the study. The last

Table 10-14 Total Pulmonary Resistance in Four People before and after Administering Hydralazine

| | Hydralazine | | | | | |
| | Before (control) | | 48 h after | | 3–6 mo after | |
Person	Units	Rank	Units	Rank	Units	Rank
1	22.2	3	5.4	1	10.6	2
2	17.0	3	6.3	2	6.2	1
3	14.1	3	8.5	1	9.3	2
4	17.0	3	10.7	1	12.3	2
Rank sums for each treatment		12		5		7

Source: L. J. Rubin and R. H. Peter, "Oral Hydralazine Therapy for Primary Pulmonary Hypertension," *N. Engl. J. Med.*, **302**:69–73, 1980, table 2. Reprinted by permission.

row gives the sums of the ranks for each treatment. Since the possible ranks are 1, 2, and 3, the average rank is $(1 + 2 + 3)/3 = 2$. Since there are 4 people, if the treatments had no effect, these rank sums should all be about $4(2) = 8$. Hence, our measure of the difference between this expectation and the observed data is

$$S = (12 - 8)^2 + (5 - 8)^2 + (7 - 8)^2 = (4)^2 + (-3)^2 + (-1)^2 = 26$$

We convert S into χ_r^2 by dividing by $nk(k + 1)/12 = 4(3)(3 + 1)/12 = 4$ to obtain $\chi_r^2 = {}^{26}\!/_4 = 6.5$. Table 10-13 shows that for an experiment with $k = 3$ treatments and $n = 4$ experimental subjects there is only a $P = .042$ chance of obtaining a value of χ_r^2 as big or bigger than 6.5 by chance if the treatments have no effect. Therefore, we can report that hydralazine alters total pulmonary resistance ($P = .042$).

To isolate which treatment or treatments differ from the others, use the Wilcoxon signed-rank test with the Bonferroni correction to make the pairwise comparisons.

Effect of Secondhand Smoke on Angina Pectoris

Cigarette smoking aggravates the conditions of people with coronary artery disease, for several reasons. First, the arteries that supply blood to the heart muscle to deliver oxygen and nutrients and remove metabolic wastes are narrowed and are less able to maintain the needed flow of blood. Second, cigarette smoke includes carbon monoxide; it binds to the hemoglobin in blood and displaces oxygen that would otherwise be delivered to the heart muscle. In addition, nicotine and other chemicals in tobacco smoke act directly on the heart muscle to depress its ability to pump and deliver the blood containing oxygen and nutrients to the entire body, including the heart muscle. When the heart muscle is not adequately supplied with oxygen, the person with coronary artery disease experiences a typical chest pain called *angina pectoris*. People with coronary artery disease often feel fine when resting but develop pain when they exercise and increase the heart muscle's need for oxygen. It is well established that smoking can precipitate angina pectoris in people with severe coronary artery disease and decrease the ability of other people with milder disease to exercise. Aronow* wondered whether exposing people with coronary artery disease to someone else's cigarette smoke would produce similar effects on people with coronary artery disease, even though they were not smoking the cigarette themselves.

To answer this question, he measured how long 10 men with well-documented coronary artery disease could exercise on a bicycle. Aronow tested each subject to see how long he could exercise before developing chest pain. After obtaining these control measurements, he sent each subject to a waiting room for 2 h, where three other volunteers were waiting who either (1) did not smoke, (2) smoked five cigarettes with the room ventilator turned on, or (3) smoked five cigarettes with the room ventilator turned off. After this exposure, Aronow again measured each subject's exercise tolerance.

The experimental subjects were exposed to these different environments on different days in random order. The investigator knew whether or not they had been exposed to the secondhand smoke, but the subjects themselves did not know that the purpose of the study was to assess their response to secondhand smoke. Therefore, this is a single-blind experiment that minimizes placebo effects but not observer biases.

Table 10-15 shows the results of this experiment together with the ranks of exercise duration in each experimental subject, 1 being assigned to the shortest duration and 6 being assigned to the longest.

*W. S. Aronow, "Effect of Passive Smoking on Angina Pectoris," *N. Engl. J. Med.*, 299:21–24, 1978.

Table 10-15 Duration of Exercise until Angina in the Control Periods and after Exposure to Clean Air, Smoking in a Well-Ventilated Room, and Smoking in an Unventilated Room

Person	Clean air				Well-ventilated room				Unventilated room			
	Control		Treatment		Control		Smoke		Control		Smoke	
	Time, s	Rank	Time, s	Rank	Time, s	Rank	Time, s	Rank	Time, s	Rank	Time, s	Rank
1	193	4	217	6	191	3	149	2	202	5	127	1
2	206	5	214	6	203	4	169	2	189	3	130	1
3	188	4	197	6	181	3	145	2	192	5	128	1
4	375	3	412	6	400	5	306	2	387	4	230	1
5	204	5	199	4	211	6	170	2	196	3	132	1
6	287	3	310	5	304	4	243	2	312	6	198	1
7	221	5	215	4	213	3	158	2	232	6	135	1
8	216	5	223	6	207	3	155	2	209	4	124	1
9	195	4	208	6	186	3	144	2	200	5	129	1
10	231	6	224	4	227	5	172	2	218	3	125	1
Rank sum		44		53		39		20		44		10
Mean	231.6		241.9		232.3		181.1		233.7		145.8	

Source: W. S. Aronow, "Effect of Passive Smoking on Angina Pectoris," N. Engl. J. Med., 299:21–24, 1978, table 1.

Since there are 6 possible ranks, the average rank for each subject is $(1 + 2 + 3 + 4 + 5 + 6)/6 = 3.5$; since there are 10 people in the study, we would expect the rank sums to all be around $10(3.5) = 35$ if the different treatments all had no effect on how long a person could exercise. The rank sums at the bottom of the table appear to differ from this value.

To convert this impression to a single number, compute

$$\chi_r^2 = \frac{12}{10(6)(6+1)}(44^2 + 53^2 + 39^2 + 20^2 + 44^2 + 10^2)$$

$$- 3(10)(6+1) = 38.629$$

This value exceeds 20.517, the critical value that defines the .1 percent of largest values of the χ^2 distribution with $\nu = k - 1 = 6 - 1 = 5$ degrees of freedom (from Table 5-7), so we can report that passive smoking shortens the amount of exercise a person with coronary artery disease can do, much as if he had smoked a cigarette himself ($P < .001$).

SUMMARY

The methods in this chapter permit testing hypotheses similar to those we tested with analysis-of-variance and t tests but do not require us to assume that the underlying populations follow normal distributions. We avoid having to make such an assumption by replacing the observations with their ranks before computing the test statistic (T, W, H, or χ_r^2). By dealing with ranks, we preserve most of the information about the relative sizes (and signs) of the observations. More important, by dealing with ranks, we do not use information about the population or populations the samples were drawn from to compute the distribution of possible values of the test statistic. Instead we consider the population of all possible ranking patterns (often by simply listing all the possibilities) to compute the P value associated with the observations.

It is important to note that the procedures we used in this chapter to compute the P value from the ranks of the observations is essentially the same as the methods we have used everywhere else in this book:

   • *Assume that the treatment(s) had no effect, so that any differences observed between the samples are due to the effects of random sampling.*

  • *Define a test statistic that summarizes the observed differences between the treatment groups.*
  • *Compute all possible values this test statistic can take on when the assumption that the treatments had no effect is true. These values define the distribution of the test statistic we would expect if the hypothesis of no effect was true.*
  • *Compute the value of the test statistic associated with the actual observations in the experiment.*
  • *Compare this value with the distribution of all possible values; if it is "big," it is unlikely that the observations came from the same populations (i.e., that the treatment had no effect), so conclude that the treatment had an effect.*

The specific procedure you should use to analyze the results from a given experiment depends on the design of the experiment and the nature of the data. When the data are measured on an ordinal scale or you cannot or do not wish to assume that the underlying populations follow normal distributions, the procedures developed in this chapter are appropriate. The final chapter places all the tests we have discussed in this book in context, together with some general comments on how to assess what you read and write.

PROBLEMS

10-1 A person who has decided to enter the medical care system as a patient has relatively little control over the medical services (laboratory tests, x-rays, drugs) purchased. These decisions are made by the physician and other medical care providers, who are often unaware of how much of the patient's money they are spending. To improve awareness of the financial impacts of their decisions regarding how they use medical resources in making a diagnosis and treatment, there is an accelerating trend toward auditing how individual physicians choose to diagnose and treat their patients. Do such audits affect practice? To answer this question, Steven Schroeder and his colleagues ("Use of Laboratory Tests and Pharmaceuticals: Variation among Physicians and Effect of Cost Audit on Subsequent Use," *JAMA*, **225**:969–973, 1973, copyright 1970–1973, American Medical Association) measured the total of money a sample of physicians practicing in the George Washington University outpatient clinic spent on laboratory tests (including x-rays) and drugs for comparable patients for 3 months. The physicians were either salaried or volunteers. None received any direct compensation for the tests or drugs ordered. To be included, a patient must have been seen in the clinic for at least 6 months and have at least 1 of the 15 most common diagnoses among patients seen at the clinic. In addition, they excluded patients who were receiving a therapy that required frequent laboratory tests as part of routine management, e.g., anticoagulant therapy. They selected 10 to 15 patients at random from the people being seen by each physician and added up the total amount of money spent over a 3-month period, then computed the average annual cost for laboratory tests and drug costs for each physician. They then assigned each physician a number (unknown to the other participants in the study) and gave the physicians the results of the audit. In this way, the physicians could see how their costs compared with those of the other physicians, but they could not identify specific costs with any other individual physician. Then, unknown to the physicians, Schroeder and his colleagues repeated their audit using the same patients. Here is what they found:

Physician	Mean annual lab charges per patient		Mean annual drug charges per patient	
	Before audit	After audit	Before audit	After audit
1	$ 20	$ 20	$ 32	$ 42
2	17	26	41	90
3	14	1	51	71
4	42	24	29	47
5	50	1	76	56
6	62	47	47	43
7	8	15	60	137
8	49	7	58	63
9	81	65	40	28
10	54	9	64	60
11	48	21	73	87
12	55	36	66	69
13	56	30	73	50

Did knowledge of the audit affect the amount of money physicians spent for laboratory tests? For drugs? Is there any relationship between expenditures for laboratory tests and drugs? What are some possible explanations for these results? (Raw data supplied by Steven Schroeder of the University of California at San Francisco.)

10-2 Reanalyze the data of Prob. 4-2 on the permeability of blood vessels in normal and abnormal retinas using the appropriate nonparametric statistic. Compare your answer with the answer obtained in Prob. 4-2 and explain any differences.

10-3 The data analyzed in Probs. 4-2 and 10-2 are actually a subset of a larger study on the effects of several different retinal abnormalities on the permeability of the retina. Analyze these data using the appropriate nonparametric method.

Penetration ratio (10^{-6}/min) by status of retina

Normal	Foveal abnormality	Foveal and peripheral abnormalities
0.5	1.2	6.2
0.7	1.4	12.6
0.7	1.6	12.8
1.0	1.7	13.2
1.0	1.7	14.1
1.2	1.8	15.0
1.4	2.2	20.3
1.4	2.3	22.7
1.6	2.4	27.7
1.6	6.4	
1.7	19.0	
2.2	23.6	

10-4 Rework Probs. 4-3, 9-5, and 9-6 using methods based on ranks.

10-5 Chapter 3 discusses a study of whether or not appropriate use of drugs to treat pyelonephritis affects length of hospitalization. Deanne Knapp and her colleagues also did a study of whether appropriate use of drugs to treat pneumonia was associated with shorter hospitalizations. (Raw data supplied by David Knapp of the University of Maryland at Baltimore.) They collected data on 28 patients using a protocol similar to that discussed in Chap. 3 and found the following lengths of hospital stay:

Appropriate treatment	Inappropriate treatment			
3.7	3.8	1.7	4.8	8.6
2.5	6.8	2.5	5.3	9.0
2.8	7.9	2.9	5.5	10.3
3.0	8.8	3.0	5.8	11.0
5.5	9.0	3.4	7.1	
6.4	9.3	3.7	7.6	

Are these data consistent with the hypothesis that whether the use of drugs is appropriate or not has no effect on length of hospitalization for pneumonia?

10-6 When people exercise, the demand on the heart to pump blood increases, so that the heart muscle requires more blood to bring oxygen and remove waste products. In coronary artery disease, one or more of the arteries that serve the heart are blocked; the heart may not receive an adequate increase in blood during exercise and the heart fails to meet the demands placed upon it. As a result, blood may back up and pool in the lungs. Robert Okada and his colleagues ("Radionuclide-Determined Change in Pulmonary Blood Volume with Exercise: Improved Sensitivity of Multigated Blood-Pool Scanning in Detecting Coronary-Artery Disease," *N. Engl. J. Med.,* **301**:596–576, 1979, used by permission) infused a radioactive isotope into people thought to have coronary artery disease and used a gamma camera to measure the amount of blood pooled in the lungs during rest and when the people exercised. They computed the ratio of pulmonary blood volume during exercise to pulmonary blood volume during rest. They reasoned that if blood backed up in the lungs because of failure of the heart to meet the demands imposed on it, this ratio might be a useful diagnostic test to identify coronary artery disease. They separated the patients they studied into three groups using independent methods: people without signs of coronary artery disease, people with disease only of the right coronary artery (which provides blood to the right side of the heart, not the left side that pumps blood to the body), and people with disease of a major artery that supplies the left side of the heart (the left coronary artery) or disease of more than one artery. Here are the data:

No coronary artery disease	Right coronary artery	Left coronary artery or multiple arteries			
.83	.86	.98	1.07	1.22	
.89	.92	1.02	1.08	1.13	1.23
.91	1.00	1.03	1.10	1.32	
.93	1.02	1.04	1.15		
.94	1.20	1.05	1.12	1.18	1.37
.97		1.06	1.58		
.97		1.07			
.98					
1.02					

Is the pulmonary blood-volume ratio different in any of these groups of patients? If so, which one, and are the differences large enough for this test to be a useful diagnostic tool?

10-7 In his continuing effort to become famous, the author of an introductory biostatistics text invented a new way to test if some treatment changes an individual's response. Each experimental subject is observed before and after treatment, and the change in the variable of interest is computed. If this change is positive, we assign a value of +1 to that subject; if it is negative, we assign a value of zero (assume that there are never cases that remain unchanged). The soon-to-be-famous G test statistic is computed by summing up the values associated with the individual subjects. For example,

Subject	Before treatment	After treatment	Change	Contribution to G
1	100	110	+10	+1
2	95	96	+ 1	+1
3	120	100	−20	0
4	111	123	+12	+1

In this case, $G = 1 + 1 + 0 + 1 = 3$. Is G a legitimate test statistic? Explain briefly. If so, what is the sampling distribution for G when $n = 4$? $n = 6$? Can you use G to conclude that the treatment had an effect in the data given above with $P < .05$? How confident can you be about this conclusion? Construct a table of critical values for G when $n = 4$ and $n = 6$.

Chapter 11

What Do the Data
Really Show ?

The statistical methods we have been discussing permit you to estimate the certainty of statements and precision of measurements that are common in the biomedical sciences and clinical practice about a population after observing a random sample of its members. To use statistical procedures correctly, one needs to use a procedure that is appropriate for the experiment (or survey) and the scale (i.e., interval, nominal, or ordinal) used to record the data. All these procedures have, at their base, the assumption that the samples were selected at random from the populations of interest. If the real experiment does not satisfy this randomization assumption, the resulting P values and confidence intervals are meaningless. In addition to seeing that the individuals in the sample are selected at random, there is often a question exactly what actual populations the people in any given study represent. This question is especially important and often difficult to answer when the experimental subjects are patients in academic medical centers, a group of people hardly typical of the population as a whole. Even so, identifying the population in question is the crucial step in deciding the broader applicability of the findings of any study.

WHEN TO USE WHICH TEST

We have reached the end of our discussion of different statistical tests and procedures. It is by no means exhaustive, for there are many other approaches to problems and many kinds of experiments we have not even discussed. (For example, *two-factor* experiments in which the investigator administers two different treatments to each experimental subject and observes the response. Such an experiment yields information about the effect of each treatment alone as well as the joint affect of the two treatments acting together.) Nevertheless, we have developed a powerful set of tools and laid the groundwork for the statistical methods needed to analyze more complex experiments. Table 11-1 shows that it is easy to place all these statistical hypothesis-testing procedures this book presents into context by considering two things: the *type of experiment* used to collect the data and the *scale of measurement.*

To determine which test to use, one needs to consider the experimental design. Were the treatments applied to the same or different individuals? How many treatments were there? Were all treatments applied to the same or different individuals? Was the experiment designed to define a tendency for two variables to increase or decrease together?

How the response is measured is also important. Were the data measured on an interval scale? If so, are you satisfied that the underlying population is normally distributed? Do the variances within the treatment groups or about a regression line appear equal? When the observations do not appear to satisfy these requirements — or if you do not wish to assume that they do — you lose little power by using nonparametric methods based on ranks. Finally, if the response is measured on a nominal scale in which the observations are simply categorized, one can analyze the results using contingency tables.

Table 11-1 comes close to summarizing the lessons of this book, but there are three important things that it excludes. First, as Chap. 6 discussed, it is important to consider the power of a test when determining whether or not the failure to reject the hypothesis of no

Table 11-1 Summary of Some Statistical Methods to Test Hypotheses

Scale of measurement	Type of experiment				
	Two treatment groups consisting of different individuals	Three or more treatment groups consisting of different individuals	Before and after a single treatment in the same individuals	Multiple treatments in the same individuals	Association between two variables
Interval (and drawn from normally distributed populations*)	Unpaired t test (Chap. 4)	Analysis of variance (Chap. 3)	Paired t test (Chap. 9)	Repeated-measures analysis of variance (Chap. 9)	Linear regression and Pearson product-moment correlation (Chap. 8)
Nominal	Chi-square analysis-of-contingency table (Chap. 5)	Chi-square analysis-of-contingency table (Chap. 5)	McNemar's test (Chap. 9)	Cochrane Q†	Contingency coefficient†
Ordinal	Mann-Whitney rank-sum test (Chap. 10)	Kruskal-Wallis statistic (Chap. 10)	Wilcoxon signed-rank test (Chap. 10)	Friedman statistic (Chap. 10)	Spearman rank correlation (Chap. 8)

*If the assumption of normally distributed populations is not met, rank the observations and use the methods for data measured on an ordinal scale.
†Not covered in this text.

treatment effect is likely to be because the treatment really has no effect or because the sample size was too small for the test to detect the treatment effect. Second, Chaps. 7 and 8 discussed the importance of quantifying the size of the treatment effect (with confidence intervals) in addition to the certainty with which you can reject the hypothesis that the treatment had no effect (the P value). Third, one must consider how the samples were selected and whether or not there are biases that invalidate the results of any statistical procedure, however elegant or sophisticated. This important subject has been discussed throughout this book; we will finish with a few more comments and examples relating to it.

RANDOMIZE AND CONTROL

As already noted, all the statistical procedures assume that the observations represent a sample *drawn at random* from a larger population. What, precisely, does "drawn at random" mean? It means that any specific member of the population is as likely as any other member to be selected for study, and further that any given individual is as likely to be selected for one sample group as the other (i.e., control or treatment). The only way to achieve randomization is to use an objective procedure, such as a table of random numbers, to select subjects for a sample or treatment group. When other criteria are used that permit the investigator (or participant) to influence which treatment a given individual receives, one can no longer conclude that observed differences are due to the treatment rather than *biases* introduced by the process of assigning different individuals to different groups. When the randomization assumption is not satisfied, the logic underlying the distributions of the test statistics (F, t, χ^2, r, r_s, T, W, H, χ_r^2) used to estimate that the observed differences between the different treatment groups are due to chance as opposed to the treatment fails and the resulting P values (i.e., estimates that the observed differences are due to chance) are meaningless.

To reach meaningful conclusions about the efficacy of some treatment, one must compare the results obtained in the individuals who receive the treatment with an appropriate *control* group that is identical to the treatment group in all respects except the treatment. Clinical studies often fail to include adequate controls. *This omission generally biases the study in favor of the treatment.*

Despite the fact that questions of proper randomization and control are really distinct statistical questions, in practice these two areas are so closely related that we will discuss them together by considering two classic examples.

Internal Mammary Artery Ligation to Treat Angina Pectoris

People with coronary artery disease develop chest pain (angina pectoris) when they exercise because the narrowed arteries cannot deliver enough blood to carry oxygen and nutrients to the heart muscle and remove waste products fast enough. Relying on some anatomical studies and clinical reports during the 1930s, some surgeons suggested that tying off (ligating) the mammary arteries would force blood into the arteries that supplied the heart and increase the amount of blood available to it. By comparison with most cardiac surgery (major operations that require splitting the chest open), the procedure to ligate the internal mammary arteries is quite simple. The arteries are near the skin, and the entire procedure can be done under local anesthesia.

In 1958, Mitchell and his colleagues* published the results of a study in which they ligated the internal mammary arteries of 50 people who had angina before the operation, then observed them for 2 to 6 months; 34 of the patients (68 percent) improved clinically in that they had no more chest pain (36 percent) or fewer and less severe attacks (32 percent); 11 patients (22 percent) showed no improvement, and 5 (10 percent) died. On its face, this operation seems an effective treatment for angina pectoris.

In fact, even before this study was published, *Reader's Digest* carried an enthusiastic description of the procedure in an article entitled "New Surgery for Ailing Hearts."† (This article may have done more to promote the operation than the technical medical publications.)

Yet, despite the observed symptomatic relief and popular appeal of the operation, no one uses it today. Why not?

In 1959, Cobb and his colleagues‡ published the results of a double-

---

*J. R. Mitchell, R. Glover, and R. Kyle, "Bilateral Internal Mammary Artery Ligation for Angina Pectoris: Preliminary Clinical Considerations," *Am. J. Cardiol.,* 1:46–50, 1958.

†J. Ratcliff, "New Surgery for Ailing Hearts," *Reader's Dig.,* 71:70–73, 1957.

‡L. Cobb, G. Thomas, D. Dillard, K. Merendino, and R. Bruce, "An Evaluation of Internal-Mammary-Artery Ligation by a Double-Blind Technic," *N. Engl. J. Med.,* 260:1115–1118, 1959.

blind randomized controlled trial of this operation. Neither the patients nor the physicians who evaluated them knew whether or not a given patient had the internal mammary arteries ligated. When the patient reached the operating room, the surgeon made the incisions necessary to reach the internal mammary arteries and isolated them. At that time, the surgeon was handed an envelope instructing whether or not actually to ligate the arteries. The treated patients had their arteries ligated, and the control patients had the wound closed without touching the artery.

When evaluated in terms of subjective improvement as well as more quantitative measures, e.g., how much they could exercise before developing chest pain or the appearance of their electrocardiogram, there was little difference between the two groups of people, although there was a suggestion that the control group did better.

In other words, the improvement that Mitchell and his colleagues reported was a combination of observer biases and, probably more important, the placebo effect.

The Portacaval Shunt to Treat Cirrhosis of the Liver

Alcoholics often develop cirrhosis of the liver when the liver's internal structure breaks down and increases the resistance to the flow of blood through the liver. As a result, blood pressure increases and often affects other parts of the circulation, such as the veins around the esophagus. If the pressure reaches a high enough level, these vessels can rupture, causing internal bleeding and even death. To relieve this pressure, many surgeons performed a major operation to redirect blood flow away from the liver by constructing a connection between the portal artery (which goes to the liver) and the vena cava (the large veins on the other side of the liver). This connection is called a *portacaval shunt.*

Like many medical procedures, the early studies that supported this operation were completed without controls. The investigators completed the operation on people, then watched to see how well they recovered. If their clinical condition improved, the operation was considered a success. This approach has the serious flaw of not allowing for the fact that some of the people would have been fine (or died) regardless of whether or not they had the operation.

In 1966, more than 20 years after the operation was introduced, Grace and his colleagues* examined 51 papers that sought to evaluate

*N. Grace, H. Muench, and T. Chalmers, "The Present Status of Shunts for Portal Hypertension in Cirrhosis," *Gastroenterology,* 50:684–691, 1966.

Table 11-2   Value of Portacaval Shunt According to 51 Different Studies

Design	Degree of enthusiasm		
	Marked	Moderate	None
No controls	24	7	1
Controls			
Not randomized	10	3	2
Randomized	0	1	3

Source: Adapted from N. D. Grace, H. Muench, and T. C. Chambers, "The Present Status of Shunts for Portal Hypertension in Cirrhosis," *Gastroenterology,* **50**:684–691, 1966, table 2.

this procedure. They examined the nature of the control group, if one was present, whether or not patients were assigned to treatment or control at random, and how enthusiastic the authors were about the operation after they finished their study. Table 11-2 shows that the overwhelming majority of investigators who were enthusiastic about the procedure did studies failing to include a control group or including a control group that was not the result of a random assignment of patients between control and the operation. The few investigators who included controls and adequate randomization were not enthusiastic about the operation.

The reasons for biases on behalf of the operation in the studies that did not include controls—the placebo effect and observer biases—are the same as in the study of internal mammary artery ligation we just discussed.

The situation for the 15 studies with nonrandomized controls contains some of these same difficulties, but the situation is more subtle. Specifically, there *is* a control group that provides some basis for comparison; the members of the control group were not selected at random, however, but assigned on the basis of the investigators' judgment. In such cases, there is often a bias to treat only patients who are well enough to respond (or occasionally, hopeless cases). This selection procedure biases the study in behalf of (or occasionally against) the treatment under study. This bias can slip into studies in quite subtle ways. For example, suppose that you are studying some treatment and decide to assign patients who are admitted to the control and treatment groups alternately in the order in which they are admitted or on alternate days of the month. It then makes it easy for the investigators to decide which group a given person will be a member of by manipulating the day or time of admission to the hospital. The investigators may not even realize they are introducing such a bias.

A similar problem can arise in laboratory experiments. For example, suppose that you are doing a study of a potential carcinogen with rats. Simply taking rats out of a cage and assigning the first 10 rats to the control group and the next 10 rats to the treatment group (or alternate rats to the two groups) will not produce a random sample because more aggressive, or bigger, or healthier rats may, as a group, stay in the front or back of the cage.

The only way to obtain a random sample that avoids these problems is *consciously to assign the experimental subjects at random* using a table of random numbers, dice, or other procedure.

Table 11-2 illustrates that the four randomized trials done of the portacaval shunt showed the operation to be of little or no value. This example illustrates a common pattern:

> *The better the study the less likely it is to be biased in favor of the treatment.* *

Is Randomization of People Ethical?

Having concluded that the randomized clinical trial is the definitive way to assess the value of a potential therapy, we need to pause to discuss the ethical dilemma that some people feel when deciding whether or not to commit someone's treatment to a table of random numbers. The short answer to this problem is that *if no one knows* which therapy is better, there is no ethical imperative to use one therapy or another.

In reality, all therapies have their proponents and detractors, so one can rarely find a potential therapy that everyone feels neutral about at the start of a trial. (If there were no enthusiasts, no one would be interested in trying it.) As a result, it is not uncommon to hear physicians, nurses, and others protesting that some patient is being deprived of effective treatment (i.e., a therapy that individual physician or nurse believes in) simply to answer a sci-

*For more discussion of this and other examples, see D. Freedman, R. Pusani, and R. Purves, *Statistics,* Norton, New York, 1978, pt. I, "Design of Experiments."

entific question. Sometimes these objections are well-founded, but when considering them it is important to ask: *What evidence of being right does the proponent have*? Remember that uncontrolled and nonrandomized studies tend to be biased in favor of the treatment. At the time, Cobb and his colleagues' randomized controlled trial of internal mammary artery ligation may have seemed unethical to enthusiasts for the surgery on the grounds that it required depriving some people of the potential benefits of the surgery. In hindsight, however, they spared the public the pain and expense of a worthless therapy.

These genuine anxieties, as well as the possible vested interests of the proponent of the procedure, must be balanced against the possible damage and costs of subjecting the patient to a useless or harmful therapy or procedure. The same holds for the randomized controlled trials of the portacaval shunt. To complete a randomized trial it is necessary to assess carefully just *why* you believe some treatment to have an effect.

This situation is complicated by the fact that once something becomes acceptable practice, it is almost impossible to evaluate it, even though it is as much a result of tradition and belief as scientific evidence, e.g., the use of leeches. To return to the theme we opened this book with, a great deal of inconvenience, pain, and money is wasted pursuing diagnostic tests and therapies that are of no demonstrated value. For example, despite the fact that the provision of coronary artery bypass graft surgery has become a major American industry, there is continuing intense debate over whom, if anyone, the operation helps.

Another seemingly more difficult issue is what to do when the study suggests that the therapy is or is not effective but enough cases have not yet been accumulated to reach conventional statistical significance, that is, $P = .05$. Recall (from Chap. 6) that the power of a test to detect a difference of a specified size increases with the sample size and as the risk of erroneously concluding that there is a difference between the treatment groups (the Type I error α) increases. Recall also that α is simply the largest value of P that one is willing to accept and still conclude that there is a difference between the sample groups (in this case, that the treatment had an effect). Thus, if people object to continuing a clinical trial until the trial accumulates enough patients (and sufficient power) to reject the hypothesis of no difference between the treatment groups with $P < .05$ (or $\alpha = 5$ percent), all they are really saying is that they are willing to conclude that there is a difference when P is greater than .05.* In other words, they are willing to accept a higher risk of being wrong in the assertion that the treatment was effective because they believe the potential benefits of the treatment make it worth pursuing despite the increased uncertainty about whether or not it is really effective. Viewed in this light, the often diffuse debates over continuing a clinical trial can be focused on the real question underlying the disagreements: How confident does one need to be that the observed difference is not due to chance before concluding that the treatment really did cause the observed differences?

The answer to this question depends on personal judgment and values, not statistical methodology.

Is a Randomized Controlled Trial Always Necessary?

No. There are rare occasions, such as the introduction of penicillin, when the therapy produces such a dramatic improvement that one need not use statistical tools to estimate the probability that the observed effects are due to chance.

There are also often accidents of nature that force attentive practitioners to reassess the value of accepted therapy. For example, Ambroise Paré, a French military surgeon, followed the accepted therapy of treating gunshot wounds with boiling oil. During a battle in Italy in 1536 he ran out of oil and simply had to dress the untreated wounds. After spending a sleepless night worrying about his patients who had been deprived of the accepted therapy, he was surprised to find them "free from vehemencie of paine to have had good rest" while the conventionally treated soldiers were feverish and tormented with pain.† History does not record whether Paré then prepared a proposal to do a randomized clinical trial to study the value of boiling oil to treat gun-

---

*When one examines the data as they accumulate in a clinical trial, one can encounter the same multiple-comparisons problem discussed in Chaps. 3 and 4. Therefore, it is important to use techniques (such as a Bonferroni correction to the P values) that account for the fact that you are looking at the data more than once. See K. McPherson, "Statistics: The Problem of Examining Accumulating Data More than Once," *N. Engl. J. Med.,* **290**:501–502, 1974, and the comments on sequential analysis in the footnote at the end of Chap. 6.

†This example is taken from H. R. Wulff, *Rational Diagnosis and Treatment,* Blackwell, Oxford, 1976. This excellent short book builds many bridges between the ideas we have been discussing and the diagnostic therapeutic thought processes.

shot wounds. Should and would it be necessary if he had made his discovery today?

DOES RANDOMIZATION ENSURE CORRECT CONCLUSIONS?

The randomized controlled trial is the most convincing way to demonstrate the value of a therapy. Can you assume that it will always lead to correct conclusions? No.

First, as Chap. 6 discussed, the trial may involve too few patients to have sufficient power to detect a true difference.

Second, if the investigators require $P < .05$ to conclude that the data are incompatible with the hypothesis that the treatment had no effect, in the long run 5 percent of the "statistically significant" effects they find will be due to chance in the random-sampling process when, in actuality, the treatment had no effect, i.e., the null hypothesis is correct. (Since investigators are more likely to publish positive findings than negative findings, more than 5 percent of the published results are probably due to chance rather than the treatments.) This means that as you do more and more tests, you will accumulate more and more incorrect statements. When one collects a set of data and repeatedly subdivides the data into smaller and smaller subgroups for comparison, it is not uncommon to "find" a difference that is due to random variation rather than a real treatment effect.

Most clinical trials, especially those of chronic diseases like coronary artery disease or diabetes, are designed to answer a single broad question dealing with the effect on survival of competing treatments. These trials involve considerable work and expense and yield a great many data, and the investigators are generally interested in gleaning as much information (and as many publications) as possible from their efforts. As a result, the sample is often divided into subgroups based on various potential prognostic variables, and the subgroups are compared for the outcome variable of interest (usually survival). This procedure inevitably yields one or more subgroups of patients in whom the therapy is effective. For example, the Veterans Administration's prospective randomized controlled trial* of coronary artery bypass surgery

*M. Murphy, H. Hultgren, K. Detre, J. Thomsen, and T. Takaro, "Treatment of Chronic Stable Angina: A Preliminary Report of Survival Data of the Randomized Veterans Administration Cooperative Study," *N. Engl. J. Med.*, **297**:621–627, 1977.

did not detect a difference between the operation and medical therapy for the study group taken as a whole but did suggest that surgery improved survival in patients with left main coronary artery disease (disease of a specific artery, the left main coronary artery). This conclusion has had a major impact on the treatment physicians now recommend to their patients.

One needs to be extremely cautious when interpreting such findings, especially when they are associated with relatively large P values (of the order of 5 percent as opposed to less than 1 percent).

Another way that perfectly correct application of statistical tests of hypotheses (from an arithmetical point of view) can lead to unreliable conclusions is when they are used *after the fact*. All the procedures to test hypotheses begin with the assumption that the samples are all drawn from the same population (the null hypothesis). It is not uncommon to conduct a clinical trial—or, for that matter, any experiment—to answer a question, then notice an interesting pattern in the data that may have been totally unrelated to the original reason for the study. This pattern certainly can suggest future research. It might even be striking enough to lead you to conclude that there is actually a relationship present. *But* it is not fair to turn around and apply a statistical test to obtain a P value after you have already observed that a difference probably exists. The temptation to do this is often quite strong and, while it produces impressive P values, they are quite meaningless.

To demonstrate the difficulties that can arise when one begins examining subgroups of patients in a randomized controlled trial, Lee and his colleagues* took 1073 patients who had coronary artery disease and were being treated with medical therapy at Duke University and randomly divided them into two groups. *The "treatment" was randomization.* Therefore, if the samples are representative, one would not expect any systematic differences between the two groups. Indeed, when they compared the two groups with respect to age, sex, medical history, electrocardiographic findings, number of blocked coronary

*K. Lee, F. McNeer, F. Starmer, P. Harris, and R. Rosati, "Clinical Judgment and Statistics: Lessons from a Simulated Randomized Trial in Coronary Artery Disease," *Circulation,* 61:508–515, 1980.

arteries, or whether or not the heart exhibited a normal contraction pattern, using the methods this book describes, they found no significant differences between the two groups, except in the left ventricular contraction pattern. This result is not surprising, given that the two groups were created by randomly dividing a single group into two samples. Most important, there was virtually no difference in the pattern of survival in the two groups (Fig. 11-1A). So far, this situation is analogous to a randomized clinical trial designed to compare two groups receiving different therapies.

As already noted, after going to all the trouble of collecting such data, investigators are usually interested in examining various subgroups to see whether any finer distinctions can be made that will help the individual clinician deal with each individual patient according to the particular circumstances of the case. To simulate this procedure, Lee and his colleagues subdivided (the technical statistical term is *stratified*) the 1073 patients into six subgroups depending on whether one, two, or three coronary arteries were blocked and whether or not the patient's left ventricle was contracting normally. They also further subdivided these six groups into subgroups based on whether or not the patient had a history of heart failure. They analyzed the resulting data for the 18 subgroups (6 + 12) using life-table techniques not covered in this book.* This analysis revealed, among others, a statistically significant ($P < .025$) difference in survival between the two groups of patients who had three diseased vessels and an abnormal contraction pattern (Fig. 11-2B). How could this be? After all, *randomization was the treatment.*

This result is another aspect of the multiple-comparisons problem discussed at length in Chaps. 3 and 4. Without counting the initial test of the global hypothesis that the survival in the two original sample groups is not different, Lee and his colleagues completed 18 different comparisons on the data. Thus, according to the Bonferroni inequality, the chances of obtaining a statistically significant result with $P < .05$,

---

*For an introduction to the analysis of life tables, see T. Colton, *Statistics in Medicine,* Little, Brown, Boston, 1974, chap. 9, "Longitudinal Studies and the Use of the Life Table," or B. Brown, Jr., and M. Hollander, *Statistics: A Biomedical Introduction,* Wiley, New York, 1977, chap. 14, "Methods for Censored Data."

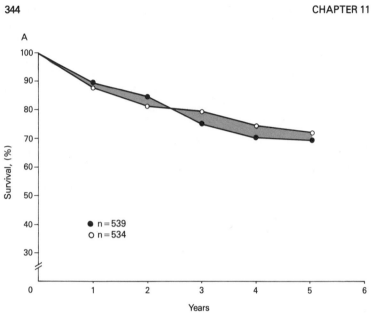

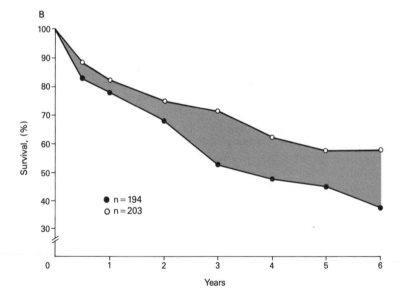

by chance is not above 18(.05) = .90.* The result in Fig. 11-1*B* is an example of this fact. When the total patient sample in a clinical trial is subdivided into many subgroups and the treatment compared within these subgroups, the results of these comparisons need to be interpreted very cautiously, especially when the *P* values are relatively large (say, around .05, as opposed to being around .001).

One approach to this problem would be to use the Bonferroni inequality (much as we used it in earlier chapters) and require that the value of the test statistic exceed the critical value for $P = \alpha_T/k$; however, this approach is too conservative when there are a large number of comparisons.

Another approach is to use more advanced statistical techniques that permit looking at all the variables together rather than just one at a time. (These methods, called *multivariate analysis,* are generalizations of linear regression, and are beyond the scope of this book.) In fact, although the patients in the two randomized groups were not detectably different when their baseline characteristics were examined one at a time, when Lee and his colleagues looked at all of them together, the

---

*When there are so many tests, the Bonferroni inequality overestimates the true probability of making a Type I error. It also increases the probability of making a Type II error. If you complete k comparisons each at the α level of significance, the total risk of making a Type I error is

$$\alpha_T = 1 - (1 - \alpha)^k$$

In the case of 18 comparisons with $\alpha = .05$, the total chance of obtaining $P < .05$ at least once by chance is

$$\alpha_T = 1 - (1 - .05)^{18} = .60$$

Figure 11-1 (*A*) Survival over time of 1073 people with medically treated coronary artery disease who were randomly divided into two groups. As expected, there is no detectable difference. (*B*) Survival in two subgroups of the patients shown in panel *A* who have three-vessel disease and abnormal left ventricular function. The two different groups were selected at random and received the same medical treatment. The difference is statistically significant (*P* < .025) if one does not include a Bonferroni correction for the fact that many hypotheses were tested even though the only treatment was randomization into two groups. (*Data for panel A from the text of K. Lee, J. McNeer, C. Starmer, P. Harris, and R. Rosati, "Clinical Judgment and Statistics: Lessons from a Simulated Randomized Trial in Coronary Artery Disease," Circulation, 61:508–515, 1980, and personal communication with Dr. Lee. Panel B is reproduced from Fig. 1 of the same paper. By permission of the American Heart Association, Inc.).*

statistical analysis showed that one of the treatment groups with three-vessel disease and abnormal contraction was slightly sicker than the other; and when these differences were taken into account, there no longer appeared to be a difference in survival between the two groups.

This exercise illustrates an important general rule for all statistical analysis: design the experiment to *minimize the total number of statistical tests of hypotheses that need to be computed.*

PROBLEMS WITH THE POPULATION

In most laboratory experiments and survey research, including marketing research and political polling, it is possible to define and locate the population of interest clearly, and then arrange for an appropriate random sample. In contrast, in clinical research, the sample generally has to be drawn from patients and volunteers at medical centers who are willing to participate in the project. This fact can make the interpretation of the study in terms of the population as a whole quite difficult. Most medical research involving human subjects is carried out on people who either attend clinics or are hospitalized at university medical centers. Yet, these groups of people are not really typical of the population as a whole or even the population of sick people. Figure 11-2 shows that, of 1000 people in a typical community, only 9 are admitted to a hospital in any given month, 5 referred to another physician (usually a specialist), and *only 1* is referred to a university medical center. It is often that one person who is available to participate in a clinical research protocol. Often the population of interest consists of people with the arcane or complex problems that lead to referral to an academic medical center; in such cases, a sample consisting of such people can be considered to represent the relevant population. However, as Fig. 11-2 makes clear, a sample of people drawn (even at random) from the patients at a university medical center can hardly be considered to be representative of the population as a whole. This fact must be carefully considered when evaluating a research report to decide just what population (that is, whom) the results can be generalized to.

In addition to the fact that people treated at academic medical centers do not really represent the true spectrum of illness in the

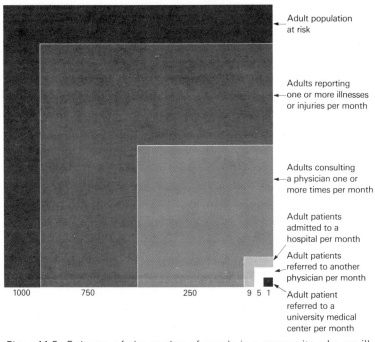

Figure 11-2 Estimates of the number of people in a community who are ill, visit a physician, or are admitted to a hospital. (*Redrawn from Fig. 1 of K. White, T. Williams, and B. Greenberg, "The Ecology of Medical Care," N. Engl. J. Med., 265:885–892, 1961. Used by permission.*)

community, there is an additional difficulty due to the fact that hospitalized patients do not represent a random sample of the population as a whole. It is not uncommon for investigators to complete studies of the association between different diseases based on hospitalized patients (or patients who seek medical help as outpatients). In general, different diseases lead to different rates of hospitalization (or physician consultation). Unless extreme care is taken in analyzing the results of such studies to ensure that there are comparable rates of including all classes of disease, any apparent association (or lack of association) between various diseases and symptoms is as likely to be due to the differential rates at which patients seek help (or die, if it is an autopsy study) as to a true association between the diseases. This problem is called *Berkson's fallacy,* after the statistician who first identified the problem.*

HOW YOU CAN IMPROVE THINGS

Using statistical thinking to reach conclusions in clinical practice and the biomedical sciences amounts to much more than memorizing a few formulas and looking up P values in tables. Like all human endeavors, applying statistical procedures and interpreting the results requires insight—not only into the statistical techniques but also into the clinical or scientific question to be answered. As Chap. 1 discussed, these methods will continue to increase in importance as economic pressures grow for evidence that diagnostic procedures and therapies actually are worth the cost both to the individual patient and to society at large. Statistical arguments play a central role in many of these discussions.

Even so, the statistical aspects of most medical research are supervised by investigators who only have heard of t tests (and, perhaps, contingency tables) regardless of the nature of the experimental design and the data. Since the investigators themselves best know what they are trying to establish and are responsible for drawing the conclusions, they should take the lead in the analysis of the data. Unfortunately, this task often falls to a laboratory technician or statistical consultant who does not really understand the question at hand or the data collected.

This problem is aggravated by the fact that investigators often go into the clinic or laboratory and collect data before clearly thinking out the specific question they wish to answer. As a result, after the data are collected and the investigators begin searching for a P value

*J. Berkson, "Limitations of the Application of Fourfold Table Analysis to Hospital Data," *Biometrics,* 2:47–53, 1946. For an additional (and less technical) discussion of Berkson's fallacy, see D. Mainland, "The Risk of Fallacious Conclusions from Autopsy Data on the Incidence of Diseases with Applications to Heart Disease," *Am. Heart J.,* 45:644–654, 1953. For an example of how the differences between considering patients in a given clinic, all hospitalized patients, and all people in the community can alter the conclusions reached in an in-hospital study, see H. Muench's comments (*N. Engl. J. Med.,* 272:1134, 1965) on H. Binder, A. Clement, W. Thayer, and H. Spiro, "Rarity of Hiatus Hernia in Achalasia," *N. Engl. J. Med.,* 272:680–682, 1965.

(often under the pressure of the deadline for submitting an abstract to a scientific meeting), they run into the fact that P values are associated with statistical *hypothesis tests* and that in order to test a hypothesis, you need a hypothesis to test. Surprisingly, very few investigators pause at the start of their work to carefully define a hypothesis; only 20 percent of the protocols approved by the committee on human research at one major health sciences center contained a clearly stated hypothesis.*

As discussed earlier in this chapter, the hypothesis (as embodied in the type of experiment) combined with the scale of measurement determines the statistical method to be used. Armed with a clearly stated hypothesis, it is relatively straightforward to design an experiment and determine the method of statistical analysis to be applied before one starts collecting the data. The simplest procedure is to make up the table to contain the data before collecting it, assume that you have the numbers, and then determine the method of analysis. This exercise will ensure that after going to the trouble and expense of actually collecting the data, it will be possible to analyze it.

While this procedure may seem obvious, very few people follow it. As a result, problems often arise when the time comes to compute the prized P value, because the experimental design does not fit the hypothesis—which is finally verbalized when a feisty statistician demands it—or the design does not fit into the paradigm associated with one of the established statistical hypothesis tests. (This problem is especially acute when dealing with more complex experimental designs.) Faced with a desperate investigator and the desire to be helpful, the statistical consultant will often try to salvage things by proposing an analysis of a subset of the data, suggesting the use of less powerful methods, or suggesting that the investigator use his or her data to test a different hypothesis (i.e., ask a different question). While these steps may serve the short-term goal of getting an abstract or manuscript out on time, they do not encourage efficient clinical and scientific investigation. These frustrating problems could be easily avoided if investigators simply thought about how they were going to analyze their data at the *beginning* rather than the end of the process. Unfortunately, most do not.

*For a complete discussion of this problem and the role that committees on human research could play in solving it, should they choose to do so, see M. Giammona and S. Glantz, "Poor Statistical Design in Research on Humans: The Role of Committees on Human Research," *Clin. Res.* **31**: 571–577, 1983.

The result is the sorry state of affairs discussed throughout this book. As a result, you and other responsible individuals can rarely take what is published or presented at clinical and scientific meetings at face value.

When evaluating the strength of an argument for or against some treatment or scientific hypothesis, what should you look for? The investigator should clearly state:

- *The hypothesis being examined (preferably, as the specific null hypothesis to be analyzed statistically)*
- *The data used to test this hypothesis and the procedure used to collect them (including the randomization procedure)*
- *The population the samples represent*
- *The statistical procedure used to evaluate the data and reach conclusions*

As Chap. 1 discussed at length, one rarely encounters this ideal. In general, however, the closer a paper or oral presentation comes to it, the more aware the authors are of the statistical issues in what they are doing and the more confident you can be of their conclusions.

One should immediately be suspicious of a paper that says nothing about the procedures used to obtain "*P* values" or that includes meaningless statements like "standard statistical procedures were used."

Finally, the issues of ethics and scientific validity, especially as they concern human and animal subjects, are inextricably intertwined. Any experimentation that produces results that are misleading or incorrect as a result of avoidable methodologic errors—statistical or otherwise—is unethical. It needlessly puts subjects in jeopardy by not taking every precaution to protect them against unnecessary risk of injury, discomfort, and, in the case of humans, inconvenience. In addition, significant amounts of time and money can be wasted trying to reproduce or refute erroneous results. Alternatively, these results might be accepted without further analysis and adversely affect not only the work of the scientific community, but also the treatment of patients in the future.

Of course, a well-designed, properly analyzed study does not automatically make an investigator's research innovative, profound, or even worth placing subjects at risk as part of the data collection process. However, even for important questions, it is clearly not ethical to place subjects at risk to collect data in a poorly designed study when this situation can be avoided easily by a little technical knowledge (such as that included in this book) and more thoughtful planning.

How can you help improve the situation?

Do not let people get away with sloppy statistical thinking any more than you would permit them to get away with sloppy clinical or scientific thinking. Write letters to the editor.* Ask questions in class, rounds, and meetings. When someone answers that they do not know how or where P came from, ask them how they can be certain that their results mean what they say. The answer may well be that they cannot.

Most important, if you decide to contribute to the fund of scientific and clinical knowledge, take the time and care to do it right.

*This procedure can be very effective when the editors of the journal are open-minded. In 1978, I wrote the editors of *Circulation Research,* a journal devoted to basic cardiovascular research, presenting the results on incorrect use of the t test described in Chaps. 1 and 4. The editors obtained an outside evaluation of my letter and revised their editorial policy to ensure adequate review of the statistical methods as well as the laboratory methods in the papers they published. Two years later, the editors reported a "marked improvement in the selection and use of statistical methods to test the [statistical] significance of results in papers published in the Journal." For the full published exchange on this question, see M. Rosen and B. Hoffman, "Editorial: Statistics, Biomedical Scientists, and *Circulation Research,*" *Circ. Res.,* 42:739, 1978; S. Glantz "Biostatistics: How to Detect, Correct, and Prevent Errors in the Medical Literature," *Circulation* 61:1–7, 1980; and S. Wallenstein, C. Zucker, and J. Fleiss, "Some Statistical Methods Useful in *Circulation Research,*" *Circ. Res.,* 47:1–9, 1980.

Computational Forms

VARIANCE

$$s^2 = \frac{\Sigma X^2 - (\Sigma X)^2/n}{n-1}$$

ONE-WAY ANALYSIS OF VARIANCE

Given Sample Means and Standard Deviations

For treatment group t: n_t = size of sample, $\bar{X}_t$ = mean, s_t = standard deviation. There are a total of k treatment groups.

$$N = \Sigma n_t$$
$$\text{SS}_{\text{wit}} = \Sigma(n_t - 1)s_t^2$$
$$\text{DF}_{\text{wit}} = N - k$$

$$SS_{bet} = \Sigma n_t \bar{X}_t^2 - \frac{(\Sigma n_t \bar{X}_t)^2}{N}$$

$$DF_{bet} = k - 1$$

$$F = \frac{SS_{bet}/DF_{bet}}{SS_{wit}/DF_{wit}}$$

Given Raw Data

Subscript t refers to treatment group; subscript s refers to experimental subject.

$$C = (\underset{t}{\Sigma}\underset{s}{\Sigma} X_{ts})^2 / N$$

$$SS_{tot} = \underset{t}{\Sigma}\underset{s}{\Sigma} X_{ts}^2 - C$$

$$SS_{bet} = \underset{t}{\Sigma} \frac{(\underset{s}{\Sigma} X_{ts})^2}{n_t} - C$$

$$SS_{wit} = SS_{tot} - SS_{bet}$$

Degrees of freedom and F are computed as above.

UNPAIRED t TEST

Given Sample Means and Standard Deviations

$$t = \frac{\bar{X}_1 - \bar{X}_2}{s_{\bar{X}_1 - \bar{X}_2}}$$

where

$$s_{\bar{X}_1 - \bar{X}_2} = \sqrt{\frac{n_1 + n_2}{n_1 n_2 (n_1 + n_2 - 2)}[(n_1 - 1)s_1^2 + (n_2 - 1)s_2^2]}$$

$$\nu = n_1 + n_2 - 2$$

Given Raw Data

Use

$$s_{\bar{X}_1 - \bar{X}_2} = \sqrt{\frac{n_1 + n_2}{n_1 n_2 (n_1 + n_2 - 2)} \left[\Sigma X_1^2 - \frac{(\Sigma X_1)^2}{n_1} + \Sigma X_2^2 - \frac{(\Sigma X_2)^2}{n_2} \right]}$$

in the equation for t above.

2 × 2 CONTINGENCY TABLES (INCLUDING YATES CORRECTION FOR CONTINUITY)

The contingency table is

A B
C D

Chi Square

$$\chi^2 = \frac{N(|AD - BC| - N/2)^2}{(A + B)(C + D)(A + C)(B + D)} \quad \text{where } N = A + B + C + D$$

McNemar's Test

$$\chi^2 = \frac{(|B - C| - 1)^2}{B + C}$$

where B and C are the numbers of people who responded to only one of the treatments.

LINEAR REGRESSION AND CORRELATION

$$SS_{tot} = \Sigma Y^2 - \frac{(\Sigma Y)^2}{n}$$

$$SS_{reg} = b \left(\Sigma XY - \frac{\Sigma X \Sigma Y}{n} \right)$$

$$s_{y \cdot x} = \sqrt{\frac{\text{SS}_{\text{tot}} - \text{SS}_{\text{reg}}}{n - 2}}$$

$$r = \sqrt{\frac{\text{SS}_{\text{reg}}}{\text{SS}_{\text{tot}}}} = \frac{\Sigma XY - n\bar{X}\bar{Y}}{\sqrt{(\Sigma X^2 - n\bar{X}^2)(\Sigma Y^2 - n\bar{Y}^2)}}$$

REPEATED-MEASURES ANALYSIS OF VARIANCE

There are k treatments and n experimental subjects.

$$A = \frac{(\underset{t}{\Sigma}\underset{s}{\Sigma}X_{ts})^2}{kn} \qquad B = \underset{t}{\Sigma}\underset{s}{\Sigma}X_{ts}^2$$

$$C = \frac{\underset{t}{\Sigma}(\underset{s}{\Sigma}X_{ts})^2}{n} \qquad D = \frac{\underset{s}{\Sigma}(\underset{t}{\Sigma}X_{ts})^2}{k}$$

$$\text{SS}_{\text{treat}} = C - A \qquad \text{SS}_{\text{res}} = A + B - C - D$$

$$\text{DF}_{\text{treat}} = k - 1 \qquad \text{DF}_{\text{res}} = (n - 1)(k - 1)$$

$$F = \frac{\text{SS}_{\text{treat}}/\text{DF}_{\text{treat}}}{\text{SS}_{\text{res}}/\text{DF}_{\text{res}}}$$

KRUSKAL-WALLIS TEST

$$H = \frac{12}{N(N + 1)} \Sigma\left(\frac{R_t^2}{n_t}\right) - 3(N + 1) \qquad \text{where } N = \Sigma n_t$$

FRIEDMAN TEST

$$\chi_r^2 = \frac{12}{nk(k + 1)} \Sigma R_t^2 - 3n(k + 1)$$

where there are k treatments and n experimental subjects and R_t is the sum of ranks for treatment t.

Answers to Exercises

2-1   Mean = 3.09, median = 2, standard deviation = 2.89, 25th percentile = 1, 75th percentile = 5. These data do not seem to be drawn from a normal distribution because the mean and median are very different; all the numbers are equal to or greater than zero, but the standard deviation is almost as large as the mean; if the population were normally distributed, it would have to contain negative values; the relationship between the percentiles and numbers of standard deviations about the mean are different from what you would expect if the data were drawn from a normally distributed population.

2-2   Mean = 244, median = 235.5, standard deviation = 43, 25th percentile = 211, 75th percentile = 246. These data appear to be drawn from a normally distributed population on the basis of the comparisons in the answer to Prob. 2-1.

2-3   Mean = 5.4, median = 2.0, standard deviation = 7.6, 25th percentile = 1.6 and 75th percentile = 2.4. These data do not appear to have been drawn from a normally distributed population because the mean is much larger than the median; in fact, the mean is greater than the 75th percentile. This result is consistent with the fact that the standard deviation is much larger than the mean, despite the fact that the observation cannot be negative. The two obvious outliers (19.0 and 23.6) skew the distribution.

2-4 There is 1 chance in 6 of getting each of the following values: 1, 2, 3, 4, 5, and 6. The mean of this population is 3.5.

2-5 The result is a sample drawn from the distribution of all means of samples of size 2 drawn from the population described in Prob. 2-4. Its mean is an estimate of the population mean, and its standard deviation is an estimate of the standard error of the mean of samples of size 2 drawn from the population in Prob. 2-4.

2-6 Given that the number of authors has to be an integer number and the size of the standard deviations compared with that of the means, the total number of authors is probably skewed toward larger numbers of authors, with a few papers containing many more authors than the rest of the population. Notice that the number of authors and spread of the population dramatically increased in 1976. The certainty with which you can estimate the mean number of authors is quantified with the standard error of the mean of each of the samples, the standard error of the mean decreasing as the precision with which you can estimate the true population means increases. The standard errors of the mean for the four different years are .11, .13, .10, .59.

3-1 $F = 15.74$, $\nu_n = 1$, $\nu_d = 40$. These observations are not consistent with the hypothesis that there is no difference in the average duration of labor between the two groups of women, and we conclude that prostaglandin E_2 gel shortens labor ($P < .01$).

3-2 $F = 64.18$, $\nu_n = 4$, $\nu_d = 995$. Mean forced midexpiratory flow is not the same, on the average, in all of the experimental groups studied ($P < .01$).

3-3 $F = 35.25$, $\nu_n = 2$, $\nu_d = 207$. At least one group of men represents a different population from the others ($P < .01$).

3-4 $F = 60.38$, $\nu_n = 6$, $\nu_d = 245$. Different amounts of smoking led to different mean percentages of bacterial inactivation ($P < .01$).

3-5 $F = 2.52$, $\nu_n = 1$, $\nu_d = 70$. This value of F is not large enough to reject the hypothesis that there is no difference between the populations of rats who received a sham injection and a THC injection with $P = .05$.

3-6 $F = 3.850$, $\nu_n = 5$, $\nu_d = 90$. Nurses in at least one unit experience more burnout than those in the others ($P < .01$).

3-7 $F = 8.12$, $\nu_n = 3$, $\nu_d = 79$. At least one of the treatment groups was drawn from a different population than the other ($P < .01$).

3-8 No. $F = 0.4088$ with $\nu_n = 5$ and $\nu_d = 102$, which does not even approach the critical value of F that defines the upper 5 percent of possible values, 2.46. Therefore, all these samples appear to be drawn from the same population.

4-1 For mean arterial pressure $t = -1.969$, and for total peripheral resistance $t = -1.286$. There are 23 degrees of freedom in each case. With 23 degrees of freedom 2.069 defines the most extreme 5 percent of the possible values of the t distribution when the treatment has no effect. Thus, these data do not provide sufficient evidence to reject the hypothesis that different anesthetic agents did not produce differences in mean arterial pressure or total peripheral resistance.

4-2 No. $t = 1.865$ with $\nu = 22$; $.05 < P < .10$.

4-3 $t = 3.846$ with $\nu = 22$. Therefore, ANF is significantly less potent in rats with cirrhotic livers.

4-4 Problem 3-1: $t = 3.967$, $\nu = 80$, $P < .01$; Prob. 3-5: $t = 1.586$, $\nu = 70$, $.2 > P > .1$, which is not sufficiently small to reject the hypothesis of no difference.

4-5 The subgroups are nonsmokers, clean environment; nonsmokers, smoky environment; light smokers; moderate smokers; and heavy smokers. Here are some of the resulting t values: nonsmokers, clean environment vs. nonsmokers, smoky environment, $t = 6.240$: light smokers vs. moderate smokers, $t = 4.715$; moderate smokers vs. heavy smokers, $t = 2.358$. Since there are a total of 10 pairwise comparisons, to keep the overall error rate at 5 percent, these values of t must be compared with the critical value corresponding to $P = .05/10 = .005$ with 995 degrees of freedom, 2.807. These data support the hypothesis that chronic exposure to other peoples' smoke affects the lung function of nonsmokers.

4-6 Inactive vs. joggers, $t = 5.616$; inactive vs. runners, $t = 8.214$; joggers vs. runners, $t = 2.598$. To maintain the overall risk of erroneously rejecting the hypothesis of no difference at 5 percent, these values of t should be compared with the critical value for $P = .05/3 = .017$ with 207 degrees of freedom, 2.44. Therefore, the three samples are drawn from distinct populations.

4-7 The subgroups are 0, 15, and 30 cigarettes; 75 cigarettes without THC and 50 cigarettes; 75 cigarettes and 150 cigarettes.

4-8 The results of the pairwise comparisons are control vs. dopamine, low dose, $t = 0$; control vs. dopamine, high dose, $t = 3.171$; control vs. nitroprusside, $t = 4.228$; dopamine, low dose, vs. dopamine, high dose, $t = 2.569$; dopamine, low dose, vs. nitroprusside, $t = 3.426$; dopamine, high dose, vs. nitroprusside, $t = .9649$. Since there are 6 comparisons, these values of t should be compared with the critical value of t corresponding to $P = .05/6 = .0083$ with 79 degrees of freedom, 2.72, to keep the total chance of erroneously reporting a difference below 5 percent. Comparing the observed values of t with this critical value shows control and dopamine, low dose, to be one subgroup and dopamine, high dose, and nitroprusside to be another. There is also sufficient evidence that control differs from both members of the second subgroup, but the value of t associated with the comparison of dopamine, low dose (in the first subgroup) and dopamine, high dose (in the second subgroup) falls short of the critical value of 2.84. This sort of ambiguity occasionally arises in multiple-comparison testing. In view of the fact that the Bonferroni t test is a conservative approach to correcting for multiple comparisons and the rest of the pattern in the observations, most investigators would report that the data support the assertion that there are two distinct subgroups.

4-9 The results of the pair-wise comparisons (in the order they should be done) are

	Difference of means	q	p
Control vs. nitro	$15 - 7 = 8$	5.979	4
Control vs. high dopa	$15 - 9 = 6$	4.485	3
Control vs. low dopa	$15 - 15 = 0$	0.000	2
Low dopa vs. nitro	$15 - 7 = 8$	4.845	3
Low dopa vs. high dopa	$15 - 9 = 6$	3.634	2
High dopa vs. nitro	$9 - 7 = 2$	1.365	2

For $\alpha_T = .05$ and $\nu_d = 79$, the critical values of q (by interpolation in Table 4-3) are 3.7 for $p = 4$, 3.4 for $p = 3$, and 2.8 for $p = 2$. All comparisons except control versus high dopamine and high dopamine versus nitroprusside are associated with values of q above the critical values. Therefore, there are two subgroups: control and high dopamine is one subgroup, and low dopamine and nitroprusside is the other. Note that in contrast to the results of multiple comparisons using Bonferroni t tests, the SNK test yields an unambiguous definition of the subgroups.

4-10 Use the SNK test for multiple comparisons because there are so many comparisons that the Bonferroni t test will be much too conservative. The results of these comparisons are

	Difference of means	q	p
G/M vs. G/S	65.2 − 43.9 = 21.3	5.362	6
G/M vs. SDU/M	65.2 − 46.4 = 18.8	4.733	5
G/M vs. ICU/S	65.2 − 49.9 = 15.3	3.852	4
G/M vs. ICU/M	65.2 − 51.2 = 14.0	3.525	3
G/M vs. SDU/S	65.2 − 57.3 = 7.9	1.989	2
SDU/S vs. G/S	57.3 − 43.9 = 13.4	3.374	5
SDU/S vs. SDU/M	57.3 − 46.4 = 10.9	2.744	4
SDU/S vs. ICU/S	57.3 − 49.9 = 7.4	1.863	3
SDU/S vs. ICU/M	57.3 − 51.2 = 6.1	1.536	2
ICU/M vs. G/S	51.2 − 43.9 = 7.3	1.838	4
ICU/M vs. SDU/M	51.2 − 46.4 = 4.8	1.208	3
ICU/M vs. ICU/M	51.2 − 49.9 = 1.3	0.327	2
ICU/S vs. G/S	49.9 − 43.9 = 6.0	1.511	3
ICU/S vs. SDU/M	49.9 − 46.4 = 3.5	0.881	2
SDU/M vs. G/S	46.4 − 43.9 = 2.5	0.629	2

For $\nu_d = 90$ and $\alpha_T = .05$, the critical values of q (by interpolation in Table 4-3) are 4.1 for $p = 6$, 3.9 for $p = 5$, 3.7 for $p = 4$, 3.4 for $p = 3$, and 2.8 for $p = 2$. Therefore, the first four comparisons in the preceding table are significant and none of the others are. Thus these results indicate that there are two groupings of units in terms of nursing burnout: One group consists of the general medical (G/M) and stepdown unit/surgical (SDU/S) units and the other group consists of both stepdown units (SDU/S and SDU/M), both intensive care units (ICU/S and ICU/M), and the general surgical unit (G/S). Note the ambiguity in the results with SDU/S appearing in both groups. This type of ambiguity arises sometimes in multiple-comparison testing, especially when there are many means (i.e., treatment) to be compared. One must simply use some judgment in interpreting the results.

4-11 a No b No c No d Yes

5-1 Yes. $\chi^2 = 17.88$, $\nu = 1$, $P < .001$. $z = 4.518$, $P < .001$.

5-2 Mother's age: $\chi^2 = 11.852$, $\nu = 1$, $P < .001$; pregnancy interval: $\chi^2 = 10.506$, $\nu = 1$, $P < .005$; pregnancy planned: $\chi^2 = 3.144$, $.1 > P > .05$; previous pregnancies: $\chi^2 = 1.571$, $\nu = 1$, $.5 > P > .25$; smoked: $\chi^2 = 17.002$, $\nu = 1$, $P < .001$; prenatal visits:

$\chi^2 = 4.527$, $\nu = 1$, $P < .05$; hemoglobin: $\chi^2 = .108$, $\nu = 1$, $P > .5$; race: $\chi^2 = .527$, $\nu = 2$, $P > .5$. The key factors seem to be age, pregnancy interval, and smoking. Whether or not the pregnancy was planned and the number of prenatal visits may also be factors, although the evidence is not nearly as strong for them. Despite the high confidence we can have in reporting these differences, they probably are not stark enough to be of predictive value in any given infant.

5-4 For the three drugs, $\chi^2 = 7.845$, $\nu = 2$, and $P < .025$, so there is evidence that is at least one difference in recurrence rates. Subdividing the table to compare just ampicillin and cephalexin yields:

	Recurrence	Nonrecurrence
Ampicillin	20	7
Cephalexin	14	1

$\chi^2 = 1.239$, $\nu = 1$, $.5 > P > .25$ (or $.1 > P > .5$ including a Bonferroni correction for the fact that we are going to do two comparisons). There is not sufficient evidence to conclude that these two drugs produce different recurrence rates. Pool the results and compare them with trimethoprim-sulfamethoxazole:

	Recurrence	Nonrecurrence
Ampicillin or cephalexin	34	8
Trimathoprim-sulfamethoxazole	24	19

$\chi^2 = 5.089$, $\nu = 1$, $P < .025$ before the Bonferroni correction or $P < .05$ after. Thus, trimethoprim-sulfamethoxazole seems to work better than either of the other two drugs.

5-5 $\chi^2 = 58.63$, $\nu = 2$; $P < 0.001$. These data suggest that the rate at which people got sick was significantly associated with water consumption.

5-6 For all the data, $\chi^2 = 48.698$, $\nu = 3$, $P < .001$. Subdividing the table does not reveal differences between 1946 and 1956 or 1966 and 1976 but reveals a significant difference between these two subgroups. In other words, things deteriorated between 1956 and 1966.

5-7 $\chi^2 = 5.185, \nu = 1, P < .025$; yes.

5-8 $\chi^2 = 2.273, \nu = 1, .25 > P > .1$; the results do change.

5-9 $\chi^2 = 8.8124, \nu = 1, P < .005$. She would not reach the same conclusion if she observed the entire population because the sample would not be biased by differential admission rates.

6-1 $\delta/\sigma = 1.1$ and $n = q$; from Fig. 6-9, power = .63.

6-2 $\delta/\sigma = .55$ and power = .80; from Fig. 6-9, $n = 40$.

6-3 For mean arterial blood pressure: $\delta = .25 \cdot 76.8$ mmHg = 19.2 mmHg, $\delta = 17.8$ mmHg (based on pooled variance estimate), so $\delta/\sigma = 1.08$. $n = 9$ (the size of the smaller sample). From Fig. 6-9, power = .63. For total peripheral resistance, $\delta/\sigma = 553/1154 = .48$, $n = 9$. From Fig. 6-9, power = .13.

6-4 Approximately 1 percent.

6-5 22 rats in each group.

6-6 *Step 1:* Let the size of each sample be n. *Step 2:* If the null hypothesis of no difference between the two groups is true, compute the standard error of the difference between the samples using the pooled estimate of the proportion $\hat{p} = (0.3 + 0.9)/2 = 0.6$. Then the standard error of the difference is

$$s_{\Delta\hat{p}} = \sqrt{\hat{p}(1 - \hat{p})\left(\frac{1}{n} + \frac{1}{n}\right)} = \frac{0.692}{n}$$

The observed change in proportion corresponding to $\alpha = 0.05$ will be the change $\Delta\hat{p}$, which yields $Z_\alpha = \hat{p}/s_{\Delta\hat{p}}$, where Z_α is the critical value corresponding to a two-tail critical value of the normal distribution with $\alpha = 0.05$; $Z_\alpha = 1.960$. *Step 3:* If the alternative hypothesis (that the proportion changes from $p_1 = 0.3$ to $p_2 = 0.9$, so $\Delta p = 0.6 \neq 0$) is true, then the standard error of the difference will be

$$s_{p_1-p_2} = \sqrt{\frac{p_1(1 - p_1)}{n} + \frac{p_2(1 - p_2)}{n}} = \frac{0.547}{n}$$

The observed change in proportion necessary to obtain a power $\pi = 0.9$ is that which corresponds to a probability of Type II error $\beta = 1 - \pi = 0.1$ and defines the lower (one tail) of the normal distribution corresponding to $Z_\beta = (\Delta p - \Delta\hat{p})/s_{p_1-p_2}$; $Z_\beta = 1.282$. *Step 4:* Set $\Delta\hat{p}$ from the two previous steps equal and solve for n

$$\Delta\hat{p} = Z_\alpha s_{\Delta\hat{p}} = \Delta p - Z_\beta s_{p_1-p_2}$$

ANSWERS TO EXERCISES

363

which yields $n = 12$ in each group. *Note on continuity correction:* To include the continuity correction, subtract $\frac{1}{n} + \frac{1}{n} = \frac{2}{n}$ from the numerators in the expressions for Z_α and Z_β as before. The resulting expression is quadratic in $\sqrt{n}$ and may be solved using the general quadratic equation to obtain $n = 15$ for each group.

7-1 90 percent confidence intervals: 1.8 to 2.2, 2.1 to 2.5, 2.6 to 3.0, 3.9 to 5.9. 95 percent confidence intervals: 1.8 to 2.2, 2.0 to 2.6, 2.6 to 3.0, 3.7 to 6.1. Answers are rounded to nearest tenth of an author; 95 percent confidence intervals are always wider than 90 percent confidence intervals.

7-2 From Fig. 7.3, for control group: 8 to 48 percent; for treatment group: 0 to 17 percent. Using the normal approximation for the difference in cesarean section rate: 2 to 53 percent. Yes.

7-3 The 95 percent confidence interval for the mean difference in duration of labor is 2.7 to 8.1 h. Yes.

7-4 For the treatment group, $\hat{p} = 0.80$ and the confidence interval is 0.60 to 0.92. For the placebo group, $\hat{p} = 0.15$ and the confidence interval is 0.03 to 0.38. Because these 95 percent confidence intervals do not overlap, we conclude that there is a significant difference between these proportions, $P < 0.05$. This result agrees with that obtained in Prob. 5-1.

7-5 Nonsmokers, clean environment: 3.03 to 3.31; nonsmokers, smoky environment: 2.58 to 2.86; light smokers: 2.49 to 2.77; moderate smokers: 2.15 to 2.43; heavy smokers: 1.98 to 2.26. Nonsmokers, smoky environment, and light smokers overlap and can be considered one subgroup, as can moderate smokers and heavy smokers. Nonsmokers, clean environment, is a third subgroup.

7-6 1946: 17 to 31 percent; 1956: 22 to 36 percent; 1966: 43 to 59 percent; 1976: 48 to 64 percent.

7-7 95 percent confidence interval for 90 percent of the population: 121 to 367 s. 95 percent confidence interval for 95 percent of the population: 108 to 380 s.

8-1 **a:** $a = 3.0$, $b = 1.3$, $r = .79$; **b:** $a = 5.1$, $b = 1.2$, $r = .94$; **c:** $a = 5.6$, $b = 1.2$, $r = .97$. Note that as the range of data increases, the correlation coefficient increases.

8-2 **a:** $a = 24.3$, $b = .36$, $r = .561$; **b:** $a = .5$, $b = 1.15$, $r = .599$. Part **a** illustrates the large effect one outlier point can have on the regression line. Part **b** illustrates that even though there are two different and distinct patterns in the data, this is not reflected when a single regression line is drawn through the data. This problem illustrates why it is very important to look at the data before computing regression lines through it.

8-3 $a = 3.0$, $b = 0.5$, $r = .82$ for all four experiments, despite the fact that the patterns in the data differ from experiment to experiment. Only data from experiment 1 satisfies the assumption of linear regression analysis.

8-4 Yes. $r = -.68$, $P < .001$.

8-5 End-diastolic volumes: $a = 15$, $b = .90$, $r = .98$. End-systolic volumes: $a = -.87$, $b = .95$, $r = .98$. The 95 percent confidence interval for angiographic volume when radionuclide volume is 150 mL: 122 to 178 mL. Compare slopes: $t = .692$; compare intercepts: $t = 2.037$. The critical value of t that defines the 5 percent most extreme values when there are 32 degrees of freedom is 2.037; thus, these data support the hypothesis that the regression lines for diastole and systole have the same slope but different intercepts.

8-6 Let B = nitrogen balance and I = nitrogen intake. For the 37 kcal/kg energy intake, $B = 0.35I - 34.8$. For the 33 kcal/kg energy intake, $B = 0.34I - 44.3$. $t_{b_1 - b_2} = 0.068$, $\nu = 20$, $P > 0.50$, so the slopes of these two regression lines are not significantly different. $t_{a_1 - a_2} = 1.205$, $n = 20$, $0.20 < P < 0.50$, so intercepts of these two regression lines are not significantly different. Therefore, the two regression lines are not significantly different.

8-7 Yes. The Spearman rank correlation r_S is 0.89; $P < .002$.

8-8 Yes. $r_S = 0.899$; $P < 0.001$. Higher clinical scores are associated with larger amounts of plaque.

8-9 $r_S = .85$, $P < .001$. These data do support the hypothesis that there is a relationship between adherence ratio and clinical severity of sickle-cell anemia.

9-1 Yes. The paired t test yields $t = 4.512$ with $\nu = 9$, so $P < .002$.

9-2 Pneumococcus: $t = 3.1738$, $\nu = 19$, $P < .01$. Streptococcus: $t = 1.849$, $\nu = 19$, $.1 > P > .05$. Pneumococcus antibody concentration appeared to change whereas streptococcus antibody concentration did not.

9-3 Use the power chart in Fig. 6-9 with δ equal to the size of the mean change (445 mg/L and 1.2 mg/L for pneumococcus and streptococcus, respectively) that corresponds to a doubling in concentration and σ equal to the size of the standard deviation of the differences before and after immunization (627 mg/L and

2.9 mg/L). There is a 5 percent chance of detecting a doubling of pneumococcus antibody concentration and a 0 percent chance of detecting a doubling of streptococcus concentration. The repeated-measures (paired) design is more powerful than the analogous design using independent samples. This can be thought of as increasing the "effective sample size."

9-4 $F = t^2$.

9-5 $F = 5.04$, $\nu_n = 2$, $\nu_d = 6$. This value falls short of 5.14, the critical value that defines the greatest 5 percent of possible values of F in such experiments. It is, however, quite close (the actual P value is .052), so one would be justified in reporting that there is a change in cardiac output associated with the drug ($P = .052$). This path would be more prudent than reporting "no significant difference," especially in view of the small samples. Multiple comparisons with paired t test (including the Bonferroni correction) will not define the subgroups with an overall confidence of 95 percent, because the analysis of variance did not reach significance at the 95 percent level.

9-6 There are significant differences between the different experimental conditions ($F = 184.50$, $\nu_n = 3$, $\nu_d = 33$). Multiple comparisons with paired t tests using the residual mean square and the Bonferroni correction show the two control conditions to be similar and different from the two interventions, which are also different from each other. Thus, both smoking and carbon monoxide alone decrease exercise capability, smoking having more of an effect than carbon monoxide alone.

9-7 Repeated measures analysis of variance yields $F = 10.61$ with $\nu_n = 2$ and $\nu_d = 12$, so $P < .01$ and the food intake appears different among the different groups. Multiple comparisons (using either Bonferroni t tests or the SNK test) reveal that food intakes at pressures of 10 and 20 mmHg are both significantly different from intake at a pressure of 30 mmHg, but they are not different from each other. The subjects were not told the true goal or design of the study in order to avoid biasing their responses.

9-8 By McNemar's test: $\chi^2 = 4.225$, $\nu = 1$, $P < .05$. No; indomethacin is significantly better than placebo.

9-9 When the data are presented in this format, they are analyzed as a 2 × 2 contingency table. $\chi^2 = 2.402$, $\nu = 1$, $P > .10$, so there is no significant association between drug and improvement of shunting. This test, in contrast to the analysis in Prob. 9-8, failed to detect an effect because it ignores the paired nature of the data, and so is less powerful.

10-1 For mean annual lab charges: $W = -80$, $n = 12$ (there is one zero in the charges), $P < .02$. For drug charges: $W = 28$, $n = 13$, $P > .048$. Therefore, the audit seemed to reduce the amount of money spent on laboratory tests but not drugs. There was not a significant relationship between money spent on laboratory tests and money spent on drugs ($r_S = .201$, $P > .5$).

10-2 $z = 3.0311$, $P < 0.005$; therefore, there is a difference between groups. In Prob. 4-2, the t test did not indicate a difference. The data from the group with retinal damage are not normally distributed (see Prob. 2-3); therefore, the parametric t test is inappropriate. The Mann-Whitney is the appropriate test.

10-3 $H = 20.64$, $v = 2$, $P < 0.001$; therefore, there is at least one difference among the groups. Multiple Mann-Whitney tests: normal versus foveal, $z_t = 3.031$ and $P < 0.02$ (after a Bonferroni correction for three comparisons); normal versus foveal and peripheral, $z_T = 3.802$ and $P < 0.005$; and foveal versus foveal and peripheral, $z_T = 2.736$ and $P < 0.05$. All groups are significantly different.

10-4 Problem 4-3: The Mann-Whitney rank-sum test yields $z_T = 3.425$, with $P < .001$, so ANF is decreased with cirrhosis. Problem 9-5: Hydralazine has a significant effect on cardiac output ($\chi_r^2 = 6.5$, $k = 3$, $n = 4$, $P = .042$). With only four cases pairwise Wilcoxon tests cannot detect differences with less than a 5 percent chance of erroneously rejecting the null hypothesis of no effect. Problem 9-6: Treatments produced different exercise durations ($\chi_r^2 = 32.4$, $v = 3$, $P < .001$). Multiple comparisons with Wilcoxon signed-rank test including Bonferroni correction yield same subgroups as before.

10-5 $T = 54$, $n_S = 6$, $n_B = 22$; $z_T = -1.848$ and $.1 > P > .05$.

10-6 $H = 18.36$, $v = 2$, $P < .001$, so there is strong evidence that the responses are different. Pairwise comparison of the groups with the Mann-Whitney rank-sum test shows the no disease and right coronary artery disease groups to be similar and both are different from the left coronary–multiple artery group.

10-7 Yes, G is a legitimate test statistic. The sampling distribution of G when $n = 4$:

G	Possible ways to get value	Probability
0	1	1/16
1	4	4/16
2	6	6/16
3	4	4/16
4	1	1/16

When $n = 6$:

G	Possible ways to get value	Probability
0	1	1/64
1	6	6/64
2	15	15/64
3	20	20/64
4	15	15/64
5	6	6/64
6	1	1/64

G cannot be used to conclude that the treatment in the problem had an effect with $P < .05$ because the two most extreme possible values (i.e., the two tails of the sampling distribution of G), 1 and 4, can occur $1/16 + 1/16 = 1/8 = 0.125 = 12.5$ percent of the time, which exceeds 5 percent. G can be used for $n = 6$, where the extreme values, 1 and 6, occur $1/64 + 1/64 = 2/64 = .033$ percent of the time, so the (two-tail) critical values (closest to 5 percent) are 1 and 6.

Index

Edward R. Stokes and Robert L. Battagin wrote the computer program used to construct the original index. Debra Brent and James Stoughton helped revise the index for the second edition.